OPHTHALMIC ESSENTIALS

Edited by

MICHAEL P. VRABEC, M.D.

Assistant Professor of Ophthalmology
The University of Vermont College of Medicine, Burlington, Vermont

Associate Editor

GEORGE J. FLORAKIS, M.D.

Associate in Clinical Ophthalmology
Edward S. Harkness Eye Institute
Columbia University College of Physicians and Surgeons, New York, New York

Medical Illustrator

DANIEL CASPER, M.D., PH.D.

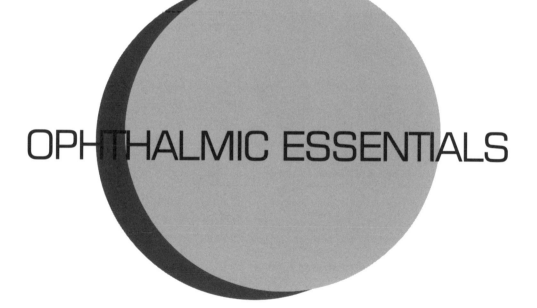

OPHTHALMIC ESSENTIALS

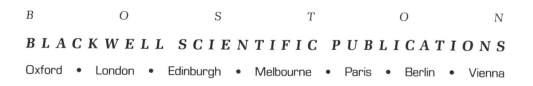

B   O   S   T   O   N

BLACKWELL SCIENTIFIC PUBLICATIONS

Oxford • London • Edinburgh • Melbourne • Paris • Berlin • Vienna

Blackwell Scientific Publications

Editorial offices:

238 Main Street, Cambridge, Massachusetts
    02142, USA

Osney Mead, Oxford OX2 0EL, England

25 John Street, London WC1N 2BL, England

23 Ainslie Place, Edinburgh EH3 6AJ,
    Scotland

4 University Street, Carlton, Victoria 3053,
    Australia

Other editorial offices:

Arnette SA, 2 rue Casimir-Delavigne, 75006
    Paris, France

Blackwell-Wissenschaft, Meinekestrasse 4,
    D-1000 Berlin 15, Germany

Blackwell MZV, Feldgasse 13, A-1238
    Vienna, Austria

Distributors:

USA

Blackwell Scientific Publications

238 Main Street

Cambridge, Massachusetts 02142

(Telephone orders: 800-759-6102)

Canada

Times Mirror Professional Publishing Ltd

5240 Finch Avenue East

Scarborough, Ontario M1S 5A2

(Telephone orders: 416-298-1588)

Australia

Blackwell Scientific Publications (Australia)
    Pty Ltd

54 University Street

Carlton, Victoria 3053

(Telephone orders: 03-347-0300)

Outside North America and Australia:

Blackwell Scientific Publications, Ltd.

c/o Marston Book Services, Ltd.

P.O. Box 87

Oxford OX2 0DT

England

(Telephone orders: 44-865-791155)

Typeset by Pine Tree Composition

Printed and bound by The Maple-Vail Book Manufacturing Group

© 1992 by Blackwell Scientific Publications

Printed in the United States of America

92 93 94 95   5 4 3 2 1

Library of Congress Cataloging-in-Publication Data

Ophthalmic essentials / edited by Michael P. Vrabec and George J.
    Florakis.
        p. cm.
    Includes bibliographical references and index.
    ISBN 0-86542-202-8
    1. Ophthalmology. 2. Eye—Diseases and defects.
    [DNLM: 1. Eye Diseases. 2. Ophthalmology—methods.   WW 140 0605]
    RE46.057 1992
    617.7—dc20
    DNLM/DLC
    for Library of Congress   91–41380
                                                            CIP

This text is dedicated to our wives, Stephanie and Catherine, for their unending love and support and to Jay H. Krachmer, M.D., our mentor, advisor, and good friend.

C O N T E N T S

C H A P T E R   T H R E E

Cornea and External Disease Sheridan Lam, M.D., Christopher J. Rapuano, M.D., Jay H. Krachmer, M.D.   50

C H A P T E R   F O U R

Glaucoma **Gregory L. Skuta, M.D.** 113

C H A P T E R   F I V E

Cataract **Thomas A. Farrell, M.D.** 164

C H A P T E R   S I X

C H A P T E R   S E V E N

C H A P T E R   E I G H T

Ophthalmic Plastics **Keith D. Carter, M.D., Gene R. Howard, M.D.** *298*

C H A P T E R   N I N E

Neuro-ophthalmology **Richard A. Appen, M.D., Michael P. Vrabec, M.D.** *336*

C   H   A   P   T   E   R   T   E   N

Pediatric Ophthalmology and Motility **Thomas D. France, M.D.** 375

C H A P T E R E L E V E N

Trauma **Michael P. Vrabec, M.D., Vincent S. Reppucci, M.D., Gregory L. Skuta, M.D., Keith D. Carter, M.D., Gene R. Howard, M.D.** *410*

CONTRIBUTORS

Richard E. Appen, M.D.
Associate Clinical Professor
  of Ophthalmology
University of Wisconsin College
  of Medicine
Madison, Wisconsin

Keith Carter, M.D.
Assistant Professor of Ophthalmology
University of Iowa College of Medicine
Iowa City, Iowa

Daniel Casper, M.D., Ph.D
Associate in Clinical Ophthalmology
Edward S. Harkness Eye Institute
Columbia University College of Physi-
  cians and Surgeons
New York, New York

Thomas R. Farrell, M.D.
Assistant Professor of Ophthalmology
University of Iowa College of Medicine
Iowa City, Iowa

R. Linsy Farris, M.D.
Professor of Clinical Ophthalmology
Edward S. Harkness Eye Institute
Columbia University College of Physi-
  cians and Surgeons
New York, New York

George J. Florakis, M.D.
Associate in Clinical Ophthalmology
Edward S. Harkness Eye Institute
Columbia University College of Phys-
  icians and Surgeons
New York, New York

Thomas D. France, M.D.
Professor of Ophthalmology
Director of Pediatric Ophthalmology
University of Wisconsin College
  of Medicine
Madison, Wisconsin

Gene R. Howard, M.D.
Assistant Professor of Ophthalmology
Medical University of South Carolina
Charleston, South Carolina

Jay H. Krachmer, M.D.
Professor of Ophthalmology
University of Iowa College of Medicine
Iowa City, Iowa

Diane Kraus, M.D.
Chief Resident
Edward S. Harkness Eye Institute
Columbia University College of Physi-
  cians and Surgeons
New York, New York

Sheridan Lam, M.D.
Assistant Professor of Ophthalmology
University of Illinois Eye and
  Ear Institute
Chicago, Illinois

Mark McDermott, M.D.
Assistant Professor of Ophthalmology
Kresge Eye Institute
Wayne State University School
  of Medicine
Detroit, Michigan

Christopher J. Rapuano, M.D.
Assistant Professor of Ophthalmology
Wills Eye Hospital
Thomas Jefferson University School
  of Medicine
Philadelphia, Pennsylvania

Vincent S. Reppucci, M.D.
Assistant Attending Ophthalmologist
Cornell University
New York, New York

Gregory L. Skuta, M.D.
Assistant Professor of Ophthalmology
Kellogg Eye Center
University of Michigan School
  of Medicine
Ann Arbor, Michigan

Michael P. Vrabec, M.D.
Assistant Professor of Ophthalmology
University of Vermont College
  of Medicine
Burlington, Vermont

Michael Weiss, M.D., Ph.D.
Assistant Professor of Clinical
  Ophthalmology
Director, Uveitis Service
Edward S. Harkness Eye Institute
Columbia University College of Physi-
  cians and Surgeons
New York, New York

P R E F A C E

In an age of ever-increasing information, texts that highlight important or "essential" knowledge become more important. Our goal was to write a text that contained the information the busy clinician could use on a day-to-day basis in an office practice or as a study guide for recertification examinations (including a section on practical optics), that an ophthalmology resident would find helpful during various rotations and as a board study guide as well, and that medical students and technicians would find useful. We felt such a text did not exist and so asked leaders in the various subspecialties of ophthalmology to contribute their knowledge. Many institutions are represented to broaden the scope of the text. The text should not be seen as a substitute for an in-depth study of various topics nor should it be considered a "standards of care" text (dosages of medications were specifically left out in many instances). It should rather be seen as a memory aide and guide for all of us to improve our evaluation and management of patients.

Michael P. Vrabec, M.D.

ACKNOWLEDGMENTS

We are indebted to the many contributors who provided us with concise well written chapters. We would like to thank Victoria Reeders, Katie Grimes, and their staff at Blackwell for assistance and patience during this project. Special acknowledgment is made to Daniel Casper, M.D., Ph.D. for his unique and invaluable illustrations. (Figures 8.1–8.9, 9.2, and 9.8–9.12 are to be published in *Orbital Disease: Imaging and Analysis* by Daniel Casper, and are printed with permission from Thieme Medical Publishers.) Finally, we are grateful to Tammy Reed for her diligent work in the preparation of the manuscript.

N O T I C E

The indications and dosages of all drugs in this book have been recommended in the medical literature and conform to the practices of the general medical community. The medications described do not necessarily have specific approval by the Food and Drug Administration for use in the diseases and dosages for which they are recommended. The package insert for each drug should be consulted for use and dosage as approved by the FDA. Because standards of usage change, it is advisable to keep abreast of revised recommendations, particularly those concerning new drugs.

OPHTHALMIC ESSENTIALS

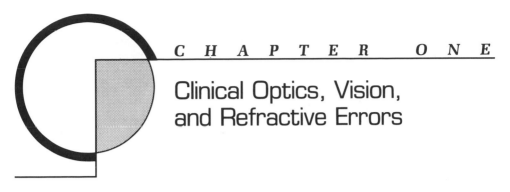

Clinical Optics, Vision, and Refractive Errors

Mark L. McDermott, M.D.

Optics: Principles and Formulae

Refractive Index

Refractive index (n) is a measure of the degree that the velocity of light of a given wavelength (λ) is *slowed* when passing through a medium.

$$n = \frac{C}{V},$$

where C is the speed of light in a vacuum, and V is the velocity of the light in the medium. Note n is wavelength (λ) dependent; for a given medium, n blue light > n red light (blue light is slowed more than red light), also n is always > 1.000. Common n, for (λ) = 555 nm (yellow):

Medium	n	Medium	n
Air	1.000	Aqueous	1.336
Tear	1.336	Lens	1.420
Cornea	1.376	Plastic	1.491
		Crown glass	1.523

Diffraction

Light traveling through an aperture produces peaks and valleys of light intensity. This intensity is related to the size of the aperture as given in the formula for the Airy disc (Fig. 1.1).

Diffraction is wavelength-dependent (longer wavelengths are diffracted more than shorter wavelengths) and determines the best size for the pupil (2.5 mm — smaller diameters limit vision due to diffraction). It also limits the resolution of all optical instruments including the eye. Diffraction is also the principle behind multifocal intraocular lens implants.

Snell's Law [Fig. 1.2]

Note that light entering a medium with a higher refractive index is bent toward the normal. For total internal reflection, r is 90° and sin 90° = 1, so solving for i gives the critical angle:

$$i \text{ crit} = \arcsin (n_r/n_i).$$

For crown glass,

$$i \text{ crit} = \arcsin (1.000/1.523) = 41°.$$

FIGURE 1.1. Diffraction

d = diameter of the central disc
f = focal length of the optical system (axial length of the eye)
λ = wavelength of light
a = diameter of aperture (pupil size)

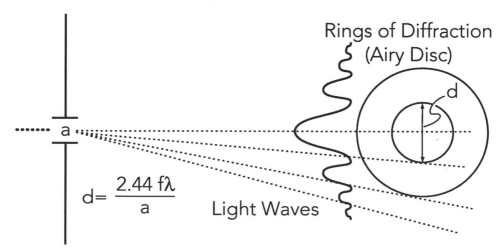

Rings of Diffraction (Airy Disc)

$$d = \frac{2.44\, f\lambda}{a}$$

Light Waves

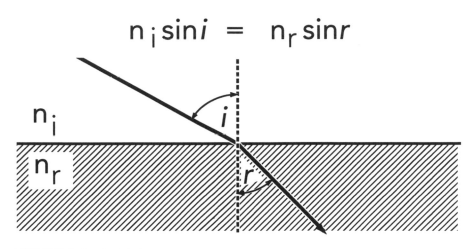

FIGURE 1.2. Snell's Law

n_i = refractive index of incident medium
i = the angle of incidence measured from the normal to the surface
n_r = refractive index of the reflecting medium
r = the angle of reflection measured from the normal to the surface

Total internal reflection can only occur when light rays traveling in a medium of higher n encounter a medium of lower n. (The converse is not true.) This is why total internal reflection occurs when light rays attempt to leave the cornea, but it also suggests how it can be overcome: replace the n cornea/n air interface with n cornea/n glass or n methylcellulose, whose refractive index exceeds n cornea (e.g., gonioscopy).

Total internal reflection is the basis for the operation of light pipes, and prisms used in the slit lamp, operating microscope, and indirect headset.

Vergence

Vergence represents the curvature of the wavefront of light emanating from a light source. By convention light always travels from left to right in nature. Curvature changes as a function of the distance from its source; at its point of origin the curvature is very steep with high (infinite) vergence, at a point distant from the source the curvature is nil, indicating zero vergence (see Table 1.1). All rays from natural sources are divergent and have negative vergence. Convergent rays have plus vergence and imply the presence of lens systems.

TABLE 1.1

Diopter/vergence equivalents

Distance from Source (m)	Vergence (D)
0	$(-)$ Infinity
$\frac{1}{4}$	-4
$\frac{1}{3}$	-3
$\frac{1}{2}$	-2
1	-1
2	$-\frac{1}{2}$
5	$-\frac{1}{5}$
Infinity	0

Vergence Formula

The vergence formula assumes thin ideal lenses surrounded by the same medium on both sides (Fig. 1.3). D is positive for plus lenses and negative for minus lenses. For object and image calculation problems, think of a single lens system as a number line with negative $(-)$ values to the left and positive $(+)$ values to the right of the lens (Table 1.2).

Ray Tracing Definitions [Fig. 1.4]

Note that an image is upright if on the same side as the object, or linear magnification is $(+)$, and is inverted if it is on the opposite side, or linear magnification is $(-)$.

Transverse [Linear] Magnification

$$M\ \text{trans} = \frac{\text{image height}}{\text{object height}} = \frac{\text{image distance}}{\text{object distance}}$$

$$M\ \text{trans} = \frac{I}{O} = \frac{v}{u} = \frac{U}{V}$$

If $|V| > |U|$ or $|u| > |v|$ the image is minified.
If $|U| > |V|$ or $|v| > |u|$ the image is magnified.

Reduced Vergence Formula

This is a more general formula which still requires thin lenses. It can account for different values of n.

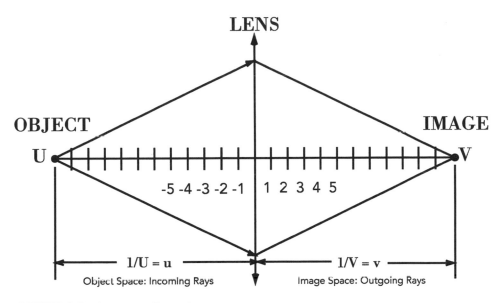

FIGURE 1.3. Vergence Formula

$U + D = V$

U = vergence of object [diopters]
D = vergence of intervening lens [diopters]
V = vergence of image [diopters]

Taking the reciprocal of U, D, and V, one determines

$1/U$ = u: object distance in meters
$1/V$ = v: image distance in meters
$1/D$ = d: focal length of lens in meters

TABLE 1.2

Object and image signs

Location	Nature	Sign
Object on same side of incoming rays	Object real	u is $(-)$
Object on opposite side of incoming rays	Object virtual	u is $(+)$
Image on same side of outgoing rays	Image real	v is $(+)$
Image on opposite side of outgoing rays	Image virtual	v is $(-)$

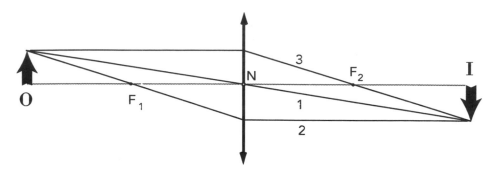

FIGURE 1.4. Ray Tracing Diagram

   O = object height.
   I = image height.
   N = nodal point: the point in the lens system where rays pass undeviated; in a
        thin lens, it is in its center.
   1 = central ray: any ray passing through the nodal point.
   F_1 = primary focal point: the object point where the image point is at infinity.
   F_2 = secondary focal point: the image point where the object at infinity is imaged.

$$\frac{n_1}{u} + \frac{n_1 - n_2}{r} = \frac{n_2}{v},$$

where n_1, n_2 are different refractive indices, and r is the radius of curvature in meters. One must use this formula in calculations involving lenses in fluid media (intraocular lens calculations).

Power of a Spherical Refracting Lens Surface [Fig. 1.5]

To determine if the lens formed is convergent or divergent observe if the surface of the lens is convex toward the medium of lower refractive index. If so, the lens formed is a convergent, or plus lens. If the surface is convex toward the medium of higher refractive index, a minus lens is formed.

Reduced Schematic Eye [Fig. 1.6]

From knowing the central ray and the distance from the nodal point to the retina (17 mm), one can determine the sizes of retinal images from distant objects using similar triangles (Fig. 1.7).

Reflecting Power of a Spherical Mirror [Figs. 1.8 and 1.9]

The primary and secondary focal points of a mirror are identical.

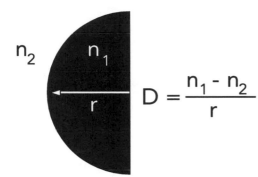

$$D = \frac{n_1 - n_2}{r}$$

FIGURE 1.5. Spherical Refracting Surface

n_1, n_2 are different refractive indices
r is the radius of curvature of the surface in meters
D is the power of the lens in diopters

FIGURE 1.6. Reduced Schematic Eye

N = nodal point
f_a = anterior focal length
f_p = posterior focal length
radius of curvature of the cornea = 5.65 mm
total refractive power of the eye = 60 D

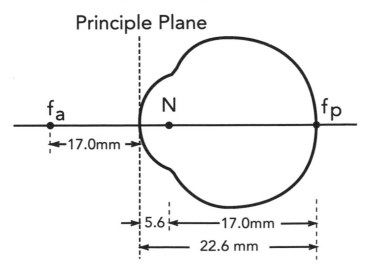

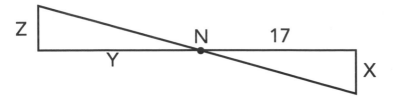

FIGURE 1.7. Retinal Image Size Using Similar Triangles

$x/17\ mm = z/y$

where

x = retinal image size
y = distance to object
z = object size

Telescopes

The optical principle is to create a system resulting in angular magnification of parallel light rays, and consists of two lens systems. The first, or objective, lens creates an image located in space at the primary focal point of the second lens or eyepiece.

In an astronomic telescope, both lenses are plus and an inverted magnified image results. In a Galilean telescope, the objective is a small plus lens, and the eyepiece is a relatively large minus lens, which creates an erect image. Surgical loupes consist of either type of telescope with an additional plus lens, called a working add, to establish an acceptable working distance.

Angular Magnification

This is the ratio of the angle of parallel light rays leaving a telescope (0 out) to that of the parallel rays entering (0 in). It can be approximated by the ratio of D eyepiece to D objective.

$$M\ ang = \frac{\theta\ out}{\theta\ in} = \frac{f\ obj}{f\ eye} = \frac{D\ eyepiece}{D\ objective}$$

Axial Magnification

$$M\ axial = (M\ transverse)^2$$

$$where\ M\ transverse = \frac{image\ height}{object\ height} = \frac{image\ distance}{object\ distance}$$

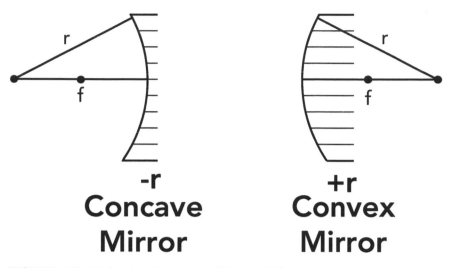

-r
Concave Mirror

+r
Convex Mirror

FIGURE 1.8. Reflecting Power of a Spherical Mirror

$$U + D = V$$

where D reflecting $= -\dfrac{1}{r/2} = -\dfrac{2}{r} = -\dfrac{1}{f}$ and $f = \dfrac{r}{2}$. Note the negative sign in the formula due to the reversal of direction of the light rays.

FIGURE 1.9. Ray Tracing with Mirrors; $r =$ the radius of curvature of the mirror in meters and $f =$ the focal length of the mirror in meters. In ray tracing with mirrors:

1. The central ray passes through r, *not* the center of the mirror.
2. A ray parallel to the axis is reflected through f.
3. A ray directed toward f is reflected back parallel to the axis.

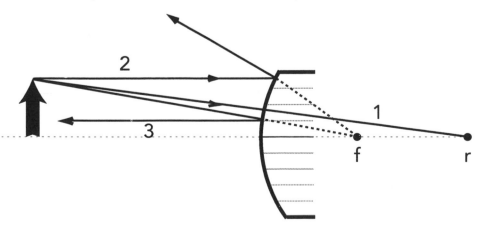

Magnification of a Simple Magnifier [Angular Magnification]

This technique uses as a standard the image size of an object held 25 cm from the eye.

$$M \text{ angular} = \frac{D}{4}$$

where D is the power of the lens.

Accommodation Through a Telescope [AT]

$$AT = Ad \, (M \text{ transverse})^2$$

where Ad = the diopters of accommodation required to image the object without the telescope's presence.

Optical Instruments

Lensmeter

1. Examples are Lensometer (A-O Scientific), Vertometer (Bausch & Lomb), and Vertex Refractionmeter (Zeiss). All are telescopes.

2. In their simplified operation a light source illuminates a movable target. A fixed power convex lens is situated such that when the dial attached to the movable target is at the "zero" setting the vergence supplied by the lens is equal and opposite in sign to the vergence of the light entering the lens; hence the light rays leaving the lens are parallel and have zero vergence. This design is an illustration of the optometer principle.

3. Addition of a spectacle lens supplies another source of vergence to the zero vergence, parallel light rays, thus creating a telescope. To balance the additional vergence supplied by the spectacle lens an equal and opposite amount can be supplied by moving the target. If the target moved farther away from the condensing lens, net plus vergence is generated, which would balance a *minus* spectacle lens. If it is moved closer to the condensing lens, net minus vergence is generated, which would balance a *plus* spectacle lens.

4. Proper use of the lensmeter for determination of a distance spectacle prescription is with the spectacle bows away from examiner with a posterior surface of the lens against the nosecone of the lensmeter.

5. The following formula will assist in the transposition of plus cylinder to minus cylinder prescriptions:

$$S + C \times A = (S+C) - C \times (A \pm 90°),$$

where

> S = sphere
> C = cylinder
> A = axis

6. The bifocal add is properly calculated by determining the distance and segment powers with the *anterior* lens surface against the nosecone of the lensmeter. Failure to do this results in significant error in the add determination in high-power prescriptions.

7. Images formed in the lensmeter are real, and if prism is present, the target is deviated toward the *base* of the prism.

8. Lensmeters measure the vertex power of the surface *against* the nosecone (usually posterior vertex power).

Geneva Lens Clock

1. The clock comprises a dial calibrated in diopters with a foot plate consisting of three pins in a line. The central pin is mobile in the vertical plane while the two peripheral pins are fixed. The vertical motion of the central pin moves the pointer along the dial scale.

2. It is calibrated for a specific refractive index (usually crown glass). If one uses the glass-calibrated lens clock on a plastic lens, it will be erroneous.

3. It can be used to determine on which surface of the spectacle lens the cylinder is ground.

Keratometer (Ophthalmometer)

1. Principle involves the determination of the *size* of a reflected image of a mire projected on the corneal surface. The size of the mire is inversely proportional to the power of the cornea as a convex mirror.

2. From the size of the image one can determine the power (P) of the cornea as a convex mirror by comparing the ratio of the size of the mire projected to its reflected image.

3. From the power of the convex mirror one can determine the radius (r) of curvature (in meters) from the formula $P = 2/r$.

4. From r and using the reduced vergence formula,

$$D = \frac{n_1 - n_2}{r},$$

where $n_1 = 1.3375$ and $n_2 = 1.000$, one can calculate $D =$ the power in diopters of the anterior corneal surface (this calculation assumes a specific corneal refractive index which has been normalized to 1.3375). The standardized formula becomes

$$\text{Dcornea} = \frac{337.5}{r \text{ (mm)}}.$$

5. Circular mires (Bausch & Lomb Keratometer) become oval if asphericity is present. The shorter radius of the oval is at the steeper meridian; the longer radius of the oval is at the flatter meridian.

6. Keratometry measures only the central 3 mm and assumes a smooth surface in that area.

Slit Lamp

1. Light source projects an *image* of the light filament at the same point in space as observation system focal point.

2. Observation system is a low-power astronomic telescope containing Porro prisms to reinvert the image and reduce the pupillary distance.

Direct Ophthalmoscope

1. Light source illuminates an area of interest.

2. Uses the lens of the patient's eye as a simple magnifier. In an emmetrope whose net cornea/lens power is 60 diopters (D), the magnification would be 60/4 or 15×.

3. In a myopic patient, the additional plus in the patient's lens creates a Galilean telescope resulting in image magnification.

4. In a hyperopic patient, the loss of plus (or addition of minus) power creates a reverse Galilean telescope creating image minification.

5. The patient's and the observer's retinas are conjugate points.

Indirect Ophthalmoscope

1. Utilizes the Gullstrand principle; the illuminating and observation rays pass through different portions of the patient's pupil to avoid reflections.

2. A bright source of light is passed through the pupil to illuminate the retina, making it a luminous object. Light rays emerging, if from an emmetropic eye, are parallel and are imaged by a condensing lens (usually 20 D).

3. The image formed is real, inverted, magnified (60/20 = 3×), and aerial.

4. The viewing system consists of prisms to reduce the pupillary distance and a series of plus lenses to prevent accommodative convergence.

5. The observer's pupil and patient's pupil are conjugate planes; the patient's retina, the aerial image, and the observer's retina are conjugate planes.

6. The fundus camera uses identical principles to image the retina. Conjugate points are the patient's pupil and the holed mirror in the camera.

Operating Microscope

1. Contains a light source that may or may not be coaxial (important in locating visual axis in refractive procedures).

2. Observation system is an astronomic telescope with inverting prisms.

Visual Acuity

Visual function can be expressed in a variety of formats. The two most important forms are minimum angle of resolution (the basis for Snellen acuity) and Vernier acuity.

Snellen Acuity

1. Snellen acuity is expressed as a fraction whose numerator is the distance of the patient to the chart, and whose denominator represents the smallest line of characters discernible at that distance.

2. A "20/20" character subtends a total arc of 5 minutes of a degree with a minimum angle of resolution of 1 minute.

3. There is a linear relation between the size of a character and its Snellen notation. A 20/40 letter is twice the size of a 20/20 letter and half the size of a 20/80 letter.

4. To check calibration of projected charts use the following relation: size of 20/400 character (in millimeters) = testing distance (in millimeters) × 0.0291, where distance denotes distance from *patient* to chart (not projector to chart).

5. The ratio of optotype sizes varies with the acuity level tested and is greater with larger letters. This can be a problem with patients who could see the 20/200 letter but not the 20/100 letter and are therefore "legally blind." Newer charts, such as those used in the Early Treatment for Diabetic Retinopathy Study (ETDRS), keep a constant ratio between lines based on a 0.1 log geometric series.

Vernier Acuity

1. Vernier acuity records the ability of the eye to detect spatial misalignment.

2. It typically measures 8 seconds of arc.

3. Examiners rely on Vernier acuity to determine the end points in Goldmann tonometry, keratometry, optical pachymetry, and in the use of the lensmeter.

4. Alterations in Vernier acuity form the basis of Amsler grid testing.

Contrast Sensitivity

1. Contrast sensitivity (CS) is determined by the identification of multiple grating patterns on a chart characterized by different stripe orientation, spatial frequency (the number of light/dark pairs per degree of visual angle), and the degree of contrast between light and dark stripes. Snellen optotypes are characterized by square wave gratings of uniform light and dark stripes with sharp edges. Charts of CS have sinusoidal gratings with a gradual transition from light to dark. At different frequencies, different amounts of contrast are needed to determine the grating pattern. Normal CS peaks at 5 to 10 cycles per degree and falls off gradually at lower frequencies; hence more contrast is required to see gratings at higher or lower spatial frequencies (Fig. 1.10). Cataracts may cause a significant loss of functional vision (due to loss of low- and high-frequency sensitivity from light diffusion) with near normal Snellen acuity. Loss of contrast sensitivity, however, is not specific for cataract.

2. The loss of acuity due to glare can be measured and quantitated by the brightness acuity test (BAT) devised by Holladay.

Near Vision

Accommodation

This represents an increase in plus power of crystalline lens secondary to increasing its curvature. It occurs as part of the near triad (miosis, convergence, and accommodation). Measurement is in one of three fashions:

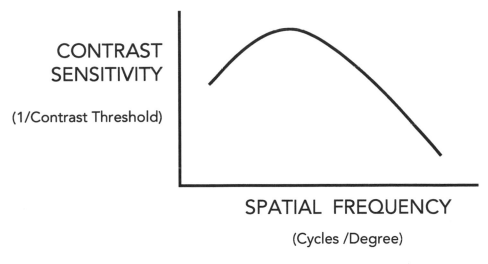

CONTRAST SENSITIVITY

(1/Contrast Threshold)

SPATIAL FREQUENCY

(Cycles /Degree)

FIGURE 1.10. Contrast Sensitivity Curve This normal curve plots CS (the inverse of threshold contrast) versus spatial frequency.

Near Point Method Patient wears best distance correction and views 6 point print, which is moved progressively closer until blurring is reported (each eye is tested separately). The reciprocal of the distance in meters at which print blurs represents the amplitude of accommodation (AOA).

Prince Rule Technique The Prince rule is a scaled ruler with gradations in centimeters and diopters. Patients are tested monocularly with best distance correction in place. A $+3.00$ sphere is added to the distance correction to bring the far point of the patient to $\frac{1}{3}$ m. A target with 6 point print is brought progressively closer from the initial point where print is clear until the print blurs. The difference in *diopters* between the two points is the diopters of accommodation.

If the patient is effectively emmetropic, the far point should be $\frac{1}{3}$ m; if that point lies closer than $\frac{1}{3}$ m, uncorrected myopia is present; if farther away, uncorrected hyperopia is present.

Spherical Adds Patients are tested monocularly with proper distance correction in place. At a fixed distance ($\frac{1}{2}$ m) patient views 4 point print. Plus sphere is progressively added to the distance spectacle correction until blurring occurs and the total amount added is noted. Plus sphere is then progressively decreased, followed by the addition of minus sphere until the image blurs, and the total amount is noted. The sum in diopters added and subtracted is calculated and represents the diopters of accommodation. If the test is begun by adding minus sphere first, the amount of accommodation calculated may be falsely low.

Deficiency States

Presbyopia   Age-related and believed secondary to lens-zonule changes:

1. General rule (for availability of diopters of accommodation based on age): age 40 = 6D (for each 4 yrs under age 40 add 1D); age 44 = 4D; age 48 = 3D (for each 4 yrs over age 48 subtract 0.50 D).
2. The add can be estimated by age, remembering not to give a first-time bifocal wearer an add of more than 1.25 D (unless for a special need) and not to add more than 0.50 D at one time, generally at a rate of 0.25 D per 5 years.
3. To calculate the add required by a patient:
   a) Calculate the dioptric demand for the task (i.e., an object at 20 cm requires 5 D).
   b) Determine the amplitude of accommodation (AOA) as previously described.
   c) Recall that a person with uncorrected myopia will have "extra diopters" available (a −3.00 myope will have 3 D). An uncorrected hyperope will have to exert accommodation to see at infinity.
   d) The patient should exert only half of his AOA, and the remaining power required is given in the add.

Other

1. Uncorrected hyperopia
2. Overminused myope
3. Spectacle-corrected myope switched to contact lenses (even with proper vertexing)
4. Contact-lens-corrected hyperope switched to spectacles (even with proper vertexing)
5. Use of topical or systemic drugs with anticholinergic effects
6. Insulin-dependent diabetes mellitus
7. Acquired immune deficiency syndrome (AIDS), diphtheria, botulism
8. Trauma to long ciliary nerves following panretinal photocoagulation

Vision Correction

Retinoscopy (Plus Cylinder Technique)

1. Observe the motion, brightness, and size of the reflex exiting the pupil at a working distance of $\frac{2}{3}$ m:
   a) Dim "pseudoneutrality" reflex indicates large degrees of ametropia. Attempt to convert to a brighter reflex by either high plus or minus sphere.
   b) If "against" motion is seen, add minus sphere to convert all meridians to "with" motion, creating a refractive state of hyperopic astigmatism.
2. With all meridians showing "with" reflexes, compare meridians at 90° to one another to determine if cylinder is present:
   a) If one meridian is brighter and broader than the other, 90° away, cylinder is present.
   b) Neutralize the brightest reflex first using plus sphere.
3. Examine the remaining "with" reflex. Attempt to determine its axis:
   a) If cylinder is high (> 1–2 D), look for the *break phenomenon* (a deviation of the streak along its length that occurs if the streak is not oriented along the patient's cylindrical axis). This is a stationary reflex.
   b) *Skew* is used when lesser amounts of cylinder are present. In this technique, the streak is moved and the relative angle of the reflex in relation to the angle of the streak is observed. The reflex will be deviated relative to the angle of the streak if the streak is off axis. Think of this as a dynamic break phenomenon.
   c) For small amounts of cylinder, use the *guideline phenomenon*. Orient the streak 45° to either side of the estimated axis and observe the reflex. If it is noticeably brighter on one side (the guideline), turn the axis slightly toward that side and recheck. When both sides are equally bright, the axis is correct.
   d) Apply plus cylinder at the determined axis until neutralization is seen.
4. Minus cylinder technique:
   a) Create simple hyperopic astigmatism by applying minus sphere.
   b) Set cylinder axis 90° from the "with" reflex.
   c) For each −0.25 of cylinder placed add +0.25 of sphere ("double click stop").
   d) When straddling the axis move cylinder away from the guideline until equal.

5. Abnormal reflexes:
   a)   Scissoring: suspect irregular corneal astigmatism, keratoconus.
   b)   Oil drop: nuclear sclerosis, posterior/anterior lenticonus.
   c)   Decreased visibility: media opacity.

Refraction

1. Begin with present spectacle prescription in phoropter or retinoscopy findings.
   a)   Irrespective of prescription attempt to add plus sphere (important in hyperopes and myopes complaining of blurred near vision).
   b)   If no improvement, add minus sphere (in myopes ask if they can see more letters or if letters are just smaller and darker). In general, each −0.25 D of additional sphere should improve a myope's vision one line on the Snellen chart.
   c)   Place Jackson cross-cylinder in position.
       i)   The power of Jackson cross used depends on patient's potential level of vision: 20/40 or better, ±0.25 D; 20/40 to 20/70, ±0.50 D; 20/70 or worse, ±1.00 D.
       ii)   Refine the axis first.
       iii) Refine the power after axis is set.
       iv)   For each +0.50 D of cylinder added, add −0.25 sphere to maintain the position of the conoid of Sturm.
       v)   Recheck the sphere power after cylinder axis and power is selected for best visual acuity.
   d)   If the refraction represents a new prescription, binocular balance both eyes.
   e)   Irregular astigmatism may prevent good vision with spectacles, and a hard contact lens over-refraction can correct this problem.
2. Postoperative cataract patients:
   a)   Perform keratometry to determine the steepest meridian.
   b)   For plus cylinder phoropters, orient the axis parallel to the steepest meridian.
   c)   Dial in two-thirds the amount of keratometric cylinder and an amount of minus sphere to create the spherical equivalent (sphere + residual cylinder/2) of plano.
   d)   Change the sphere until best visual acuity is obtained.
   e)   Refine the axis and power of the cylinder using the Jackson cross-cylinder.
   f)   Rerefine the sphere for best final visual acuity.

3. No previous prescription (cooperative patient):
   a) Add sphere (plus sphere first) to best visual acuity.
   b) Search for cylinder with Jackson cross.
      i) Begin with Jackson cross at 90° and compare flips of plus cylinder axis 90° versus axis 180°; if the patient prefers one axis over the other, add +0.50 cylinder at that axis with a −0.25 sphere.
      ii) Repeat the procedure until equal appearance.
      iii) If there is no preference, orient the axis at 45° and 135° to search for oblique cylinder. If a preference is shown, add plus cylinder in that axis and refine.
4. Binocular balancing:
   a) May use vertical prism to dissociate eyes.
   b) Add or subtract 0.25 D increments of sphere until eyes are equally clear.
5. Duochrome testing:
   a) Makes use of the chromatic interval of +1.25 D with blue light focused ahead of red light. Green is usually substituted for blue, as letters on a blue background would be more difficult to see.
   b) The goal is to place the midpoint of the interval (yellow light) on the retina such that the red and green light are *equally* defocused.
   c) This is a monocular test: ask the patient which letters are clearer, those over the green background or those over the red background.
   d) Possible responses (Table 1.3).
6. Trial lenses should be considered in the following situations:
   a) If the new prescription is more than 2 D different from previous prescription or between eyes.

TABLE 1.3

Duochrome test responses

Refractive Error	Response	Interpretation
Myopia	Red clearer	Underminused
Myopia	Green clearer	Overminused
Hyperopia	Red clearer	Overplussed
Hyperopia	Green clearer	Underplussed
Myopia or hyperopia	Equally clear	Balanced

    b) If the new prescription changes the axis of the cylinder more than 10° from the old prescription.

    c) If attempting to determine working distances for correction of presbyopia.

  7. Vertex distances:

    a) Always determine for prescriptions greater than 5 D.

    b) Use distometer (caliper) to measure.

Low Vision

1. Use the general rule: take quotient of the reciprocal of the Snellen acuity to determine the approximate power of sphere required to read J5 print. Example: a patient with a best corrected vision of 20/200 would require a 200/20 or 10 D lens to read J5.

2. Low-vision aids for near tasks:
a) Hand and stand magnifiers with and without lighting systems
b) Telescopes
c) High-power reading glasses including large (+5.00) reading adds
d) Closed-circuit television systems

The drawback of most near visual aids is their short working distance.

3. Low vision aids for distance usually involve telescopes. Telescopes are limited by their restricted field of view.

Corrective Lenses

Spectacles

To correct ametropias, spectacles are prescribed such that the secondary focal point of the spectacle is placed at the far point of the ametropic eye (Fig. 1.11).

Construction

Lens blanks are all meniscus lenses with a 5 to 6 D front curve and a variable posterior curve. By grinding a posterior curve steeper than the front curve a minus lens is formed. Similarly a flatter posterior curve generates a plus lens. Edge thickness of a minus lenses increases with higher powers, larger optic sizes, lower refractive index materials, and longer vertex distances.

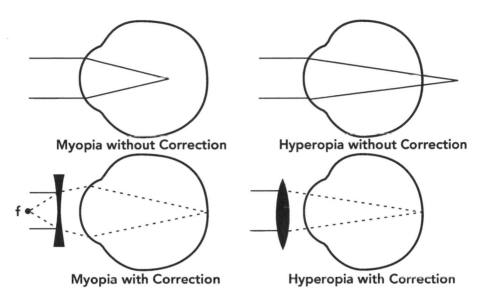

FIGURE 1.11. Simple Refractive Errors of the Eye

Induced Aberrations

1. Image size is minified by minus lenses and magnified by plus lenses.
2. Image distortion includes pincushion effect with high plus lenses, barrel distortion with high minus lenses.
3. Effects on motility deviations:
    a) Lens effects are independent of the particular type of deviation (esodeviation, exodeviation, etc.).
    b) High minus lenses increase the apparent measurement. (The measured deviation is larger than the true deviation.)
    c) High plus lenses decrease the apparent measurement.
    d) Formula to estimate effect (Scattergood, Brown, and Guyton, 1983) 2.5 × (D) = % change in the true deviation due to lens, where D = the spectacle lens power. For example, a + 10 D patient measures 30 Esotropia (ET), which is 2.5 × (10), or 25% less than the true 40 ET deviation.
4. Induced phorias or tropias:
    a) Difference in power in the vertical meridian of a spectacle correction is the most important factor.
    b) If this difference is greater than 2 D in the vertical meridian, diplopia while reading is likely.

    c) Treatment options of anisometropia in the vertical meridian:
        i)   Slab off over more minus or less plus lens.
        ii) Decenter optical centers: lower the optical center in the less myopic or more hyperopic eye.
        iii) Prescribe single vision reading glasses.
        iv) Reduce vertex distance.
        v)   Prescribe contact lenses.

5. Prismatic deviation: amount is determined by Prentice's rule (Fig. 1.12).
6. Meridional aniseikonia:
    a) Term to describe sensations (such as inclination/declination errors—tilting) resulting from disparately sized retinal images that result from meridional magnification or minification.
    b) Almost always iatrogenic (correction of ametropias, surgery such as keratoplasty or cataract, and results from the full correction of astigmatic ametropias with spherocylindrical spectacles).
    c) Generally there is a 2% change in size per diopter difference in spectacle correction, which is appreciated under binocular conditions (use trial frames).
    d) Large amounts can be corrected by contact lens–spectacle combinations that construct Galilean telescopes to alter image size. For example, to reduce the magnification of an aphakic eye, one can prescribe extra plus on the contact lens and then correct the induced myopia with a minus spectacle lens.
    e) It is also reduced by decreasing vertex distance or use of posterior curve lenses.
    f) A prescription may be changed to reduce the effect by rotating the axis of cylinder toward vertical meridian or reducing cylinder power or both.

Prismatic Deviation

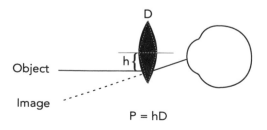

FIGURE 1.12. Prentice's Rule

P = the induced prism in prism diopters
h = the deviation in centimeters from the optical center of the lens
D = the power of the lens in diopters

$$P = hD$$

7. Lens effectivity:
   a) The general formula is

   $$D2 = \frac{1}{f2} - \frac{1}{f1-S} = \frac{D1}{1-SD1}.$$

   Or is approximated by the formula

   $$D2 = D1 + S(D1)^2,$$

   where

   $D2$ = new lens power
   $D1$ = old lens power
   S = difference in location in meters
   $f1$ = original lens focal length in meters
   $f2$ = new lens focal length in meters

   b) The secondary focal point of a spectacle moves in the same direction as the direction of the change in its vertex distance.
   c) In a hyperopic eye, the far point is posterior to the globe; if the corrective plus lens is moved closer to the eye, the secondary focal point of the lens will be moved *posterior* to the eye's far point, therefore requiring additional plus to pull the secondary focal point of the lens back to the eye's far point. Hence, a plus lens moved closer to the eye becomes less effective and requires more power to correct a given amount of hyperopia.
   d) In a myopic eye, the far point is anterior to the globe; if a correcting minus lens is moved closer to the eye, the secondary focal point will be moved *posterior* to the eye's far point, requiring a reduction in minus power to reposition the secondary focal point back to the eye's far point.
8. Pantoscopic tilt of a minus lens creates minus cylinder axis 180°; plus lens creates plus cylinder axis 180°.

Bifocals

Aberrations

Image Displacement This is due to the combined prismatic effects generated as the patient's line of sight deviates from the optical center of the distance correction and enters the bifocal segment. To illustrate, a minus lens can be simplified as two prisms, apex to apex. As a patient looks down, his line of sight deviates inferiorly from the optical center of the lens. By Prentice's rule, prism base-down will be generated and objects will appear to rise up to the patient. If a bifocal segment is then encountered with the base in the same direction base-down (a round-top bifocal), this displacement will be exaggerated by a sudden increase in further base-down prism (image jump), causing greater image displacement upward.

1. In myopic prescriptions, image displacement is minimized by flat-top bifocal segments and maximized by round-top segments.
2. In hyperopic prescriptions, image displacement is maximized by flat-top bifocal segments and minimized by round-top segments.

Image Jump   Describes a sudden shift in spatial localization of an image associated with entry into the bifocal segment where a large change due to prismatic deviation occurs.

1. Prismatic effect of a bifocal segment is a function of the decentration from its optical center (Prentice's rule). Because of this, irrespective of the distance prescription, *round-top* segments whose prismatic effect is maximal at the top of the segment *always* maximize image jump.
2. Minimized by a flat-top segment where the optical center is at the top of the segment, which therefore creates minimal prismatic deviation. (See Fig. 1.13.)

Blended Bifocals   Have corridor of clear vision at all distances. Multiple types are available.

FIGURE 1.13.   Prismatic Effects of Bifocals

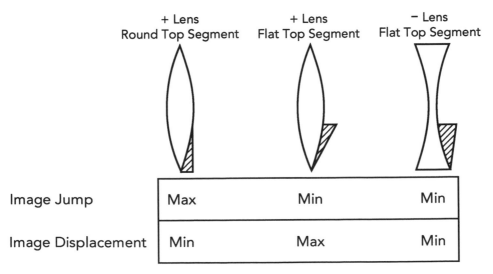

	+ Lens Round Top Segment	+ Lens Flat Top Segment	− Lens Flat Top Segment
Image Jump	Max	Min	Min
Image Displacement	Min	Max	Min

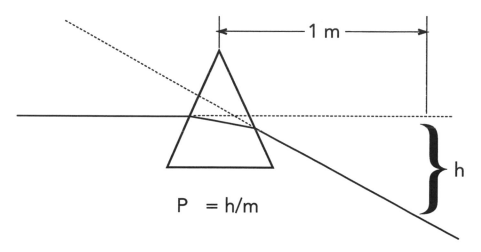

FIGURE 1.14. Prism Power *p* = power in prism diopters and *h/m*=deviation of light in centimeters at 1 m.

1. Adjacent to this area, the lens image is often optically distorted.
2. It is imperative to match the exact type and manufacturer of blended bifocal style when duplicating a prescription.

Prisms

Prisms create *virtual* images that are displaced toward the apex of the prism. Prisms displace real images and light rays toward the *base*.

Power

This is given by the formula in Fig. 1.14.

Materials

1. Glass prisms are calibrated in Prentice position.
2. Plastic prisms are calibrated in minimum angle of deviation position.

Calibration

1. Prentice position: prism is oriented with one of the prism faces perpendicular to the light rays. All the prismatic deviation occurs at second prism-air interface.
2. Minimum angle of deviation position: prism oriented so that mid-axis of prism is perpendicular to the axis of the incident light. Equal deviation occurs at each air-prism interface.

3. Frontal plane position: prism oriented so that posterior surface of the prism is parallel to the patient's forehead. This position is close to the minimum angle of the deviation position.

Prism Usage

1. Orient the apex of the prism toward the direction of the deviation.
2. In an orthophoric patient, a prism induces a phoria in the direction of its *base*.

Determination of Prism in Spectacles

1. Measured in the Prentice position in the lensometer.
2. Image observed in the lensometer is real and is displaced in the direction of the base.
3. To determine the total power of prism in spectacles cancel prisms in the same direction in each lens, and add prisms going the opposite way.

In Clinical Practice

1. Astronomic telescopes use prisms to invert images to create erect final images (slit lamp, operating microscope).
2. Prisms are also used in indirect ophthalmoscopes, Goldmann applanator (doubling prism), the keratometer, and in prismatic contact fundus lenses (McLean).
3. Stacking prisms with faces in contact with each other results in large errors in prismatic power (their prismatic effect exceeds the sum of their individual powers).

Ametropias

Myopia

1. Inheritance of high myopia tends to be dominant.

2. Acquired causes are usually refractive in nature rather than axial. For example: keratoconus, accommodative spasm, lens changes secondary to osmotic shifts (diabetes mellitus, pregnancy), drug-induced (sulfa drugs, acetazolamide [Diamox]), and nuclear sclerosis.

Hyperopia

1. Unknown inheritance; it is the usual refractive state of normal newborns (approximately 2 D hyperopia).

2. Acquired causes center on changes (reductions) in axial length. Examples are retro-orbital tumors, central serous retinopathy, choroidal elevations.

3. Total hyperopia is the sum of latent hyperopia, facultative hyperopia, and absolute hyperopia.

$$H_T = H_L + H_F + H_A,$$

where

H_T = total hyperopia
H_L = latent hyperopia, or the amount of hyperopia uncovered following cycloplegia (i.e., corrected by tone of the ciliary muscle)
H_F = facultative hyperopia, or the amount of hyperopia that can be overcome through accommodation
H_A = absolute hyperopia, or that which cannot be compensated by the eye.

4. Manifest hyperopia is the facultative hyperopia plus absolute hyperopia.

5. At young ages, total hyperopia = latent hyperopia; in the postpresbyopic age, total hyperopia = absolute hyperopia.

Astigmatism

1. Astigmatism describes a nonspherical surface. Most patients have small to moderate amounts.

2. If the steeper and flatter axes are 90° apart, it is regular; if not, it is irregular. Irregular astigmatism is uncorrectable with spectacles containing cylinders and requires the use of a contact lens to provide a regular refracting surface.

3. The term "with the rule" refers to astigmatism in which the steeper meridian lies at the vertical meridian. Cylinders create a line focus (spheres create a point focus) parallel to the cylinder's axis. The power of a cylinder is 90° from its axis.

4. Acquired causes
a) Corneal ectasia: keratoconus, keratoglobus, pellucid marginal degeneration, post ulcer, or traumatic scar.
b) Corneal lesions: pterygium—flattens the meridian aligned with the lesion.
c) Postoperative: a tight corneal or corneoscleral suture steepens the cornea in the meridian of the suture.
d) Lid lesions: masses such as large chalazia tend to cause steepening of the meridian aligned with the mass.

5. Cylinder transposition and the power cross. In astigmatic ametropias, two focal lines are formed within the eye; between these lines the conoid of Sturm is formed. As an example, consider an eye corrected with a $-2.00 + 1.00 \times 90°$ spectacle lens. The corresponding eyeball error is $+2.00 \times 180° \supset +1.00 \times 90°$ (Fig. 1.15).

a) Remember the power cross describes cylinder power that is 90° from the axis.

b) Both focal lines formed will be anterior to the retina, with the horizontal line farther into the vitreous than the vertical one. The patient should see the vertical lines more clearly than the horizontal lines.

c) A *vertically* oval blur area will be on the retina.

Correction of Ametropias

1. Correction of spherical refractive errors creates a single *point* of focus.

2. Correction of astigmatic refractive errors creates a small, sharp *circle* of focus. There is no single point of focus.

3. Correction of axial ametropias (almost all are naturally occurring) will result in similarly sized retinal images. This is Knapp's rule.

4. Attempts at correcting refractive ametropias (usually man-made, for example, surgical aphakia with spectacles) will result in disparately sized retinal images (approximately 2% change per 1 D difference in correction).

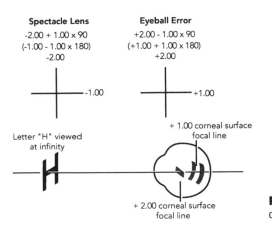

Spectacle Lens
-2.00 + 1.00 x 90
(-1.00 - 1.00 x 180)
-2.00

Eyeball Error
+2.00 - 1.00 x 90
(+1.00 + 1.00 x 180)
+2.00

-1.00

+1.00

+ 1.00 corneal surface focal line

Letter "H" viewed at infinity

+ 2.00 corneal surface focal line

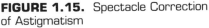

FIGURE 1.15. Spectacle Correction of Astigmatism

Selected Readings

Milder B, Rubin ML. The fine art of prescribing glasses without making a spectacle of yourself. Gainesville, Florida: Triad Publishing Company, 1978.

Reinecke RD, Herm RJ. Refraction: a programmed text. Norwalk, Connecticut: Appleton-Century-Crofts, 1983.

Rubin ML. Optics for clinicians. Gainesville, Florida: Triad Publishing Company, 1974.

Sadun AA, Brandt JD. Optics for ophthalmologists. New York: Springer-Verlag, 1987.

Scattergood KD, Brown MH, Guyton DL. Artifact introduced by spectacle lenses in the measurement of strabismic deviations. Am J Ophthalmol 1983;96:439–88.

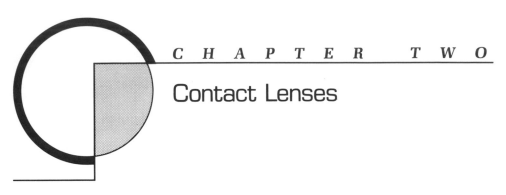

R. Linsy Farris, M.D.

General Considerations

Patient Selection

A complete ophthalmic examination is required before contact lenses are discussed in any depth. Special attention should be directed toward the following points:

1. Patient expectations regarding contact lenses, including any prior experience of the patient with contact lenses personally or through the experience of a friend or relative. One can consider starting with a different type or brand of contact lens if a previous experience was extremely negative.

2. The eye examination should emphasize the following:
  a) Careful distance and near refraction.
  b) Keratometry.
  c) Corneal diameters.
  d) External eye problems. For example, look for oily lid margins,

allergic conjunctivitis, mucus in the tear film, prominent limbal vasculature, folliculosis, and dry eyes.
e) The evaluation for dry eyes is particularly important. Only when tears cannot be produced as a result of reflex tearing will significant ocular surface intolerance to contact lenses develop. This is because increased evaporation of tears during contact lens wear is the result of tear film disruption (Farris 1986). A careful Schirmer's test (lid margins should be cleaned of meibomian oils, which can permeate the filter paper and slow fluid migration, and insertion should be at the junction of the middle and lateral lower lid margin to avoid touching the cornea when the patient looks up) without anesthetic, with a value of 5 mm of wetting or greater in 5 minutes, is adequate.

3. After the examination, patients are informed of the findings and their suitability as candidates for contact lens wear. Patients should be encouraged to obtain a pair of spectacles with a current prescription. Hence, they will have a back-up system and be less tempted to overwear the contact lens if they begin to have problems. The caution, to be repeated many times, is to remove the contact lens if it does not begin to feel right, to clean the lens, and insert it again only after the eye feels normal. If the problem continues and persists, the patient is to remove the lens and come in for an examination even as an emergency.

Patient Discussion: Risks and Benefits

An initial conversation about contact lenses with patients should include informing them about the advantages (including the lack of frame discomfort and cosmesis) and disadvantages of various types of contact lenses, as well as the risks and the inexact nature of the fitting process, which may involve trial and error. As with any elective procedure, the physician should indicate lenses as one solution to their vision problem. There are two goals in fitting contact lenses:

1. First and foremost, protect the eye.
2. Satisfy the patient with the most comfortable lens possible with clear vision.

A patient should be aware that these goals may not always be achieved. This should be documented in the medical record. Some practitioners have patients sign a statement that they accept the risk of contact lens fitting and that they have been instructed in the proper care in wearing the lenses.

The inherent risks of contact lens wear must also be discussed. Patients should be told that contact lens wear may lead to permanent scarring and decreased vision. The following complications should be discussed (see Changes and Complications Induced by Contact Lens Wear, below, for other problems).

1. Corneal abrasion: direct trauma from lens insertion or removal, anoxia producing decompensation of the corneal epithelium, or from a foreign body under the lens.
2. Conjunctivitis: usually a minor complication that clears without sequela after the patient discontinues contact lens wear and is treated with antibiotic drops, preferably one effective against pseudomonas.
3. Corneal ulceration: again, pseudomonas is of concern as it can destroy vision within hours if treatment is not instituted.

Patients are told these risks will be minimized or avoided by careful fitting and follow-up care (examinations, instruction, and reinforcement of appropriate lens cleaning, insertion, and removal techniques).

Material Selection

Soft Lenses   The advantages include comfort, a shorter adaptation period, and flexible wearing time. Disposable extended-wear lenses avoid contact with potentially contaminated solutions and lens storage cases. Disposable contact lenses are one of the greatest advances in the past two to three decades, perhaps even exceeding the introduction of gas-permeable materials. Most patients will be able to wear the lens safely 1 to 2 weeks before discarding it. The actual length of time should be based on the amount of film deposition, which provides a foothold for bacteria (Stern and Zam 1986; Aswad et al. 1990). The only truly clean lens is a new lens.

Disposable soft contact lenses are not markedly different from daily or extended-wear soft contact lenses except for reduced cost due to computerized quality control techniques. Disposable lens costs are currently slightly higher than conventional daily-wear soft contact lenses (even when factoring in the cost of solutions) and the limited power availability and size may limit their applicability.

Epidemiologic studies of lens complications suggest great care must be taken in the fitting of disposable extended-wear contact lenses because of the increased risk of serious eye infections (Schein et al. 1989; Poggio et al. 1989).

However, some studies suggest that bathing contact lenses in sterile tears resting on the ocular surface is much safer than transferring them repeatedly across a bacteria-laden lid margin. (Hart et al. 1990).

Disadvantages of soft contact lenses are a shorter life, higher risk of complications such as hypoxia and infection, less reproducibility, and variable vision.

Rigid Lenses   In general, a rigid gas-permeable (RGP) material is preferable over polymethyl methacrylate (PMMA) because of superior oxygen transport capabilities. RGP material allows for larger-diameter lenses, which move less and are more comfortable. Extended-wear rigid lenses have been made possible by increased oxygen permeability (Garcia et al. 1990) but are not as safe as soft lenses.

1. Advantages: better vision compared with soft lenses, easier handling, greater durability, and lower maintenance cost with better correction of astigmatism, keratoconus, and aphakia. They are generally better tolerated in the dry-eye patient.
2. Disadvantages: initial discomfort and a longer adaptation time than with soft lenses.

Patients who are doing well with PMMA are not switched to an RGP lens unless they are having problems that require a refitting. The evidence regarding PMMA and endothelial polymegathism at this time is not significant.

Contact Lens Fees

Contact lenses can be a losing proposition economically unless the physician considers the additional time and costs involved. A firm policy for collecting the total fee before the lens is ordered and certainly before the patient receives any lens is mandatory. This will avoid the patient's refusal to pay if the lenses do not feel right or work out. Prior payment will motivate the patient to be a successful lens wearer, and physicians will be encouraged, as compensation for the lenses and time has already been received.

The fee structure should allow a separate charge for the contact lens trial visit, which is credited to the fitting fee. A provision for a refund of unused portions of the fitting fee or returned contact lens at any time after the lenses are ordered will reduce the pressure to fit everyone successfully. A list of fees for various types of contact lens fittings and replacements should be provided.

Contact Lens Terminology

Contact lens terminology is presented in Figure 2.1.

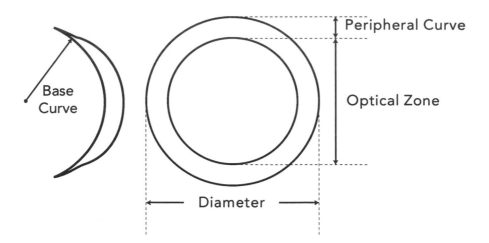

FIGURE 2.1. Contact Lens Terminology Base curve (in millimeters) = radius of curvature of the central posterior optical portion of the contact lens. Diameter = edge-to-edge length in millimeters.

Trial Lens Fitting

The goal of the trial lens fitting is to provide both the patient and fitter with information that will ensure greater success. Key factors are the feel and fit of the contact lens and best correctable vision. An adequate inventory of lenses is required to achieve these goals, and the first lens ordered should be considered a trial lens. Lenses returned can be added to the inventory to quickly build a good selection. The trial period to find the most satisfactory lens possible may last for 2 to 3 months.

Again, the patient should be involved in the decision of which lens will be fit (see above, General Considerations, Material Selection). With 1 D or less of corneal astigmatism, a soft disposable contact lens is a first option. If the degree of astigmatism is greater than 1 D, and the patient is not satisfied with the vision achieved using a spherical soft contact lens, a toric soft lens is chosen. If the vision is still unsatisfactory, then a rigid gas-permeable lens is chosen. If this lens is unsuitable due to discomfort, then one usually returns to a toric soft lens. If the patient still has problems, then spectacles are recommended.

Soft Lens Fitting

1. Determine the spherical equivalent (sph. eq. = sph + $\frac{1}{2}$ cyl) of the refraction, preferably in minus cylinder.

2. Correct for vertex distance for powers of ± 4.50 D (see Table 2.1). Note: fine-tuning of the power is best performed after the patient is wearing the contact lens regularly (best if the lens has been in 4 h to allow settling of the lens on the cornea and equilibration of the tears, but at the very least 15 min).

3. Choose a soft lens with a specific diameter and base curve guided by the manufacturer's recommendations. Most lenses have varying parameters, and in most cases three base curves are available. Soft lenses have considerable flexure, so that a range of corneal curvatures may be fit with one base curve. The *Ophthalmology Physicians' Desk Reference* (*PDR*) is an excellent source of information on the various lens manufacturers, and it is best to have several companies to choose from. There are two basic ways that soft contact lenses are manufactured:

a) Spin cast (Bausch & Lomb)
b) Lathe cut (Hydrocurve)

The water content of soft lenses varies from 38% to 78%; 55% is borderline for extended wear, but no contact lens should be worn in extended-wear fashion if it is not approved by the Food and Drug Administration for this purpose. In general, the drier the eye, the lower

TABLE 2.1

Vertex distance conversions at 12 millimeters

5.00 – 4.75	7.00 – 6.50	9.00 – 8.25	12.75 – 11.00	17.00 – 14.00
5.12 – 4.87	7.12 – 6.62	9.25 – 8.37	13.00 – 11.25	17.25 – 14.25
5.37 – 5.00	7.37 – 6.75	9.50 – 8.62	13.50 – 11.50	17.62 – 14.37
5.50 – 5.12	7.50 – 6.87	9.75 – 8.75	12.75 – 11.75	18.00 – 14.50
5.62 – 5.25	7.62 – 7.00	10.00 – 9.00	14.00 – 12.00	18.12 – 14.75
5.75 – 5.37	7.75 – 7.12	10.25 – 9.12	14.25 – 12.25	18.50 – 15.00
5.87 – 5.50	7.87 – 7.25	10.50 – 9.25	14.50 – 12.37	18.75 – 15.25
6.00 – 5.62	8.00 – 7.37	10.75 – 9.37	14.75 – 12.50	19.00 – 15.50
6.12 – 5.75	8.12 – 7.50	11.00 – 9.62	15.00 – 12.75	19.50 – 15.75
6.37 – 5.87	8.25 – 7.62	11.25 – 9.75	15.50 – 13.00	20.00 – 16.00
6.50 – 6.00	8.50 – 7.75	11.50 – 10.00	15.75 – 13.25	
6.62 – 6.12	8.75 – 8.00	11.75 – 10.25	16.25 – 13.50	
6.75 – 6.25		12.00 – 10.37	16.75 – 13.75	
6.87 – 6.37		12.50 – 10.75		

Plus spectacle lens power must be increased at the corneal plane; read numbers from right to left. Minus spectacle lens power must be decreased at the corneal plane; read numbers from left to right.

the water content of the lens should be, as a lens with higher water content requires more tears to remain hydrated.

Soft lenses should be fit as flat as possible (approximately 1 mm flatter than the flattest keratometry reading) to avoid vaulting (and its accompanying variation in vision produced by blinking) and to allow greater tear circulation beneath the lens. Place the lens in the eye.

4. Contact lens insertion. An adaptation of 15 minutes for soft lenses and 5 minutes for hard lenses is required. The initial insertion should be done by the fitter rather than the patient to save time and avoid distortion of the cornea that can confuse the examination. A sturdy hand rest makes this task much easier. Upper lid control is necessary, and one should wait until the patient can give full cooperation so that the insertion is the least traumatic as possible. The patient may also look from side to side to ensure proper lens placement. If the lens falls out, rinse with sterile saline and repeat the insertion. Reassurance and persistence are often necessary to make this a success. After the lens has had time to equilibrate, its fit should be assessed. In general, a good soft lens should

    a) center well, covering the cornea completely;

    b) move slightly (less than 1 mm with a good blink); and

    c) not have any air bubbles under its surface.

Rigid Lens Fitting

In general, more precise calculations are required with rigid lenses because they do not flex in the same way as soft lenses.

1. Refract in minus cylinder, and obtain keratometry (K) readings. Convert K values from diopters to millimeters (see Table 2.2).

2. Convert refraction to the spherical equivalent, correcting for the vertex distance (see Table 2.1). Again, power is secondary as it can be modified later with an over-refraction.

3. Choose the lens's base curve "on K," that is, the same as the flattest keratometry reading or slightly steeper than K (if the astigmatism is 1 D or greater, the base curve is made to be one-fourth of the corneal astigmatism steeper than the flattest K). When a lens is fit steeper than the flattest K, a "plus" tear lens is created, which must be compensated by adding more "minus" in the contact lens power. In a similar fashion, a lens that is flatter than the flattest K will create a "minus" tear lens and have to be compensated with addition of "plus" power. Hence the mnemonic SAM/FAP, for steeper add minus/flatter add plus.

4. The diameter is the least important value of the parameters to be chosen. Most often, it is 9.0 ± 0.5 mm (for RGP material) compared with 8.0 ± 0.5 mm for PMMA.

TABLE 2.2

Diopter – millimeter radius conversion table

56.00 – 6.03	53.00 – 6.37	50.00 – 6.75	47.00 – 7.18	44.00 – 7.67	41.00 – 8.23	38.00 – 8.88
55.87 – 6.04	52.87 – 6.38	49.87 – 6.77	46.87 – 7.20	43.87 – 7.69	40.87 – 8.26	37.87 – 8.91
55.75 – 6.05	52.75 – 6.40	49.75 – 6.78	46.75 – 7.22	43.75 – 7.71	40.75 – 8.28	37.75 – 8.94
55.62 – 6.07	52.62 – 6.41	49.62 – 6.80	46.62 – 7.24	43.62 – 7.74	40.62 – 8.31	37.62 – 8.97
55.50 – 6.08	52.50 – 6.43	49.50 – 6.82	46.50 – 7.26	43.50 – 7.76	40.50 – 8.33	37.50 – 9.00
55.37 – 6.10	52.37 – 6.44	49.37 – 6.84	46.37 – 7.28	43.37 – 7.78	40.37 – 8.36	37.37 – 9.03
55.25 – 6.11	52.25 – 6.46	49.25 – 6.85	46.25 – 7.30	43.25 – 7.80	40.25 – 8.39	37.25 – 9.06
55.12 – 6.12	52.12 – 6.48	49.12 – 6.87	46.12 – 7.32	43.12 – 7.83	40.12 – 8.41	37.12 – 9.09
55.00 – 6.14	52.00 – 6.49	49.00 – 6.89	46.00 – 7.34	43.00 – 7.85	40.00 – 8.44	37.00 – 9.12
54.87 – 6.15	51.87 – 6.51	48.87 – 6.91	45.87 – 7.36	42.87 – 7.87	39.87 – 8.47	36.87 – 9.15
54.74 – 6.16	51.75 – 6.52	48.75 – 6.92	45.75 – 7.38	42.75 – 7.89	39.75 – 8.49	36.75 – 9.18
54.62 – 6.18	51.62 – 6.54	48.62 – 6.94	45.62 – 7.40	42.62 – 7.92	39.62 – 8.52	36.62 – 9.22
54.50 – 6.19	51.50 – 6.55	48.50 – 6.96	45.50 – 7.42	42.50 – 7.94	39.50 – 8.54	36.50 – 9.25
54.37 – 6.21	51.37 – 6.57	48.37 – 6.98	45.37 – 7.44	42.37 – 7.97	39.37 – 8.57	36.37 – 9.28
54.25 – 6.22	51.25 – 6.59	48.25 – 6.99	45.25 – 7.60	42.25 – 7.99	39.25 – 8.60	36.25 – 9.31
54.12 – 6.24	51.12 – 6.60	48.12 – 7.01	45.12 – 7.48	42.12 – 8.01	39.12 – 8.63	36.12 – 9.34
54.00 – 6.25	51.00 – 6.62	48.00 – 7.03	45.00 – 7.50	42.00 – 8.04	39.00 – 8.65	36.00 – 9.38
53.87 – 6.27	50.87 – 6.63	47.87 – 7.05	44.87 – 7.52	41.87 – 8.06	38.87 – 8.68	
53.75 – 6.28	50.75 – 6.65	47.75 – 7.07	44.75 – 7.54	41.75 – 8.08	38.75 – 8.71	
53.62 – 6.29	50.62 – 6.67	47.62 – 7.09	44.62 – 7.56	41.62 – 8.11	38.62 – 8.74	
53.50 – 6.31	50.50 – 6.68	47.50 – 7.11	44.50 – 7.59	41.50 – 8.13	38.50 – 8.77	
53.37 – 6.32	50.37 – 6.70	47.37 – 7.12	44.37 – 7.61	41.37 – 8.16	38.37 – 8.80	
53.25 – 6.34	50.25 – 6.72	47.25 – 7.14	44.25 – 7.63	41.25 – 8.18	38.25 – 8.82	
53.12 – 6.35	50.12 – 6.73	47.12 – 7.16	44.12 – 7.65	41.12 – 8.21	38.12 – 8.85	

A larger diameter generally provides a more comfortable fit because of less lens movement, upper lid entrapment, and touch to the lid margin.

5. To summarize with an example:
  a) Refraction in minus cylinder (and correct for vertex distance, Table 2.1) → −2.00/−1.00 × 180.
  b) Obtain K readings (D) → 43.00/44.00 × 90.
  c) Convert K values to millimeters (Table 2.2) → 7.84, 7.67.
  d) Choose base curve of lens → 43.25 = 7.80 ($\frac{1}{4}$ of the total astigmatism, in this case 1 D).
  e) Calculate power:

$$
\begin{array}{lll}
\text{Sphere, vertex corrected} & = & -2.50 \text{ D} \\
\text{"SAM" (steeper add minus)} & = & \underline{-.25 \text{ D}} \\
 & & -2.75 \text{ D}
\end{array}
$$

  f) Choose diameter: = 9.0 mm. Lens parameters:

$$
\begin{array}{lll}
\text{Power} & = & -2.75 \text{ D} \\
\text{Diameter} & = & 9.0 \text{ mm} \\
\text{Base curve} & = & 7.80 \text{ mm}
\end{array}
$$

  g) Choose color: the chief purpose is to aid in the location of the lens and not impart color to the eye, as rigid lenses do not usually cover the entire cornea.

The lens is placed on the eye and allowed to equilibrate. The fit of the lens should then be evaluated. A rigid lens should move several millimeters with a blink and recenter after each blink. Distance and near check of vision and an over-refraction should be performed. Please refer to Figure 2.2 for diagrams of an acceptable fluorescein pattern for a hard lens fit and of a lens that is too steep and one that is too flat. Based on the fluorescein pattern, movement and comfort, adjustments will then have to be made.

Special Contact Lenses

The fitting of special lenses is beyond the scope of this text. However, certain fundamental principles will be covered.

Aphakia Generally, aphakia is best corrected with rigid contact lenses, as they are easier to handle and better tolerated due to decreased corneal sensation after surgery. Such rigid lenses are usually of a lenticular design to decrease weight for better movement and centering. Problems may occur with chipping of a thin lens and distortion of vision when the lenticular portion moves over the pupil. Extended-wear

Fluorescein Pattern for Rigid Lenses

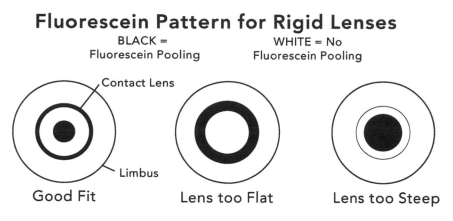

BLACK =
Fluorescein Pooling

WHITE = No
Fluorescein Pooling

Contact Lens

Limbus

Good Fit   Lens too Flat   Lens too Steep

FIGURE 2.2.

soft lenses are a better option in those patients unable to handle lenses on a daily basis.

Patients are generally best fit by trial and error with a trial set. A spectacle overcorrection for any uncorrected astigmatism and presbyopia is used.

In these patients, it is often advantageous to have two lenses, especially when soft lenses are being used, with one lens being cleaned, perhaps by a professional company (such as Vision Systems, telephone: 1-800-874-7546), while the other lens is being worn.

Keratoconus   For mild keratoconus, a standard spherical lens may be sufficient. However, with increasing disease, a set of rigid trial lenses with progressively different base curves in similar or identical diameters is required. The lenses are fit in succession until an even distribution of forces is observed across the cornea. Fluorescein patterns, movement, centration, and the presence and location of an air bubble beneath the contact lens are observed. It is best to start with a steep spherical lens and vary the diameter.

After the best lens is inserted, leave it in place for 15 minutes and then over-refract. The 15-minute wait is necessary to allow for patient adjustment and to make sure the lens will stay in the eye. One must frequently accept a lens which gives less than ideal appearance and which, although flat, will be stabilized by the upper lid and have lower edge lift with a small air rim at the lower edge portion.

Keratometry readings are a guide but are not as useful in keratoconus fitting as in routine contact lens fitting.

With more severe keratoconus, specially designed lenses with apical clearance are necessary. These lenses are bicurved with a coned out central portion to allow the periphery of the lens to come closer to the normal peripheral cornea and produce less baring on the cone.

Posttraumatic Corneal Scars   These are best fit by trial set.

Postkeratoplasty   Patients generally are not fit for 6 to 9 months after surgery and then with a trial set.

Corneal Astigmatism with a Soft Toric Lens   These lenses will generally not give as good a result as a rigid contact lens and must be prism balanced to prevent rotation. In general, a trial set is used to determine the closest fit. Select a lens with slightly less astigmatic power and the same axis as the spectacle refraction written in minus cylinder form and corrected for vertex distance. The lens is observed on the eye. If there is a change in orientation of the 6 o'clock astigmatism mark on the contact lens, the final astigmatic axis must be changed. The mnemonic LARS for left add, right subtract, is used to remember that if a trial toric contact lens rotates counter clockwise (to the practitioner's left), this amount of rotation must be added to the axis of the spectacle refraction when ordering the lens. Likewise, if the lens rotates clockwise (to the practitioner's right), this amount of rotation must be subtracted from the spectacle refraction. One clock hour of rotation is approximately 30°.

Presbyopia   Bifocal contact lenses have not become as simple and as satisfactory as monovision lenses. This approach involves one contact for near vision and one for distance work. A third contact lens for distance vision with reading glasses should also be considered for patients who will be performing prolonged close work.

Pediatric Cases   Typically an aphakic lens is required after cataract surgery. A willing and determined parent is the key to success. Again, trial lens fitting is necessary with keratometry readings if available. Changes in the base curve and power are often required in the first year because of marked changes in corneal curvature (Enoch 1979). Lens material options include RGP lenses, which are easier to handle than silicone or hydroxyethyl methacrylate (HEMA) lenses. Again, extended-wear soft lenses are an option in cases where handling is a problem.

Bandage Contact Lenses   Not all soft contact lenses are approved by the FDA for bandage purposes. Informed consent for use of non-FDA-approved lenses should be obtained (Table 2.3).

TABLE 2.3

Bandage contact lenses

Lens	Sagittal Depth	% Water	Diameter	Base Curve
Low Water Content				
B&L B3	2.7738	38.6	13.5	9.6
B&L U3	3.2711	38.6	13.5	8.6
CSI	3.63	40.0	14.8	9.36
B&L U4	3.6673	38.6	14.5	9.0
Plano T	4.69	38.6	14.7	8.1
Medium Water Content				
Softcon*	3.53	56	14	8.7
Hydrocurve II*	2.81	55	14.5	8.8
High Water Content				
Permalens*	4.0251	71	15	9
Sauflon PW*	4.0733	79	14.4	8.4

Note: (1) a higher water content contact lens requires more tears to work well, and is thinner (more oxygen permeable); (2) as one increases diameter, the sagittal depth increases, and the lens will fit tighter; (3) must see patient next day to make sure lens does not tighten, resulting in iritis or other complications.
*FDA-approved for bandage purposes.

Contact Lens Delivery

After the initial trial fit has been performed and lenses are ordered, the patient is ready to pick up the contact lens.

Contact Lens Verification

The dimensions of the lenses that have been received must be verified with what was actually ordered. This information should be entered in the medical record and is extremely important for lens replacement. The power of a soft lens can be checked at the office by blotting the lens with a facial tissue and using a lensometer, with less than 0.5 D error. The diameter of the soft lens can be verified with a measuring magnifier with a 0.2 mm error.

A hard lens can be verified with a lensometer or radioscope to check the power. Also, the Con-Ta-Chek (Wesley Jessen Division, Schering Corp., Chicago, Illinois) can fit on a keratometer to check the power. A trough gage is helpful for measuring diameter. The acceptable tolerance for hard lens manufacturing is 0.25 D for the base curve and power and 0.2 mm for diameter and center thickness.

Contact Lens Care and Follow-up

General Points

The instruction session should include advice regarding the length of wear and which disinfectant and cleaning solutions the patient should use. This information should be entered in the medical record. Select one method and stay with it. Reinforce points made at each follow-up visit. Give free samples, kits, and cases every return visit. Tell patients to discard old solutions and cases every 3 months in order to avoid bacterial contamination. Old solutions, cases, and certain preservatives may cause more problems than a poor contact lens fit. Patients should apply mascara to the tips of lashes only after a contact lens is inserted, and clean the lid margins of oils and mascara before insertion with a dry, tightly wound, cotton-tipped applicator.

Rigid Lenses

All rigid materials can be cared for by using solutions for RGP materials. Clean lenses with a cleaner, rinse with tap water, dry with a tissue, and soak overnight in a disinfecting or conditioning solution. Insert lenses directly into the eye from the conditioning solution. After at least a 2-hour soak, rinse the case with tap water and leave open to dry. Many systems are available; good results are usually obtained with the Advance Boston (Polymer Technology, Inc., Wilmington, Massachusetts) cleaning and wetting solutions. "All-in-one" solutions may create a hydrophobic surface on the contact lens and should be avoided.

Account Settlement

Please refer above to General Considerations, Contact Lens Fees.

Teaching Insertion and Removal

Ophthalmic residents should practice teaching, insertion and removal in training to gain experience, especially in this age of malpractice. Many doctors starting out in practice will not have all the technical support that was once available to them during their training. Thorough hand washing is critical, and insertion and removal of lenses must be done away from sinks and wet areas, which are known to harbor pseudomonas.

Insertion Spread the lids by pressing lashes against the orbital rim with fingers in a "V" fashion. Center lens with the tip of a moist index finger after it is cleaned and moistened. Slight side-to-side movement of the finger will help keep the lens on the cornea. Gentle blinks are then required; large blinks will cause the lens to decenter. After, the patient should be observed and allowed to practice with a towel and a mirror.

Removal A hard lens can be removed by a "scissors method." Place the fingers on the lid margin against the opposite upper and lower lens edges, and press the lids together until the lens ejects. The use of a small suction cup is an alternative. To remove soft lenses, place the tip of the index finger against the lens while it is in the eye, and drag the lens to one side or downward off the cornea while pinching and folding the lens between the thumb and index finger. After removal, place the lens in a case emersed in fresh contact lens conditioning solutions or nonpreserved saline.

Contact Lens Adjustments

Evaluate the lens fit for comfort, movement, and fluorescein pattern (for rigid lenses). (See above, Trial Lens Fitting, Soft Lens Fitting, and Rigid Lens Fitting.) Some adjustments may be required after an adequate equilibration period.

1. A lens that rides low may be
   a) too heavy (consider a smaller or thinner lens) or
   b) too flat (steepen the lens) or
   c) the lid may push the lens down, in which case lenticular construction is necessary.
2. A lens may ride too high because the upper lid pulls it up. This can be altered by thinning the edge, enlarging the lens diameter, or steepening the lens.
3. A loose lens can be tightened by increasing its diameter, decreasing its base curve, or sagittal depth. If the lens rides laterally, a larger or steeper lens is usually required.
4. The patient notices excessive blurring of vision:
   a) If the vision is blurry and the patient blinks and then the vision clears, the lens was probably too steep.

b) If the vision is good and with a blink the vision blurs, then the lens is probably too flat.

Soft Lenses

With daily-wear lenses, a nonpreserved hydrogen peroxide system or Polyquad (Farris et al. 1989) preserved solutions are good. For extended wear, the lenses are removed at least weekly then cleaned and disinfected overnight with hydrogen peroxide or Polyquad. The FDA recommends that extended-wear lenses be worn no longer than 1 week continuously. Note that heat is considered by some to be more effective against *Acanthamoeba* (Moore et al. 1985; Lindquist et al. 1988); however, it can cause protein deposits to stick to the lens, like eggs to a frying pan. Enzymes may be necessary, but patients may confuse these enzymes with the disinfecting process, and residues can cause red eyes.

Disposable weekly replacement lenses would not require any cleaning solutions. In a patient with a low tendency to form deposits, it should be possible to use the lenses for 2 weeks, with removal of the lens overnight after 1 week to clean and disinfect the lens with hydrogen peroxide or Polyquad solution.

Wearing Schedules

1. The wearing schedule is generally individualized and written in the chart. A gradual increase in wearing time is necessary as a precaution, and the patient is told to remove the lens if any discomfort or redness persists for more than 5 to 10 minutes and is not relieved by blinking and increased tearing. A nonpreserved artificial tear or saline solution can be used up to six times a day for discomfort. However, overusing these drops can cause an increase in tear evaporation from rinsing away of the normal tear film, creating a situation not unlike "dishpan hands."

2. Rigid contact lens wear should start at 8 to 10 hours the first day and increase 2 hours per day for a period of 4 days until the lenses are worn during full waking hours.

3. For soft contact lenses, one can begin at 10 to 12 hours per day and increase 2 hours each day until full waking hour wearing time is achieved. Extended-wear lenses must be checked in the first 24 hours and then 1 week later.

Follow-up Visits

After the first visit, a recheck in 1 week is necessary for daily-wear lenses, and in 1 day for extended-wear and bandage lenses, but sooner if there are any problems. If a lens was fit elsewhere, more time and effort will be required to determine the safety and effectiveness of the present lens. The lens should be in at least 4 hours before the visit. On this follow-up visit, patients should be asked how their distance and near vision is and how the contact lens feels. Details of how the lens is handled and cared for should be entered in the medical record. If the patient does have significant problems, consider alternatives such as a change in the lens material, wearing time, solutions, or as a last measure, discontinuation of contact lenses.

On examination, an over-refraction should be performed if necessary, with a check of lens centration and movement, a check for lens deposits, and slit lamp evaluation of the conjunctiva including the upper lid and cornea for staining and edema. Note that on the first visit, mild staining, foreign body sensation, and edema are expected and do not necessarily mean the contact lens needs to be adjusted. Sometimes, "blinking exercises" consisting of 10 blinks in each of five directions of gaze four times a day may be of help.

Further visits will depend on the needs of the patient and the findings of the examination. Emphasis on compliance and compulsiveness in the care and wear of lenses with assurance of the physician's availability is required.

In general, patients with extended-wear lenses should be followed every 3 months for approximately a year and then every 6 months. Rigid lens wearers should be seen at 2 months, 6 months, then once a year unless any problems arise. For aphakic patients with soft contact lenses, a follow-up at least every 4 months is necessary, with lenses removed at least every 2 months for cleaning or as needed to replace and clean the lens any time discrete deposits are visible.

Changes and Complications Induced by Contact Lens Wear

Any contact lens resting on the cornea produces changes in the tears, lids, and cornea. These changes depend on the contact lens shape, material, and lens care and may lead to clinically recognized complications. A few of the more important changes and complications are described.

Corneal Changes

Oxygen Deprivation Oxygen needed for metabolic processes in the epithelium of the cornea comes directly from the atmosphere (partial pressure of 155 mmHg). Oxygen in the anterior chamber is 55 mmHg. An oxygen-impermeable contact lens of PMMA reduces the amount of oxygen available to the epithelium, which cannot obtain adequate amounts from the anterior chamber (Farris et al. 1971). This can result in the following:

> *Corneal edema:* results from an increased permeability of the epithelium, leading to stromal swelling, increased corneal thickness, and corneal curvature alterations, detectable on keratometry (Holden and Mertz 1984). Patients may see halos around lights or notice changes in their spectacle refraction called spectacle blur. Rigid gas-permeable contact materials and soft lenses have increased the amount of oxygen available to the cornea (an amount similar to that of sleep with lid closure) to decrease this problem.
>
> *Polymegathism* (variation in corneal endothelial cell size): has been noted more frequently in contact lens wearers than in those who do not wear contact lenses (MacRae et al. 1985; Carlson et al. 1988). The significance of this finding is unclear at this time, but the concern is that this would place a patient at a higher risk of endothelial decompensation if intraocular surgical procedures are performed in the future. Using a contact lens material of high oxygen transmission does not, however, guarantee adequate oxygen availability in the tears flowing around and beneath the edges of the lens, due to considerable patient variation of corneal shape, lens and lid movement, and tear secretion.
>
> *Corneal neovascularization:* can be superficial or deep, an isolated vessel, or part of a pannus.

Tear Film Changes   The tear film is a complex and kinetic fluid and contact lenses result in excessive evaporation. What might seem to be adequate tear production during an examination may in fact be reflex tearing. Hence, signs of drying (corneal superficial keratitis, tight lens fit) must be carefully sought.

Upper Tarsal Conjunctival Changes   Only the cornea comes in more continual contact with a lens than the upper tarsus. (See Allansmith 1989; Allansmith and Ross 1990.) Changes include the following:

1. Giant papillae are greater than 1 mm and are also seen with exposed nylon sutures or plastic prostheses (Srinivasan et al. 1979).
2. Papillae are 0.1 to 1 mm conjunctival elevations, diffusely distributed on the tarsus, graded on a scale of 1 to 4+, and may be seen by some individuals not wearing contact lenses.

Vision Variation   A small amount of variation is unavoidable to safely fit a contact lens that allows enough movement to permit adequate oxygenation. This tendency is greater in soft lenses (but to a lesser degree with toric lenses) than in rigid lenses as a result of lens flexure and lack of a tear lens.

Complications of Lens Wear

Lens Discomfort   A positive attitude on the part of the ophthalmologist is required, as many times the lens will become more comfortable with time. The differential diagnosis of an uncomfortable lens includes the following:

1. An oily lens.
2. A tight-fitting lens.
3. A lens with a rough edge (detected by a shadow graph such as the Profile Analyzer [Gulf Coast Contact Lens Inc., New Orleans, Louisiana]). Such lenses can be refinished; however, any modification of an older lens has a risk of breakage requiring a new and possibly less comfortable lens.
4. Inadequate tearing: this should be evaluated under normal room lighting conditions, as slit lamp illumination may produce reflex tearing.
5. Intolerance of a rigid lens in a patient who previously wore a soft lens: the patient may need to go back to a soft lens.
6. Hyperchondriasis: especially in a low myope wearing disposable contact lenses with a white and quiet eye.

Red Eye   Do not forget other causes of a red eye unrelated to contact lenses such as uveitis or glaucoma. Contact lenses can also make pre-existing problems worse. For example, patients of fair complexion are more likely to demonstrate dilation of their conjunctival vessels after any stimulation, including that by contact lenses. The most feared complication is that of a corneal ulcer. The management is discussed in the Ulcers section in Chapter 3. Note that patients who wear contact lenses and have a corneal abrasion should not be patched, as this creates an environment more conducive to corneal ulcer.

Blepharitis   Oils can build up on the lenses, aggravating this condition and possibly leading to other complications such as a stye. A thin profile lens will avoid excessive lid contact and may lessen this problem. (See the Blepharitis section in Chapter 3.)

Allergic Tendencies   See the Conjunctivitis section in Chapter 3. Cromolyn may be needed indefinitely to control symptoms from upper tarsal plate papillae. Steroid use is not indicated, as the risks of infection are too great.

Excessive Tearing   This could be due to rough edges, dry eyes with reflex tearing, or a foreign body present under the lid. Careful examination, possibly with a Schirmer's test, should reveal the etiology (see the Dry Eye section in Chapter 3).

Selected Readings

Allansmith MR. Immunologic effects of extended-wear contact lenses. Ann Ophthalmol 1989;21:465–74.

Allansmith MR, Ross RN. Contact lens wear and ocular allergy. In: Stein HA, Slatt BJ, Stein RM, eds. Contact Lens Wear and Ocular Allergy. St. Louis: CV Mosby, 1990, pp. 482–88.

Aswad MI, John T, Bvarza M, Kenyon K, Baum J. Bacterial adherence to extended wear soft contact lenses. Ophthalmology 1990;97:296–302.

Carlson KH, Bourne WM, Brubaker RF. Effect of long-term contact lens wear on corneal endothelial cell morphology and function. Invest Ophthalmol Vis Sci 1988;29:185–93.

Cohen EJ. CLAO Journal. New York: Kellner/McCaffrey, 1990.

Contact lenses: challenges, controversies, and opportunities. Cornea 1990;9 (Suppl 1).

Contact lens update. Columbus, Ohio: Anadem, 1990.

Dabezies OH. Contact Lenses: The CLAO guide to basic science and clinical practice, 2nd ed. Boston: Little, Brown, 1989. An excellent two-volume looseleaf series updated regularly. CLAO membership is another way to keep abreast of changes in basic and advanced lens care.

Enoch JM. Fitting parameters which need to be considered when designing soft contact lenses for the neonate. Contact Intraocular Lens Med J 1979;5:31–37.

Farris RL. The dry eye: its mechanisms and therapy, with evidence that contact lens is a cause. CLAO J 1986;12:234–46.

Farris RL, Donshik PC, Nelson JD, Tripathi BJ, Rashid R. Protecting corneal epithelial cell growth in the treatment of dry eye. Alcon Roundtable Monograph 1989.

Farris RL, Kubota Z, Mishima S. Epithelial decompensation with corneal contact lens wear. Arch Ophthalmol 1971;85:651–60.

Garcia GE, Aucoin J, Gladstone G. Extended wear rigid gas permeable lenses used for correction of aphakia. CLAO J 1990;16:195–99.

Hart ED, Farris RL, Hosmer M. A bacterial assay of contact lens wearers. Presented at the International Contact Lens Research Conference, Monaco, Monte Carlo, Sept. 1990.

Holden BA, Mertz GW. Critical oxygen levels to avoid corneal edema for daily and extended wear contact lenses. Invest Ophthalmol Vis Sci 1984;25:1161–67.

Lindquist TD, Sher NA, Doughman DJ. Clinical signs and medical therapy of
   early *Acanthamoeba* keratitis. Arch Ophthalmol 1988;106:73–77.
Lowther GE, Ghormeley NR. Internal contact lens clinic. Stoneham,
   Massachusetts: Butterworth, 1990.
MacRae S, Matusuda M, Yee R. The effect of long-term hard contact lens
   wear on the corneal endothelium. CLAO J 1985;11:322–26.
Moore MB, McCulley JP, Luckenbach M. *Acanthamoeba* keratitis associated
   with soft contact lens wear. Am J Ophthalmol 1985;100:396–403.
Poggio EC, Glynn RJ, Schein OD, et al. The incidence of ulcerative keratitis
   among users of daily-wear and extended-wear soft contact lenses. N
   Engl J Med 1989;321:779–83.
Schein OD, Glynn RJ, Poggio EC, Seddon JM, Kenyon KR. The relative risk
   of ulcerative keratitis among users of daily-wear and extended wear soft
   contact lenses. N Engl J Med 1989;321:733–78.
Srinivasan BD, Jakobiec FA, Iwamoto T, DeVoe AG. Giant papillary
   conjunctivitis with ocular prosthesis. Arch Ophthalmol 1979;97:892–95.
Stein HA, Slatt BJ. CLAO home study course for contact lens technicians.
   New Orleans: CLAO, 1990.
Stein HA, Slatt BJ, Stein RM. Fitting guide for rigid and soft contact lenses.
   St. Louis: CV Mosby, 1990.
Stern GA, Zam ZS. The pathogenesis of contact lenses associated
   Pseudomonas aeruginosa corneal ulceration: I. The effect of contact lens
   coatings on adherence of *Pseudomonas aeruginosa* to soft contact lenses.
   Cornea 1986;5:41–45.
Weinstock FJ. Contact lens fitting. A clinical text atlas. Philadelphia: JB
   Lippincott and Gower, 1989.

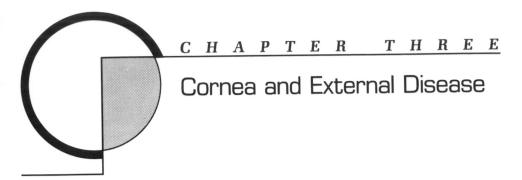

C H A P T E R   T H R E E

Cornea and External Disease

Sheridan Lam, M.D.
Christopher J. Rapuano, M.D.
Jay H. Krachmer, M.D.

Bacteria and Gram Stains

Aerobic Gram-Negative Cocci

1. *Staphylococcus*
   a) Usually present in singles, pairs, or clusters.
   b) *S. aureus* is coagulase-positive; *S. epidermidis* is coagulase-negative.
   c) Common pathogens of corneal ulcers and blepharitis.
2. *Streptococcus*
   a) Usually in chains and can be classified by pattern of hemolysis on blood agar (α, β, and γ); *S. pneumoniae* is encapsulated and usually found in pairs.
   b) Can cause corneal ulcers and conjunctivitis; common pathogens in infected conjunctival blebs; *S. viridans* can cause infectious crystalline keratopathy.

Aerobic Gram-Positive Rods

1. *Corynebacterium*
   a) Resembles Chinese characters.
   b) Can invade intact corneal epithelium.
2. *Bacillus*
   a) Rarely causes corneal infections; can cause fulminant and devastating endophthalmitis and panophthalmitis.
   b) Clindamycin and gentamicin are antibiotics of choice.
3. *Nocardia asteroides*
   a) Can lead to keratitis and endogenous endophthalmitis, especially in alcoholics and immunocompromised patients.
   b) Acid-fast (must be differentiated from mycobacteria).

Aerobic Gram-Negative Cocci

1. *Neisseria*
   a) Usually seen in pairs; may be present in polymorphonuclear leukocytes.
   b) Can invade intact corneal epithelium.
   c) Can lead to hyperacute purulent keratoconjunctivitis.
2. *Branhamella*

Aerobic Gram-Negative Rods

1. *Hemophilus*
   a) May exist as a bacillus or as a coccobacillus.
   b) *H. aegyptius* (Koch-Weeks bacillus): common cause of bacterial conjunctivitis in warm climate.
   c) *Hemophilus* can invade intact corneal epithelium.
2. *Moraxella*
   a) Resemble "boxcars" and present as pairs.
   b) Can cause corneal ulcers and angular blepharitis.
3. *Pseudomonas*
   a) Usually in singlets.
   b) Common pathogen of corneal ulcers.
4. *Enterobacter*: rarely reported pathogen in eye infections.
5. *Shigella, Klebsiella, Serratia, Escherichia coli,* and *Salmonella* are relatively rare as pathogens of ocular infections.

Anaerobic Gram-Positive Cocci

1. *Peptococcus*
2. *Peptostreptococcus*

Anaerobic Gram-Negative Cocci

1. *Veillonella*
2. *Acidaminococcus*
3. *Megasphaera*

Anaerobic Gram-Positive Rods

1. *Clostridium*
   a)   Produces gas.
   b)   Can cause panophthalmitis and endophthalmitis, which may be exogenous (e.g., trauma) or endogenous (e.g., septicemia).
2. *Actinomyces israelii*
   a)   Filamentous (falsely classified as a fungus in past).
   b)   Common pathogen in canaliculitis.
3. *Propionibacterium*: can cause chronic endophthalmitis.

Anaerobic Gram-Negative Rods

1. *Bacteroides fragilis*: seldom seen in corneal infections.
2. *Fusobacterium*: seldom seen in corneal infections; not to be confused with *Fusarium*, a fungus.

Blepharitis

Definition and Symptoms   Inflammation of the eyelids; can be caused by infections, seborrhea, or rosacea.

Signs and Etiology

1. Lids and lashes
   a)   Erythema and telangiectasia at lid margins.
   b)   Scaly and oily skin; cutaneous pustules may be present; comedones (in acne) never occur in rosacea.
   c)   Meibomianitis: chalazion; hordeolum; plugging of meibomian gland orifices.
   d)   Deposits (scurf, collarettes, and sleeves) on lashes.
       i)   Scurf, scaly deposits on the shafts of lashes, indicate seborrhea.
       ii)   Collarettes at the bases of lashes indicate staphylococcal etiology.
       iii) Sleeves indicate presence of *Demodex folliculorum*.
   e)   Angular blepharitis: inflammation and scaling of the lid in the lateral canthal area, commonly caused by *Staphylococcus* or *Moraxella*.

    f)   Trichiasis, lash loss, or poliosis.

    g)   Rosacea: telangiectasis and erythema of the forehead, cheeks, and nose; rhinophyma may occur in late stage.

2. Tear film: unstable (faster breakup time); foaming.
3. Cornea: pannus formation; superficial punctate keratopathy (usually inferiorly); peripheral corneal infiltrates; phlyctenulosis.

Workup   Cultures and sensitivities in serious cases; conjunctival or lid biopsy, or both, if sebaceous cell carcinoma is suspected.

Differential Diagnosis   Sebaceous cell carcinoma should be suspected if blepharitis persists despite extensive treatment, if there is thickening of lids, or if blepharitis is unilateral; patients with recurrent chalazion should undergo biopsy to rule out sebaceous cell carcinoma.

Treatment

1. Warm compresses for 10 to 15 minutes, every day to twice a day.
2. Lid hygiene, including lid scrubs with baby shampoo or glyceryl monotallowate (e.g., Eagle Vision Lid Cleaners), every day to four times a day, according to patient's symptoms.
3. Topical antibiotics (bacitracin or erythromycin eye ointments) or antibiotic and steroid combinations (Blephamide) applied directly to the eyelid and adjusted according to culture and sensitivity results.
4. Tetracycline (250 mg p.o. q.i.d.), doxycycline (100 mg p.o. b.i.d.), or erythromycin (250 mg p.o. q.i.d.) given to thin meibomian gland secretions; usual course is 6 weeks and then tapered according to signs and symptoms; some patients may need to be on maintenance treatment indefinitely.

    a)   Tetracycline should be taken on an empty stomach, 1 hour before meals or 2 hours after meals; doxycycline does not have to be taken on an empty stomach.

    b)   Warn patient about sensitivity to sunlight while on tetracycline or doxycycline.

    c)   Tetracycline is contraindicated in children under the age of 8, pregnant women, nursing mothers, and patients allergic to tetracycline.

4. For concomitant dry eyes: artificial tears; temporary or permanent punctal occlusion (see Dry Eye Section, below).

Follow-up   Initially, weekly or biweekly; after course stabilizes, every 3 to 12 months.

Course   If untreated, blepharitis may result in hordeolum, chalazion, or corneal infiltrates. Chronic irritation by meibomian gland secretions in blepharitis may lead to sebaceous cell carcinoma.

Conjunctivitis

History and Etiology   Inflammation of conjunctiva has many causes; when the cornea becomes involved, it is called keratoconjunctivitis.

1. Infectious: bacterial, viral, chlamydia
2. Noninfectious
   a) Chemical burns (see Chemical and Thermal Burns, in Adnexal and Orbital Trauma section, Chapter 11.)
   b) Hypersensitivities
      i) Conjunctivitis associated with contact dermatitis
      ii) Vernal keratoconjunctivitis (VKC)
      iii) Atopic keratoconjunctivitis (AKC)
      iv) Hay fever conjunctivitis
      v) Giant papillary conjunctivitis (GPC)
   c) Drug-induced (e.g., topical epinephrine)

Bacterial Conjunctivitis

Hyperacute Conjunctivitis

Etiology   *N. gonorrheae* or *N. meningitides*; can penetrate intact corneal epithelium; rapid onset, usually within 24 hours.

Signs

1. Copious purulent discharge; lid edema and mattering.
2. Severe conjunctival injection and chemosis.
3. Corneal infiltrates or ulcers may be present.
4. Bilateral or unilateral (which may become bilateral).

Workup

1. Conjunctival scraping for gram and giemsa stains.
2. Conjunctival cultures and sensitivities.

3. Corneal cultures if there is corneal involvement.
4. VDRL or rapid plasma region (RPR) test; fluorescent treponemal antibody-absorption (FTA-ABS) test.
5. Chlamydial cultures or immunologic tests.
6. May have to be reported to health authorities.

Treatment

1. Topical and systemic; systemic treatment is the mainstay.
2. Adults:
   a) Conjunctival involvement: ceftriaxone, 1.0 g intramuscularly, or spectinomycin, 2.0 g intramuscularly, once (if allergic to cephalosporins or penicillin).
   b) Conjunctival and corneal involvement: ceftriaxone, 1.0 g intravenously every 12 hours for 3 days, or spectinomycin, 2.0 g intravenously every 12 hours for 2 days (if allergic to cephalosporins or penicillin).
   c) Topically: saline lavage and antibiotic eye ointment four times a day (erythromycin; gentamicin; bacitracin).
   d) Empirically treat for chlamydial infection: tetracycline, 250 mg orally four times a day for 2 to 3 weeks; or doxycycline, 100 mg orally twice a day for 2 to 3 weeks; or erythromycin, 250 mg orally four times a day for 2 to 3 weeks.
   e) Sexual partners contacted and treated as needed.
3. Neonates
   a) Conjunctival involvement: ceftriaxone, 50 mg/kg intramuscularly once, or gentamicin, 2 to 2.5 mg/kg intravenously every 8 hours for 3 days (if allergic to penicillin or cephalosporin).
   b) Conjunctival and corneal involvement: ceftriaxone, 25 to 40 mg/kg intravenously every 12 hours for 3 days, or gentamicin, 2 to 2.5 mg/kg intravenously every 8 hours for 3 days (if allergic to penicillin or cephalosporin).
   c) Topical treatment: lavage with normal saline; topical antibiotic ointment four times a day (erythromycin, gentamicin, or bacitracin).
   d) Empirically treat for chlamydial infection: erythromycin syrup, 50 mg/kg daily in four divided doses for 2 weeks.
4. Consultation with a specialist in infectious disease may be helpful.

Acute Conjunctivitis

Etiology *S. pneumoniae* (cooler climate); *H. influenzae*; *H. aegytius* (warmer climate); *Staphylococcus*.

Signs   Conjunctival hyperemia; subconjunctival hemorrhage (especially on the upper lid); mild to moderate mucopurulent discharge; sticky eyelids on awakening; corneal infiltrate or ulceration.

Workup

1. Conjunctival scraping for gram and giemsa stains.
2. Conjunctival cultures and sensitivities.
3. Corneal scraping and cultures if cornea is involved.

Treatment

1. Sulfacetamide 10% eyedrops every 2 hours while awake or polymyxin B and trimethoprim (Polytrim) eyedrops every 3 hours while awake for 7 days.
2. Erythromycin or bacitracin ointment at bedtime.
3. Adjust regimen according to culture and sensitivities.

Chronic Conjunctivitis

Etiology   *Moraxella* (often seen in alcoholics or immunosuppressed patients); *S. aureus*; chlamydia.

Signs

1. Conjunctival hyperemia; scanty mucoid discharge.
2. Blepharitis: angular blepharitis (e.g., *Moraxella*); collarettes at the base of lashes (e.g., *Staphylococcus*).
3. Cornea: infiltrates or ulceration (usually in peripheral cornea); phlyctenulosis; inferior superficial punctate keratopathy (SPK).

Workup

1. Conjunctival scraping for gram and giemsa stains.
2. Lid and conjunctival cultures and sensitivities.

Treatment

1. Topical antibiotic ointment at bedtime (e.g., erythromycin or bacitracin).
2. Topical antibiotic and steroid in phlyctenulosis and sterile peripheral corneal infiltrates.
3. Lid hygiene.
4. Oral antibiotics (e.g., doxycycline, tetracycline, or erythromycin) in severe cases of staphylococcal blepharoconjunctivitis or meibomianitis.

Membranous and Pseudomembranous Conjunctivitis

Etiology Beta-hemolytic *Streptococcus*; *S. pneumoniae*; *Corynebacterium diphtheriae* (rare).

Signs

1. Fibrin/exudate membrane on the conjunctiva; pseudomembrane if it can be peeled off without bleeding; a membrane bleeds when peeled off.
2. Lid edema; conjunctival hyperemia.
3. In chronic cases, conjunctival scarring and symblepharon formation.
4. Corneal infiltrates and ulceration may be present.
5. Nasopharynx and larynx affected in *C. diphtheriae.*

Workup Conjunctival scraping for gram and giemsa stains; conjunctival cultures and sensitivities; ear, nose, and throat consultation if *C. diphtheriae* is suspected.

Differential Diagnosis Adenovirus keratoconjunctivitis; neonatal inclusion conjunctivitis; gonococcal keratoconjunctivitis.

Treatment

1. If organism is unknown, a broad spectrum topical antibiotic (sulfacetamide or erythromycin) should be used until the sensitivity results are available.
2. Systemic penicillin and topical erythromycin in cases of beta-hemolytic *Streptococcus.*
3. Antitoxin is necessary in *C. diphtheriae* (infectious disease specialist should be consulted).

Phlyctenulosis

Phlyctenulosis is a hypersensitivity reaction (probably type IV) caused commonly by *Staphylococcus* and *Mycobacterium tuberculosis.*

Clinical Characteristics

1. Phlyctenules start as a localized elevated conjunctival nodule, often at the limbus; later phlyctenules may ulcerate.
2. Scarring and corneal vascularization may occur if the phlyctenule invades the cornea.
3. Spontaneously resolves in 2 to 3 weeks.

Workup

1. Conjunctival scraping for gram, giemsa, and acid-fast stains.
2. Conjunctival cultures and sensitivities.
3. Purified protein derivative (PPD) skin test and chest x-ray if tuberculosis is suspected.

Treatment

1. Corticosteroid eyedrops three to four times daily.
2. Warm soaks, lid hygiene, and topical antibiotic ointment in staphylococcal cases.
3. Antibiotic therapy in cases of tuberculosis.

Chlamydial Conjunctivitis

Depending on the serotypes, chlamydial infection of the eye results in either inclusion conjunctivitis or trachoma.

Inclusion Conjunctivitis

This is a chronic ocular infection caused by *Chlamydia trachomatis* (serotypes D through K). It is transmitted sexually or during delivery (in neonatal cases). Organisms can be found in the respiratory tract, the cervix in women, and the urethra in male.

Clinical Features

1. Conjunctival hyperemia; mucopurulent discharge.
2. Pseudoptosis; photophobia.
3. Papillary reaction, mainly in the upper palpebral conjunctiva; follicles present in upper and lower palpebral conjunctiva.
4. Preauricular nodes: enlarged, tender, and palpable.
5. Micropannus located along either the upper or the lower limbus.
6. Superficial punctate staining of cornea.
7. Subepithelial corneal stromal infiltrates.

Workup

1. Giemsa stain shows intracytoplasmic basophilic inclusions ("cap on the nucleus")—Leber cells.
2. Immunofluorescent assay (IFA) or complement fixation test or a chlamydial culture.

Treatment

1. Adults (sexual contacts should be treated also):
    a) Doxycycline (100 mg p.o. b.i.d. 3–6 wks); or tetracycline or erythromycin (250 mg p.o. q.i.d. 3–6 wks; systemic

tetracycline is contraindicated in children under 8 yrs of age, pregnant women, and nursing mothers).

b) Topical tetracycline or erythromycin ointment four times a day for 3 weeks.

2. Neonates:
   a) Prophylaxis when born to infected mothers: topical tetracycline or erythromycin ointment twice a day for a week.
   b) With active ocular infection: erythromycin syrup, 50 mg/kg a day in four divided doses for 2 to 3 weeks (to prevent chlamydial pneumonitis); and topical tetracycline or erythromycin ointment, four times a day for 2 to 3 weeks.
   c) Asymptomatic mothers and their sexual partners should also be treated: tetracycline or erythromycin (250 mg p.o. q.i.d. for at least 2–3 wks); tetracycline is contraindicated if mother breast-feeds.

Trachoma

This is a chronic ocular infection caused by *Chlamydia trachomatis* (serotypes A, B, and C). It is transmitted through person-to-person contact or flies carrying chlamydial organisms. One of the most common ocular infections in the world, it is prevalent in developing countries, also in some Indian tribes in Southwest United States.

Physical Findings

1. Conjunctival findings:
   a) Pannus: classically at the superior limbus.
   b) Conjunctival follicles (papillary reaction may also be present).
   c) Arlt's lines (horizontal scarring lines on the upper tarsus); conjunctival scarring; forniceal foreshortening; symblepharon formation.
   d) Herbert's pits: limbal depressions left by resolved limbal follicles.
2. Lids may show trichiasis, entropion, and ectropion.
3. Corneal findings: SPK; superior corneal infiltrates; secondary corneal infections (e.g., ulcers).

MacCallan's Classification (This is based on the findings of upper palpebral conjunctiva).

Stage 1: immature follicles
Stage 2: mature follicles
Stage 3: follicles and cicatrization
Stage 4: no follicles, only cicatrization

Treatment

1. Adults:
   a) Doxycycline (100 mg p.o. b.i.d. for 3–4 wks); or tetracycline (250 mg p.o. q.i.d. for 3–4 wks); or erythromycin (250 mg p.o. q.i.d. for 3–4 wks).
   b) Topical erythromycin or tetracycline ointment (q.i.d. for 3–4 wks).
   c) Systemic tetracycline is contraindicated in children under the age of 8, pregnant women, and nursing mothers.
2. Children: topical erythromycin or tetracycline ophthalmic ointment (b.i.d. for 6–8 wks); or erythromycin (40 mg/kg q.d. for 3 wks).
3. World Health Organization (WHO) recommendations for mass treatment in endemic areas: tetracycline ointment twice a day for the first 5 days of month for 6 months or tetracycline ointment twice a day for 2 months.
4. Surgical repair of trichiasis and lid abnormalities.

Course   Patient can be reinfected, and repeated treatments may be necessary; trachoma patients are prone to superinfections. If left untreated or inadequately treated, trachoma can result in

1. conjunctival shrinking, forniceal shortening, and symblepharon formation;
2. dry eye secondary to destruction of accessory lacrimal glands and conjunctival goblet cells; and
3. lid abnormalities—trichiasis, ectropion, entropion.

Viral Conjunctivitis

Adenovirus Conjunctivitis: Epidemic Keratoconjunctivitis (EKC)

Caused by adenovirus types 8 and 19.

Symptoms and Signs

1. Sudden onset of redness and watery discharge.
2. Follicular conjunctivitis.
3. Preauricular nodes: enlarged and tender.
4. A pseudomembrane or membrane may be present.
5. Keratitis (four different types):
   a) Diffuse epithelial keratitis (first week)
   b) Focal epithelial keratitis (second week)

    c) Subepithelial opacities (after second week)
    d) Gray epithelial infiltrates (after second week)
6. Bilateral or unilateral; second eye may become infected within 10 days.

Course Self-limited; conjunctivitis usually resolves within 2 to 3 weeks after onset; subepithelial infiltrates may last months to years.

Transmission Hand-to-eye contact or contaminated ophthalmic instruments; meticulous handwashing and instrument cleaning are important.

Treatment Mainly supportive:

1. Antiviral eyedrops ineffective.
2. Artificial tears; cool compresses.
3. Vasoconstrictor or antihistamine for itching.
4. Topical steroids in patients severely debilitated by subepithelial infiltrates (glare or decreased vision); steroids may prolong the presence of subepithelial infiltrates.

Prevention

1. Meticulous handwashing and cleaning of ophthalmic instruments (with alcohol or chlorine bleach).
2. Infected persons: avoid contact for 2 weeks.

Adenovirus Conjunctivitis: Pharyngoconjunctival Fever (PCF)

Caused by adenovirus types 3 and 7.

Clinical Presentation

1. Acute-onset follicular conjunctivitis and conjunctival hyperemia.
2. Concomitant fever and pharyngitis.
3. Enlarged and tender preauricular nodes.
4. A pseudomembrane or membrane may be present.
5. Subepithelial infiltrates may occur; usually not as severe and do not last as long as in EKC.

Course Self-limited; lasts about 2 weeks.

Transmission Usually through airborne droplets; virus is shed in tears, respiratory secretion, and feces.

Treatment Mainly supportive (see EKC).

Prevention   See EKC.

Acute Hemorrhagic Conjunctivitis

Caused by Coxsackie virus and enterovirus.

Clinical Presentation   Acute follicular reaction; subconjunctival hemorrhages; watery discharge; enlarged preauricular nodes.

Transmission   Through hand-to-eye contact.

Course   Self-limited; resolves in 2 to 3 weeks.

Treatment   Supportive (see EKC).

Prevention   See EKC.

Molluscum Contagiosum

Etiology   A poxvirus.

Clinical Presentation
1. Elevated nodular lesion with umbilicated center on the eyelid.
2. Chronic follicular conjunctivitis.
3. Superficial punctate staining; pannus formation.

Treatment   Excision of lid lesion; cryotherapy; curettage of the center of the molluscum lesion.

Noninfectious (Hypersensitivity) Conjunctivitis

Vernal Keratoconjunctivitis (VKC)

This has IgE-mediated type I hypersensitivity and possibly basophil cutaneous hypersensitivity.

Clinical Signs
1. Stringy and purulent discharge.
2. Itching; irritation (it has been stated, "no itching, no vernal").
3. Children and young adolescents; male predominance.
4. More prevalent in warm climates; more severe in spring and summer.

Clinical Findings

1. Two forms:
   a) Palpebral VKC; typically affects the superior tarsal conjunctiva.
   b) Limbal VKC; affects mainly the limbus (Trantas's dots); more common in nonwhites.
2. Giant papillae on tarsal conjunctiva (may exhibit a cobblestone pattern).
3. Conjunctival shrinkage does not occur in vernal patients (in contrast to atopic patients).
4. Shield corneal ulcer: usually located in the superior half of the cornea.
5. Trantas's dots: collections of eosinophils at the limbus; characteristic of limbal VKC.
6. Conjunctival scrapings show eosinophils, mast cells (mostly degranulated), and basophils.

Treatment

1. For mild cases, cool compresses and topical vasoconstrictors.
2. Topical steroids (prednisolone acetate or phosphate 1%) during periods of exacerbation; "pulse" therapy with frequent topical steroid drops (one drop every 2 h while awake) for 2 to 4 days during exacerbations and for treating shield ulcers; taper according to clinical course.
3. Cromolyn (Opticrom 4% eyedrop) prevents degranulation of mast cells; a preventive measure; takes about 2 to 4 weeks for Cromolyn to be effective.
4. Mucolytic agents (e.g., N-acetylcysteine or Mucomyst 10% eyedrops q.i.d.) to break up mucus strands; Mucomyst eyedrops should be refrigerated and replaced every 3 weeks; Mucomyst has unpleasant odor (like rotten eggs).
5. Systemic steroids may be required in difficult cases.
6. Topical cyclosporine effective in recalcitrant cases (as a last resort).

Course   Resolves (burns out) on its own within 10 years. There may be residual superficial corneal scarring. Keratoconus may develop in some patients with VKC.

Atopic Keratoconjunctivitis (AKC)

This is characterized by lack of seasonal variation (in contrast to VKC); ropy purulent discharge, itching, and irritation; and older patients (>20 yrs of age).

Clinical Findings

1. May have atopic dermatitis.
2. Usually affects the inferior palpebral conjunctiva, in contrast to VKC (which involves mainly the superior conjunctiva).
3. Conjunctival scarring, forniceal foreshortening, and symblepharon (vernal conjunctiva does not show scarring or shrinkage).
4. Fewer eosinophils than VKC on conjunctival scraping.
5. Cataracts.
6. Cornea: pannus formation; corneal vascularization; SPK; arcus formation; keratoconus.

Treatment   Similar to VKC.

Course   Longer than VKC; may extend into adulthood.

Hay Fever Keratoconjunctivitis

This involves a type I hypersensitivity reaction. It is characterized by recurrence with exacerbations during early summer. Some patients may have asthma.

Clinical Findings   During exacerbations:

1. Lid edema; conjunctival hyperemia and chemosis.
2. Sudden onset.

Treatment   Cold compresses; topical vasoconstrictors; topical Opticrom 4% four times day (as prophylaxis); oral antihistamines.

Giant Papillary Conjunctivitis (GPC)

This is caused by chronic contact lens wear (usually soft contact lenses), exposed sutures, or prostheses. It is characterized by irritation, ropy discharge, itching, and decreased contact lens tolerance.

Clinical Findings

1. Giant papillae (> 1 mm in diameter) on the superior tarsal conjunctiva.
2. Conjunctival scraping: eosinophils, mast cells, and basophils; most of the mast cells are not degranulated (in contrast to VKC); fewer eosinophils in GPC than in VKC.

Treatment   Remove any exposed sutures or clean the prosthesis; if secondary to contact lens, then note the following:

1. Replace old contact lens or change to gas-permeable contact lenses; contact lenses may have to be cleaned enzymatically more frequently or replaced more often.
2. Reduce wearing time or discontinue contact lens for a short period of time.
3. Topical cromolyn and steroids may be used.
4. Discontinue contact lens use permanently in recalcitrant or severe cases.

Toxic Conjunctivitis (Drug-Induced or Medicomentosa)

Chronic use of eye medications can lead to conjunctivitis:

1. Preservatives in eyedrops (e.g., thimerosal and benzalkonium)
2. Antiviral medications (e.g., idoxuridine, arabinoside A, trifluorothymidine)
3. Antibiotic medications (e.g., neomycin, gentamicin, tobramycin)
4. Glaucoma medications (e.g., epinephrine, propine, pilocarpine)
5. Atropine

Degenerations

Definition Nonheritable corneal changes due to exogenous factors (e.g., trauma, chronic sunlight exposure, age).

Arcus

1. Termed arcus senilis if seen in elderly.
2. Termed arcus juvenilis if seen in the young.
3. Gray-white deposits in the peripheral cornea, parallel to the limbus with a lucid zone separating the arcus from the limbus; the outer border is sharp; the inner border is ill-defined.
4. Consists of lipid depositions in the corneal stroma.
5. May indicate hypercholesterolemia or hyperlipidemia.
6. Asymmetry may suggest occlusion of the carotid artery ipsilateral to the cornea with less arcus.

Cornea Farinata

1. Deep stromal punctate opacities anterior to Descemet's membrane; best seen with retroillumination.
2. Commonly seen in elderly; not visually significant.
3. Differential diagnosis: pre-Descemet's dystrophy; X-linked ichthyosis; polymorphic stromal dystrophy.

Pinguecula

1. Yellow-white subepithelial deposits of the bulbar conjunctiva; typically in the interpalpebral zone, most often nasally.
2. Due to chronic actinic exposure.
3. Histopathology: elastotic degeneration of subconjunctival collagen fibers; stains positive for elastic fibers but indigestible by elastase.
4. Can be resected for cosmesis, chronic irritation, or interference with contact lens wear.
5. Pinguecula-like lesions may occur in Gaucher's disease.

Pterygium

1. Extension of vascular tissue from a pingueculum into the cornea, usually nasally.
2. Iron line (Stocker's line) may be anterior to pterygium.
3. Cause and histopathology (see pingueculum).
4. Resection for cosmesis, astigmatism, or if the visual axis is threatened or involved.
5. May recur; beta-irradiation, thiopeta eyedrops, mitomycin eyedrops, or conjunctival transplant to prevent recurrences.
6. Pseudopterygia can be differentiated from true pterygia by passing a rod underneath the pseudopterygium (this cannot be done with a true pterygium); pseudopterygia are usually the results of trauma.

Salzmann's Degeneration

1. Bluish gray nodular elevation secondary to exuberant subepithelial scarring.
2. Usually the result of trauma or other corneal disorders (e.g., dry eye, trachoma, and phlyctenulosis).
3. Treatment: artificial tears in mild cases, superficial keratectomy in more severe cases; Salzmann lesions may recur after surgical removal.

Spheroidal (Labrador) Degeneration

1. Fine, golden-yellow deposits under corneal epithelium.
2. Result of prolonged actinic exposure or previous corneal trauma or pathology.
3. Hyalin deposits in Bowman's layer and anterior stroma.
4. In severe cases, superficial keratectomy is indicated.

Limbal Girdle of Vogt

1. In the aging cornea; small white deposits beneath the corneal epithelium typically at 3 o'clock and 9 o'clock positions near limbus.

2. Pathology: subepithelial elastotic degeneration.
3. No treatment is usually needed.

Crocodile Shagreen

1. Anterior or posterior; anterior type is at the level of Bowman's membrane; posterior type is at the level of Descemet's membrane.
2. Polygonal mosaics with clear intervening areas.
3. Rarely reduces visual acuity.

Band Keratopathy

1. Chalky crystalline white to grayish deposits; usually begins near limbus at 3 o'clock and 9 o'clock and can cross the cornea; typically a clear (lucid) zone of cornea between limbus and band keratopathy.
2. Histopathology: calcium on Bowman's layer.
3. Associated with chronic iridocyclitis (e.g., juvenile rheumatoid arthritis), renal failure, hyperparathyroidism, excessive vitamin D intake, sarcoidosis, dry eye, interstitial keratitis, chronic glaucoma, chronic bullous keratopathy, phthisis bulbi.
4. Treatment: visually significant band keratopathy can be removed with EDTA; remove epithelium before applying EDTA.

Hassall-Henle Warts

1. Small round dark areas seen with the slit lamp at Descemet's membrane in the periphery of cornea.
2. Focal areas of thickening of Descemet's membrane; identical to cornea guttata (which are located in the central cornea).
3. Normal variant in an aging cornea or part of Fuchs' endothelial dystrophy.

Polymorphic Amyloid Degeneration

1. Punctate or filamentous glassy deposits in deep stroma.
2. Can be confused with corneal lattice dystrophy.
3. In contrast to lattice dystrophy, polymorphic amyloid degeneration is not a heritable condition.
4. Histopathology: deposits are amyloid.

Dellen

1. Focal corneal thinning due to drying or poor wetting by tear film; most commonly in peripheral cornea.
2. Corneal epithelium is intact; no fluorescein staining; however, fluorescein pooling may occur.

3. Common etiologies:
   a) Perilimbal tissue swelling or irregularities: eye surgeries (e.g., muscle surgery, cataract surgery, conjunctival blebs); pterygium; or pingueculum.
   b) Contact lens; dry eye; lagophthalmos.
4. Treatment: ocular lubrication; pressure patching.

Terrien's Degeneration

Noninflammatory progressive thinning (guttering) of peripheral cornea; usually begins superiorly or superonasally.

Clinical Features

1. Usually bilateral.
2. Guttering process spreads perilimbally.
3. Male predominance.
4. Intact corneal epithelium.
5. Vascular pannus may traverse the gutter, and lipid deposition may occur on the leading edge of pannus.

Course   Progressive worsening of astigmatism. Spontaneous perforation does not usually occur.

Treatment   Protective glasses if thinning is severe. Lamellar graft to reinforce areas of severe thinning. Penetrating keratoplasty may be needed.

Pellucid Marginal Degeneration

Noninflammatory progressive thinning of inferior peripheral cornea with high against-the-rule astigmatism.

Clinical Features

1. Frequently diagnosed between ages 20 and 40.
2. Bilateral inferior thinning from 4 to 8 o'clock; 1 to 2 mm from the limbus and 1 to 2 mm in width.
3. Cornea adjacent to limbus appears normal.
4. Irregular against-the-rule astigmatism.
5. Intact corneal epithelium.
6. Descemet's folds (stress lines) may develop.

Treatment   In mild cases spectacles or contact lenses. Large corneal graft in severe cases to restore vision; results are usually excellent.

Dry Eye (Keratoconjunctivitis Sicca)

History and Etiology   Dry eye causes ocular surface changes from decreased tear production or instability of tear film; dryness in mucous membranes other than the conjunctiva (buccal and vaginal mucosa) may also be present; causes of dry eye can be divided as follows:

1. Decreased production of the aqueous layer in tear film:
   a) Idiopathic (may be age-related).
   b) Sjögren's syndrome.
      i) Primary Sjögren's syndrome (dry eye and mouth).
      ii) Secondary Sjögren's syndrome: dry eye and dry mouth with collagen-vascular diseases (e.g., rheumatoid arthritis [RA] and systemic lupus erythematosus [SLE]).
      iii) Indeterminate: dry eye and dry mouth with positive laboratory findings (e.g., antinuclear antibody [ANA] and rheumatoid factor [RF]) but no clinical evidence of collagen-vascular diseases.
   c) Infiltrative or inflammatory lesions in the lacrimal glands (e.g., lymphoma, dacryoadenitis, tuberculosis, sarcoidosis, syphilis).
   d) Riley-Day syndrome and congenital alacrima.
   e) Anorexia nervosa (not related to vitamin A deficiency).
   f) Postradiation (irradiation of lacrimal glands or face).
2. Decrease in mucin production resulting from loss of conjunctival goblet cells: chemical burns; Stevens-Johnson syndrome; vitamin A deficiency; ocular cicatricial pemphigoid; trachoma.
3. Decrease in lipid production is rare; can occur in anhidrotic ectodermal dysplasia.
4. Disturbance in oil production of the meibomian glands (e.g., blepharitis and meibomianitis).
5. Abnormal lid function and anatomy (e.g., Bell's palsy, lid coloboma).
6. Medication-induced (e.g., antihistamines, birth-control pills, beta-blockers, and phenothiazines).

Physical Findings

1. SPK, usually inferior and within palpebral fissure
2. Unstable tear film; shortened tear breakup time (TBUT)
3. Decrease in the height of tear meniscus
4. Debris or foam in tear film
5. Increased mucus discharge
6. Loss of conjunctival luster

7. Bitot's spots (keratinization of paralimbal conjunctival epithelium in triangular patches) in vitamin A deficiency
8. Blepharitis and meibomianitis may be present

Workup   Tailored according to clinical suspicion.

1. Schirmer's test:
   a) After the application of topical anesthesia, the inferior fornices are dried with a cotton-tipped applicator. A strip of filter paper is placed in the inferior cul-de-sac and over the lateral lower lid margin (without touching the cornea) for 5 minutes.
   b) Normal value is between 10 and 15 mm or greater; some normal patients may have values less than 10 mm.
2. Rose Bengal test: stains devitalized epithelial cells; may sting.
3. Tear breakup time (TBUT):
   a) TBUT is assessed by having patient hold the eye open (eyelids should not be held open with fingers), while the fluorescein pattern of the tear film is observed at the slit lamp.
   b) Tear breakup is seen as dark areas in the tear film; normal TBUT is 10 seconds or more.
4. Rheumatoid factor, ANA, SSA and SSB (for collagen-vascular diseases).
5. PPD, FTA-ABS (for tuberculosis and syphilis).
6. Chest x-ray, angiotensin-converting enzyme (ACE) test, serum lysozyme test, and/or conjunctival biopsy (for sarcoidosis).
7. Labial biopsy (for Sjögren's syndrome or lymphoma).
8. Tear osmolarity and tear levels of lysozyme and lactoferrin levels (these tests are not routinely used clinically).
9. Conjunctival impression cytology (not for routine clinical use).

Treatment

1. Artificial tears: if used less than four times a day tears with preservatives are well tolerated; if used more than four times a day consider nonpreserved tears (e.g., Refresh).
2. Occlusion of puncta: temporarily with plugs or permanently with cautery.
3. Warm compresses, lid hygiene, and antibiotic ointment or medications in cases of blepharitis and meibomianitis.
4. Stop birth control pills, phenothiazines, beta-blockers or antihistamine medications if possible.
5. Mucomyst 10% eyedrop four times a day for excessive mucus discharge; Mucomyst should be kept refrigerated and replaced every 3 weeks.

6. Goggles, moist chamber glasses, and tarsorrhaphy in severe or recalcitrant cases.
7. Conjunctival or buccal mucous membrane graft if there is extensive loss of conjunctiva from chemical burns.
8. Vitamin A supplement if patient is vitamin A deficient.
9. Topical retinoic acid and cyclosporin (experimental and currently under investigation).
10. Parotid duct transposition (rarely done).

Course and Prognosis   In most patients, dry eye is a chronic condition that will last a lifetime, with periods of exacerbation, depending on weather and seasonal changes; prognosis in most patients is good; in severe cases, if left untreated, dry eye may lead to corneal infiltrates, band keratopathy, and secondary corneal and conjunctival infections, stromal melt, and corneal perforations.

Dystrophies

Anatomy   For normal corneal anatomy, see Figure 3.1.

Definition   Corneal dystrophies are hereditary conditions in which the cornea is genetically predisposed to develop certain pathologic changes; corneal dystrophies are autosomal dominant except for macu-

FIGURE 3.1 Normal Corneal Anatomy

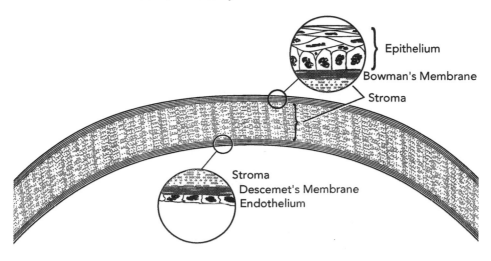

lar dystrophy and congenital hereditary endothelial dystrophy, which can be autosomal recessive; corneal dystrophies are bilateral, although there can be asymmetry; systemic disorders may be associated with some corneal dystrophies.

Epithelium

Map-Dot-Fingerprint (MDF) Dystrophy (Anterior Basement Membrane Dystrophy)

1. Recurrent erosion present in 10% of cases of MDF dystrophy; MDF dystrophy present in 50% of recurrent erosion cases.
2. Erosions most commonly occur upon awakening.
3. The defect is in the basement membrane of epithelium.
4. Histopathology: map (extensions of basement membrane); dot (intraepithelial cysts); fingerprint (reduplication of basement membrane).
5. Treatment
   a) Mechanical debridement of loose epithelium.
   b) Pressure patch or bandage contact lens.
   c) Antibiotic prophylaxis and cycloplegia.
   d) Hypertonic sodium chloride (5%) to prevent recurrent erosions after reepithelialization.
   d) Anterior stromal puncture for recalcitrant cases.
6. With scarring of the epithelial basement membrane, the frequency of erosions decreases.

Meesmann's Dystrophy

1. Multiple tiny epithelial vesicles, best seen with retroillumination.
2. Histopathologically, intracytoplasmic inclusion bodies contain yet-to-be-identified "peculiar substance."
3. Symptoms: transient blurred vision, photophobia, and intermittent irritation or foreign body sensation.
4. In most cases, treatment is not needed; superficial keratectomy reported to be curative; epithelial lesions disappear with soft contact lens wear but recur when the contact lens is stopped.

Bowman's Membrane

Reis-Bückler's Dystrophy

1. Characterized by recurrent spontaneous erosions.
2. Fishnet-like subepithelial opacities in the Bowman's membrane of the central cornea.
3. Histopathology shows replacement of normal Bowman's membrane with fibrocellular tissue.

4. Treatment for recurrent erosions: pressure patching; soft bandage contact lens; hypertonic sodium chloride drops or ointment; superficial keratectomy or excimer surface ablation and penetrating keratoplasty (PK) necessary in severe cases; Reis-Bückler's dystrophy recurs in corneal grafts.

Stroma

Granular Dystrophy

1. Characterized by gradual decrease in visual acuity; epithelial erosions seldom occur.
2. White "bread-crumb" deposits in the superficial central corneal stroma may extend into mid-stroma; the areas between the deposits remain clear, as does the peripheral cornea.
3. Histopathology: corneal deposits are hyaline that stain red with Masson trichrome.
4. Penetrating keratoplasty in patients with significant decreased vision due to corneal opacification; may recur in graft.

Macular Dystrophy

1. Autosomal recessive.
2. Characterized by progressive decrease in vision; epithelial erosions occur infrequently.
3. Diffuse stromal haziness with focal gray-white opacities with ill-defined borders, extending to the corneal periphery and through the entire stroma.
4. Histopathologically corneal deposits are glycosaminoglycans (principally precursors of keratan sulfate) that stain positive with alcian blue and colloidal iron.
5. Treatment is PK when vision is severely limited by corneal changes; can recur in corneal graft, but less frequently than lattice or granular dystrophies.

Lattice Dystrophy

1. Characterized by recurrent erosions and progressive decreased vision.
2. Clinical features: refractile lines, white dots, and central stromal haze.
3. Histopathologically amyloid (stains positive with Congo red and thioflavin T); shows metachromasia with crystal violet; shows birefringence and polarizes lights.
4. Treatment
   a) Pressure patching or bandage contact lens for epithelial erosions.

  b) Penetrating keratoplasty for visual loss due to corneal changes.
  c) Lattice dystrophy can recur in graft; recurs more frequently than granular or macular dystrophies.

Central Crystalline Dystrophy (of Schnyder)

1. Characterized by minute stromal crystals, diffuse central corneal opacification, and arcus formation.
2. Histopathology: lipid (stains with Sudan black and oil red O).
3. Associated with hyperlipidemia, hypercholesterolemia, and genu valgum.
4. Treatment: screen for hyperlipidemia and hypercholesterolemia; PK in severe cases.

Fleck Dystrophy

1. Does not affect vision; no treatment required.
2. Diffuse deposits of small dandruff-like material in stroma, distributed through the entire stroma.
3. Histopathology lipids and glycosaminoglycans.

Pre-Descemet's Dystrophy

1. Minute discrete opacities in stroma, just anterior to Descemet's membrane.
2. Occur as isolated ocular findings or can be associated with aging (cornea farinata) or X-linked ichthyosis.
3. Histopathology: lipids.
4. Differential diagnosis: see cornea farinata.

Congenital Hereditary Stromal Dystrophy

1. Rare bilateral congenital diffuse stromal haze; nonprogressive; nystagmus may develop.
2. Differential diagnosis: congenital hereditary endothelial dystrophy; congenital glaucoma; mucopolysaccharidoses; posterior polymorphous dystrophy.
3. Treatment: PK; amblyopia may limit the visual outcome.

Endothelium

Fuchs' Endothelial Dystrophy

Characteristics

1. Bilateral
2. Decreased vision; visual acuity tends to be worse in the morning and improves throughout the day

3. Pain; foreign body sensation; or photophobia
4. Female predominance (3:1); most patients older than 50
5. Autosomal dominant in some pedigrees.

Clinical Signs

1. Cornea guttata that are densest centrally
2. Thickening of Descemet's membrane
3. Stromal thickening and edema
4. Descemet's folds (striate keratopathy)
5. Microcystic epithelial edema (bedewing)
6. Subepithelial bullae (bullous keratopathy) and subepithelial
   fibrosis

Stages

1. Endothelial dystrophy (stage I): degeneration of corneal
   endothelium leading to thickening of Descemet's membrane,
   usually with the presence of cornea guttata, although cornea
   guttata do not necessarily have to be present; no evidence of
   edema at this stage.
2. Fuchs' dystrophy (stage II): endothelial degeneration leading to
   failure of endothelial pump; aqueous percolates into the stroma
   and epithelium leading to stromal thickening, Descemet's folds,
   microcystic epithelial edema, bullous keratopathy, and
   subepithelial fibrosis; vascularization rarely occurs.

Histopathology Excrescences on Descemet's membrane located centrally (guttata) and similar to Hassall-Henle warts located in corneal
periphery; Descemet's membrane is thickened; endothelial cells are attenuated.

Workup Endothelial cell count shows decreased density of endothelial cells; corneal thickness measurement with pachometry demonstrates increased central corneal thickness.

Differential Diagnosis

1. Pseudoguttata in inflammatory conditions (iridocyclitis, syphilitic
   interstitial keratitis, and disciform keratitis) or from contact lens
   wear.
2. Surgically induced corneal edema (aphakic and pseudophakic
   bullous keratopathies).
3. Posterior polymorphous dystrophy.

Treatment

1. Hypertonic sodium chloride (5%) eyedrops and ointment in mild cases of corneal edema.
2. Warm air from a hair dryer in morning to reduce corneal edema (used in mild cases).
3. Ruptured bullae can be treated with pressure patch or bandage soft contact lens.
4. Penetrating keratoplasty in severe cases.
5. If patient is not a surgical candidate, cautery of Bowman's membrane may be considered.

Congential Hereditary Endothelial Dystrophy

This is either autosomal dominant or recessive. The recessive type is nonprogressive, present at birth, and associated with nystagmus; the dominant type is progressive, appears in first decade of life, and is associated with pain and photophobia (not nystagmus).

Characteristics

1. Bilateral stromal haze; epithelial edema.
2. Gray and thickened Descemet's membrane.
3. Band keratopathy (in chronic cases).

Histopathology   Collagen fibrils posterior to Descemet's membrane; the endothelium is attenuated.

Differential Diagnosis   Congenital glaucoma; mucopolysaccharidosis; forceps corneal injury; posterior polymorphous dystrophy (especially if the inheritance appears autosomal dominant).

Treatment   Penetrating keratoplasty.

Posterior Polymorphous Dystrophy (PPMD)

Clinical Signs

1. Vesicles and bands in endothelium
2. Thickened Descemet's membrane
3. Iridocorneal adhesions, usually peripheral
4. Stromal and epithelial edema
5. Elevated intraocular pressure in 15% of cases

Histopathology   Epithelial transformation of the endothelium.

Differential Diagnosis   Iridocorneal endothelial (ICE) syndromes (essential iris atrophy; Chandler's syndrome; Cogan-Reese syndrome); unlike PPMD, ICE syndromes are not hereditary, almost always unilateral and predominantly female. (See Glaucoma chapter.)

Treatment   Hypertonic sodium chloride; bandage contact lens; PK in severe cases.

Edema

Definition   Corneal edema usually means increased stromal thickening (due to epithelial breakdown or endothelial dysfunction); edema of the epithelium (e.g., microcystic edema) and endothelium (e.g., pseudoguttata) can also occur. The stroma consists of glycosaminoglycans that have an affinity for water; this tendency is counterbalanced by the pump action of endothelium and the barrier function of epithelium. Corneal edema can lead to decreased vision, foreign body sensation, pain, and photophobia. Corneal edema can be subdivided as follows.

Epithelial Edema

Clinical Presentation

1. Microcystic edema best seen with slit lamp by using sclerotic scatter
2. Subepithelial bullae; rupture of subepithelial bullae can cause foreign body sensation and pain
3. Subepithelial fibrosis may occur in chronic cases

Causes

1. Elevated intraocular pressure (IOP), usually exceeding 50 mmHg; typically the rise of IOP is acute
2. Hypoxia secondary to ill-fit contact lenses
3. Endothelial dysfunction (e.g., Fuchs' dystrophy; PPMD; ICE syndromes)

Treatment

1. Hypertonic sodium chloride drops or ointments
2. Warm air from a hair blow-dryer in the mornings

Stromal Edema

Characteristics

1. Increased stromal thickness; measure with ultrasonic pachometry
2. Stromal haze
3. Descemet's folds (striate keratopathy)

Causes

1. Epithelial defects
2. Endothelial dysfunction
   a) Fuchs' endothelial dystrophy
   b) Congenital hereditary endothelial dystrophy
   c) Posterior polymorphous dystrophy (PPMD)
   d) Forceps injury, resulting in disruption of Descemet's membrane and corneal endothelium
   e) Hydrops associated with keratoconus or trauma
   f) Iridocorneal endothelial (ICE) syndromes
3. Inflammation (e.g., herpetic disciform keratitis; syphilitic interstitial keratitis; *Acanthamoeba* keratitis; corneal ulcer)

Treatment   See Fuchs' dystrophy.

Endothelial Edema

Intracellular swelling of endothelial cells can be clinically seen as pseudoguttata. Specular microscopy can also be used to assess the density of endothelial cells. Causes include:

1. Fuchs' endothelial dystrophy
2. Keratouveitis (e.g., herpes simplex; herpes zoster)
3. Iridocyclitis (anterior uveitis)
4. Contact lens wear

Epithelial Defects

History and Etiology   Corneal epithelial defects result from the breakdown of corneal epithelium; the causes of epithelial defect include the following:

1. Trauma (e.g., foreign body, fingernail injury, and chemical burn)
2. Spontaneous (e.g., anterior basement membrane dystrophy, lattice dystrophy, Reis-Bückler's dystrophy, Fuchs' endothelial dystrophy, or recurrent erosions from previous trauma, such as fingernail injury)
3. Dry eye
4. Part of a corneal ulcer (e.g., herpes simplex keratitis, herpes zoster keratitis, or bacterial corneal ulcer)

Physical Examination

1. Fluorescein staining of epithelial defects.
2. Heaped-up epithelium at the margin of the ulcer (may be indicative of damage to basement membrane).

3. Underlying stromal infiltrates (infectious or sterile) may be present.
4. Stromal thickening and Descemet's folds may be present.

Workup Depending on the underlying cause.

1. look for foreign body on upper or lower tarsal conjunctiva
2. perform corneal scraping and obtain culture if infection is suspected.

Differential Diagnosis Fluorescein pooling in areas of corneal depression (healed corneal ulcer or dellen) may mimic fluorescein staining.

Treatment

1. For most cases, pressure patching will suffice. A bandage contact lens may be needed if the epithelial defect takes a longer time to heal, if patient has to take eye medications, or if the patient cannot tolerate a pressure patch. Pressure patches or bandage contact lens should not be used in infections.
2. Cycloplegia and topical antibiotic ointment or drops.
3. In recalcitrant cases, anterior stromal puncture, cautery of Bowman's membrane, tarsorrhaphy (temporary or permanent), or conjunctival flap.
4. Fortified antibiotic eyedrops or antiviral eyedrops are indicated in cases of infected corneal ulcers (see Ulcers section, below).

Course Highly variable depending on the extent and the nature of epithelial defect; a damaged anterior basement membrane may prolong the resolution of epithelial defects.

Prognosis

Variable, depending on the nature of underlying cause; delay in re-epithelialization may lead to infection, progressive stromal thinning, or perforation.

Episcleritis/Scleritis

Episcleritis

History and Etiology Can be divided into two forms, simple and nodular. Female predominance of 2:1; peak incidence in fourth decade; etiology is usually unknown, although syphilis, gout, rheumatoid arthritis, and systemic lupus erythematosus can cause episcleritis. Discomfort (not pain) is characteristic of episcleritis.

Physical Examination

1. In the simple form: diffuse edema of the episcleral tissue, which is best seen with red-free slit beam; there is usually bright red discoloration.
2. In the nodular form: localized elevation of episcleral tissue with concomitant edema; the nodule is moderately mobile and may be tender to touch.

Workup   Depending on clinical suspicion, perform tests for ANA, RF, FTA-ABS, and serum uric acid level.

Differential Diagnosis   Scleritis. Episcleritis may accompany scleritis, but in pure episcleritis there is no scleral inflammation; congested episcleral vessels in episcleritis will blanch with topical 10% phenylephrine, whereas the congested deep scleral vessels in scleritis will not blanch; the nodules in episcleritis can be moved with a cotton-tipped applicator (in scleritis, nodules are immobile).

Treatment

1. Observation, if the inflammation is not severe.
2. Nonsteroidal anti-inflammatory drugs (NSAID): indomethacin (25–50 mg p.o. b.i.d.) with food or antacid.
3. Corticosteroids if the inflammation is moderately severe or unresponsive to NSAID:
   a) Topical steroids (dexamethasone 0.1%; prednisolone phosphate or acetate 1%) hourly until the inflammation starts to subside and then taper.
   b) Systemic steroids if unresponsive to topical steroids and NSAID.

Course   Exacerbations and remissions.

Prognosis   Excellent; no visually significant sequelae, if adequately treated during exacerbations.

Scleritis

History and Etiology   Inflammation of the sclera characterized by photophobia, tearing, and ocular pain, which may be associated with eye movements and be severe enough to wake the patient from sleep. Scleritis usually involves middle-aged patients (predominance of women) and may be unilateral or bilateral. Common causes include syphilis, tuberculosis, SLE, RA, sarcoidosis, and vasculitides (Wegener's granulomatosis, polyarteritis nodosa, Behçet's disease, and relapsing polychondritis); scleritis has also been reported after cataract extraction and in Lyme disease.

Physical Examination   Scleritis can be categorized as follows.

Anterior Scleritis (Anterior to Equator)
1. Diffuse and nodular:
   a) The most benign forms of scleritis.
   b) Unilateral or bilateral.
   c) Clinical signs:
      i) Dilatation and displacement of overlying conjunctival and episcleral vessels (blanch with 10% phenylephrine eyedrops).
      ii) Dilatation of deep scleral vessels (do not blanch with 10% phenylephrine eyedrops).
      iii) Severe pain with palpation of the globe.
      iv) Scleral edema best seen with a red-free narrow beam on the slit lamp or natural light.
      v) Nodules of nodular scleritis are immobile, in contrast to nodules of nodular episcleritis.
      vi) Concomitant corneal changes include acute stromal keratitis, sclerosing keratitis, and peripheral corneal melt.
2. Necrotizing (characterized by necrosis of sclera, with or without signs of inflammation):
   a) Congested scleral vessels and avascular scleral areas.
   b) Necrotizing scleritis without inflammation (scleromalacia perforans) shows scleral thinning, staphyloma, or uveal prolapse; associated with RA.

Posterior Scleritis   Clinical signs and symptoms are the following:
1. Severe pain
2. Limited extraocular movements
3. Exudative retinal detachment; choroidal folds; optic disc edema; cystoid macular edema
4. Proptosis
5. Hyperopia
6. May or may not have signs of anterior scleritis

Posterior scleritis may belong to the spectrum of orbital pseudotumor, myositis, and dacryoadenitis. Usually patients with posterior scleritis have no associated systemic disease.

Workup

1. Laboratory studies (according to clinical suspicion) may include complete blood count, erythrocyte sedimentation rate (ESR), ANA, RF, FTA-ABS, Lyme titers, PPD and anergy panel, and antineutrophilic cytoplasmic antibody (ANCA; useful in Wegener's granulomatosis and polyarteritis nodosa).
2. Imaging studies:
   a) Chest x-ray.
   b) Orbital ultrasound: best means to confirm posterior scleritis; "T" sign at the optic nerve head may be seen in posterior scleritis.
   c) Orbital computed tomography (CT) or magnetic resonance imaging (MRI); CT may be superior to MRI.
   d) Fluorescein angiogram may be useful.
3. Rheumatology consultation (if a collagen-vascular disease is suspected as an underlying cause).

Differential Diagnosis

1. Anterior scleritis can mimic nearly all the other causes of conjunctival hyperemia; distinguishing features in scleritis are scleral inflammation, thinning, and necrosis.
2. Posterior scleritis can mimic any condition that may lead to choroidal mass, or a retinal or choroidal detachment.

Treatment

1. In mild cases, nonsteroidal anti-inflammatory drugs:
   a) Salicylate (600 mg p.o. q. 4–6 h).
   b) Indomethacin (25–50 mg p.o. b.i.d.).
   c) Ibuprofen (400–600 mg p.o. q.i.d.).
2. Corticosteroids:
   a) Systemic steroid (prednisone, 80–120 mg p.o. q.d.) in severe cases (taper according to clinical course).
   b) Periocular injection of corticosteroids is contraindicated; may lead to scleral thinning and perforation, especially in necrotizing scleritis.
3. Cyclosporin and immunosuppressives (e.g., cyclophosphamide, chlorambucil, and azathioprine) in severe and recalcitrant cases; side effects from these include bone marrow suppression and possibly inducing neoplasms.

4. Any underlying causes (e.g., syphilis and tuberculosis) should be treated.

Course   Exacerbations and remissions.

Prognosis   Complications include corneal changes (see Physical Examination), anterior uveitis, glaucoma, and cataract; the latter two may be the result of chronic steroid use. Of patients with necrotizing anterior scleritis with inflammation 21% will die within 8 years.

Eye Banking

Eye banking is a collaborative system in which whole globes or part of the globe (cornea or sclera) are preserved for surgical use; this section discusses eye banking in its relationship to corneal transplantation.

Donor Suitability

The following criteria are currently used by the Corneal Service at the University of Iowa Hospitals and Clinics; these criteria may differ from those of other institutions.

1. Absolute exclusion criteria (causes of donor death that may threaten the health of the recipient): unknown cause of death; Creutzfeldt-Jakob disease; recipients of human pituitary-derived growth hormone during the years from 1963 to 1985 (these patients may have been exposed to Creutzfeldt-Jakob disease); subacute sclerosing panencephalitis; congenital rubella; progressive multifocal leukoencephalopathy; Reye's syndrome; cytomegaloviral (CMV) encephalitis; septicemia; hepatitis or hepatitis seropositivity; rabies; acquired immune deficiency syndrome (AIDS); human immunodeficiency virus (HIV) positivity; blast form of leukemia; Hodgkin's disease; lymphosarcoma.

2. Conditions of the eye that make it unsuitable for corneal transplantation: corneal diseases (e.g., keratoconus or pterygium); conjunctivitis; previous ocular surgery; retinoblastoma; tumor of anterior segment.

3. Relative contraindications (diseases or conditions that may be unsuitable): age (donors between 2 and 70 inclusive are acceptable for corneal transplant); multiple sclerosis; Parkinson's disease; amyotrophic lateral sclerosis; jaundice; chronic lymphocytic leukemia; diabetes; syphilis; chronic immunosuppression; mechanical respiratory support for more than 72 hours; previous blood transfusions.

Processing

1. Enucleation should take place within 4 hours of death and must be performed sterilely by qualified personnel.

2. The cornea should be examined for epithelial defects, stromal haze and edema, presence of arcus, Descemet's folds, presence of guttata, and condition of endothelium.

3. Rate the condition of the donor cornea as excellent, very good, good, fair, or not suitable for surgery.

4. The cornea should be preserved within 15 hours of death.

Preservation

1. Preservatives (M-K, Dexsol, or Optisol) are most commonly used; corneas are stored in preservatives at 4°C and are suitable for transplantation for up to 4 to 5 days.

2. Less frequently used methods:
  a) Moist chamber storage at 4°C is good for up to 48 hours.
  b) Cryopreservation (infrequently used) is technically complex and expensive but is good for up to a year.
  c) Organ culture (storage at 37°C (infrequently used) is good for up to 35 days.

3. Nonviable material (for lamellar or patch grafts) should be stored either frozen or in glycerin.

Herpes Simplex Virus

Definition   Ubiquitous virus, part of the herpes group (including herpes simplex virus (HSV), herpes zoster virus (HZV), Epstein-Barr virus (EBV), and CMV). HSV can lead to blepharitis, conjunctivitis, keratitis, uveitis, and retinitis. HSV keratitis is a recurrent disorder; while inactive, the virus resides in the sensory ganglia (trigeminal ganglion).

Physical Examination

1. Lids: erythema, crusting, and vesicles (especially in primary infection).
2. Conjunctival hyperemia; follicles in primary infection.
3. Cornea:
    a)   Decreased corneal sensation or asymmetry of corneal sensation; HSV keratitis is unilateral in 98% of cases.
    b)   Epithelium may show dendrites or geographic epithelial defects (indicating active viral replication); HSV dendrites

stain with fluorescein and have terminal bulbs; there may be mild stromal infiltrates beneath them.

c) Necrotizing stromal keratitis is characterized by loss of stromal substance, stromal infiltration, and overlying epithelial defect.

d) Disciform keratitis is characterized by localized stromal edema without overlying epithelial defect.

e) Keratic precipitates are seen with endotheliitis, disciform keratitis, or HSV keratouveitis.

f) Metaherpetic epithelial defect is a result of damage to anterior basement membrane and has no active viral replication, in contrast to dendrites and geographic lesions.

4. Anterior chamber reaction (keratouveitis).
5. Elevated intraocular pressure due to trabeculitis.
6. Retinal necrosis.

Workup Diagnosis usually made clinically; viral cultures or immunologic studies can confirm clinical suspicion; corneal scraping may show multinucleated giant cells and intranuclear inclusion bodies with Papanicolaou stain.

Differential Diagnosis

1. Dendrites: tyrosinemia type II, herpes zoster, trauma, contact lens, and Darier's disease (keratosis follicularis).
2. Disciform keratitis may also develop in mumps, measles, herpes zoster, vaccinia, chemical keratitis, local bullous keratopathy, and corneal graft rejection (in the postoperative patient).

Treatment

1. For dendrites: trifluorothymidine (F_3T) 1% every 2 hours while awake; idoxuridine and vidarabine are alternatives; cycloplegia with or without mechanical debridement of the diseased epithelium.
2. No topical steroids in the presence of dendrites.
3. Topical steroids and cycloplegics for necrotizing keratitis, disciform keratitis, and keratouveitis; F_3T should be prescribed, one drop for every drop of steroid (up to four to six times daily) for antiviral coverage.
4. Oral acyclovir may be used (400 mg p.o. five times a day for 7–14 d).
5. Penetrating keratoplasty may be considered for corneal scarring if the eye has remained quiet for 6 months.

6. Corneal perforation may be treated with cyanoacrylate glue, patch graft, or PK.

Course   Herpetic keratitis is a recurrent disease; about 50% of patients will have recurrence in about 2 years.

Prognosis   Prompt treatment lessens the amount of corneal scarring; delayed treatment may result in corneal scarring, stromal thinning, and even corneal perforation.

Herpes Zoster Ophthalmicus

Definition   Herpes zoster virus (HZV) is acquired primarily during childhood as chickenpox (varicella). The virus remains latent in sensory ganglia; it may become activated spontaneously or during immunosuppression (e.g., from AIDS, chemotherapy, steroids).

Physical Examination

1. Skin eruptions in the distributions of sensory nerves:
   a) Trigeminal nerves are the second most frequently involved (after thoracic nerves); ophthalmic division is most commonly involved.
   b) Hutchinson's sign: skin eruption at the tip of the nose; indicates nasociliary nerve involvement (higher chance of ocular involvement).
2. Eye:
   a) Lid: vesicular or ulcerative skin eruptions (may have bacterial superinfection); lash loss; lid necrosis.
   b) Canaliculitis; occlusion of puncta or canaliculi.
   c) Myositis; episcleritis and scleritis.
   d) Conjunctivitis: papillary or follicular.
   e) Cornea:
      i) Decreased corneal sensation.
      ii) HZV dendrites: no terminal bulbs and stain with rose Bengal (but not with fluorescein); HZV dendrite consists of heaped-up epithelium.
      iii) Stroma: nummular, interstitial, disciform keratitis.
      iv) Trophic and recurrent epithelial defects.
      v) Corneal stromal melt.
   f) Iridocyclitis or keratouveitis.
   g) Elevated intraocular pressure due to trabeculitis or iridocyclitis.

h) Other: vitritis, retinal vasculitis, retinal necrosis, choroiditis, occlusion of central retinal or ophthalmic arteries, and optic neuritis.

Treatment

1. Topical antiviral medications are ineffective against HZV; acyclovir, 800 mg orally five times daily for 10 to 14 days (started within 5–7 days after the appearance of cutaneous lesions).
2. Oral steroids may reduce postzoster neuralgia; if given during first 3 to 5 d after the appearance of skin eruptions, oral steroids may cause systemic zoster dissemination.
3. Cycloplegic agents and analgesics as needed.
4. Topical steroids: the mainstay of ocular treatment for nummular, disciform, and interstitial keratitis, iridocyclitis, and glaucoma secondary to uveitis.
5. Persistent epithelial defects: treated with pressure patching, bandage contact lenses or collagen shield with frequent lubrication; tarsorrhaphy, conjunctival flap, or corneal transplantation may be needed in severe cases.
6. Mild corneal melt: managed the same way as for mild persistent epithelial defects.
7. Acute retinal necrosis: intravenous acyclovir.

Interstitial Keratitis (IK)

Definition and Symptoms   Inflammation of the corneal stroma without primary involvement of the epithelium or the endothelium. This is probably a hypersensitivity response (immune-complex-mediated or delayed-type hypersensitivity). During the acute stage of IK, symptoms include decreased vision, photophobia, and pain.

Etiology

1. Syphilis (congenital or acquired); tuberculosis; leprosy.
2. Cogan's syndrome (consists of IK, nerve deafness, vertigo, and systemic vasculitis, which typically is polyarteritis nodosa).

Physical Examination

1. During active inflammation: stromal haze, infiltrates, and active corneal neovascularization; iris hyperemia with pink nodules; epithelial edema; anterior chamber reaction.
2. During quiet stage: stromal scars and ghost vessels.
3. Corneal epithelium is usually intact; Descemet's membrane is thickened.

Workup   VDRL and FTA-ABS tests, chest x-ray, PPD, ESR, ANA, and urinalysis.

Treatment

1. Systemic antibiotics for syphilis (consult infectious disease specialists as necessary) if there is
   a) active inflammation (e.g., iridocyclitis and chorioretinitis) secondary to syphilis;
   b) positive FTA-ABS and the patient has not been treated for syphilis in the past or is unsure about past treatment; or
   c) VDRL did not decline significantly after treatment for syphilis—this may indicate that previous treatment was inadequate.
2. If tuberculosis is suspected, refer to internist or infectious disease specialist.
3. If Cogan's syndrome is suspected, consult ear, nose, and throat specialist.
4. Acute IK is treated with topical steroids and cycloplegics.
5. Penetrating keratoplasty may be needed to replace the scarred cornea; postoperative course often complicated by severe inflammation.

Follow-up   Follow according to the severity of IK; weekly during acute attacks, otherwise semiannually or annually.

Course   Chronic; marked by recurrences with varying severities and intervals.

Prognosis   With prompt treatment, patients do fairly well; delay in treatment or no treatment will result in corneal scarring.

Keratoconus (KCN)

History and Etiology   This is a condition in which the corneal topography becomes distorted, resulting from progressive thinning of the central or pericentral corneal stroma. Keratoconus patients can be seen in the following clinical settings:

1. Idiopathic.
2. Contact-lens-induced (especially hard contact lenses).
3. Familial.
4. Associated with systemic or ocular conditions: Down syndrome; atopic diseases; Ehlers-Danlos syndrome; Leber's

congenital amaurosis (many of these are associated with chronic eye rubbing).

Physical Examination

1. Central or inferocentral stromal thinning.
2. Fleischer's ring (see Pigmentation section, below).
3. Irregular mires and inferior corneal steepening on keratometry; irregular astigmatism and retinoscopic streaks.
4. Acute corneal edema (hydrops) occurs when Descemet's membrane breaks.
5. Prominent corneal nerves; apical corneal scars.
6. Descemet's folds and Vogt's striae.

Workup   Usually not necessary, except when an associated systemic or ocular condition is suspected (see above).

Differential Diagnosis   Keratoglobus (characterized by generalized thinning of the corneal stroma to the periphery); pellucid marginal degeneration.

Treatment

1. Corrective lenses (glasses and contact lenses) are first choices; rigid (gas-permeable) contact lenses can correct mildly to moderately irregular astigmatism; "piggyback" contact lenses (rigid gas-permeable contact lens fitted over a soft contact lens) or combination hard and soft contact lens (Saturn lenses) may also be used.
2. Surgery considered if satisfactory visual acuity can no longer be obtained with contact lenses or if a patient is intolerant to contact lens wear.
   a) Penetrating keratoplasty (most common treatment):
      i)   Large graft may be necessary to encompass the cone.
      ii) Acute hydrops is not an indication for PK and usually resolves within 2 months.
      iii) Recurrence of KCN in graft is rare.
      iv) Permanent mydriasis may occur after PK in KCN.
   b) Epikeratophakia: its role in KCN is unclear at present.

Course   KCN is a chronic progressive disease; its progression is most rapid during the teens and twenties.

Prognosis   Results of PK are generally excellent.

Neoplasms and Premalignant Lesions

Neoplasms and premalignant lesions involve primarily the conjunctiva; the cornea may become secondarily involved with local extension. Malignant lesions of conjunctiva may metastasize through lymphatics and blood vessels.

Benign Neoplasms and Premalignant Lesions

Papilloma

Viral Papilloma This is caused by papilloma virus and usually appears pedunculated and multiple; eyelid may be involved.

1. Usually affects younger individuals.
2. Most resolve spontaneously and are left untreated; incomplete surgical removal may result in the dissemination of virus and multiple recurrences.
3. Complete surgical excision with cryotherapy to the base is the usual surgical treatment.
4. Has no potential for malignant transformation.

Nonviral Papilloma This is caused by dysplastic transformation of conjunctival epithelium; lesions usually are sessile.

1. Age of the patient is older than in viral type.
2. Potential for malignant transformation.
3. Treatment is complete surgical removal with cryotherapy to the base.

Primary Acquired Melanosis (PAM)

1. PAM usually occurs during middle age as patchy flat pigmentation of conjunctiva; the edges of PAM are feathery; the size of the lesion may enlarge or shrink with time.

2. PAM may be classified into two types: with or without atypia. Atypia is defined as presence of atypical melanocytes in the conjunctival epithelium, indicating a higher chance (20%–30%) of malignant transformation.

3. Differential diagnosis: racial melanosis; secondary acquired melanosis (e.g., Addison's disease and pregnancy).

4. PAM should be observed closely; obtain biopsy specimen of any suspicious lesions. PAM with atypia may be excised or treated with cryotherapy or both.

Nevus

1. Conjunctival nevi usually appear flat or mildly elevated, with brown to black discoloration, although some conjunctival nevi may completely lack pigment (amelanotic). Conjunctival nevi often contain small cysts, since some of them may contain goblet cells.

2. Conjunctival nevi usually have been present since childhood or early adolescence and rarely demonstrate any changes with time, except that they can enlarge during adolescence and pregnancy.

3. Conjunctival nevi can be moved with a cotton-tipped applicator, in contrast to ocular melanosis (nevus of Ota), which is not movable because its pigmentation is deep in the episclera and sclera.

4. Conjunctival nevi may be classified as junctional, compound, or subepithelial; only junctional and compound nevi have any potential for malignant transformation into melanoma.

Conjunctival Intraepithelial Dysplasia (CID)

1. Conjunctival epithelium can undergo dysplastic changes, similar to cervical epithelium. CID is characterized by a loss of the normal progression of maturation of conjunctival epithelium from the basal layer to the surface. CID usually begins at the basal layer; when the entire epithelium is involved (without violation of basement membrane), it is called carcinoma-in-situ.

2. Clinically, conjunctival dysplasia may appear thickened and gelatinous; dysplastic cells may extend into the corneal epithelium and form "fronds."

3. CID has the potential of transformation into squamous cell carcinoma; prolonged actinic exposure may contribute to the development of conjunctival dysplasia.

4. Obtain biopsy specimen or excise lesions suspicious of malignant changes; the dysplastic cells in the corneal epithelium should be removed without damaging Bowman's layer (which is a barrier to the spread of tumor cells).

Limbal Dermoid

1. Clinically, this is an elevated white nodular firm lesion, most frequently at the inferotemporal limbus.

2. Histopathologically, limbal dermoid consists of keratinizing dermal tissue with dermal appendages.

3. Limbal dermoid may be part of Goldenhar's syndrome.

4. When necessary, surgical excision is the usual treatment; at times a limbal dermoid may extend into the anterior chamber.

Ocular Melanosis/Oculodermal Melanosis (Nevus of Ota)

1. This is a congenital pigmentation of episclera and sclera; it is unilateral, often with concomitant involvement of ipsilateral eyelids, orbital tissue, and meninges; the iris and choroid may also be hyperpigmented ipsilateral to the side of pigmentation. The pigmentation is termed ocular melanosis if there is only ocular involvement and oculodermal melanosis (nevus of Ota) if there is both ocular and dermal involvement.

2. Histopathologically, there are blue nevi in the dermis or sclera.

3. Clinically, the pigmented lesions are not movable.

4. There is potential for malignant transformation into melanoma, which may develop in choroid, lid, orbit, and central nervous system; white patients are more prone to develop melanoma.

Malignant Neoplasms

Malignant Melanoma (MM)

1. Can arise de novo (30% of the cases), from nevi (40%), or from primary acquired melanosis (30%).
2. Appears thickened and elevated with dark brown or black discoloration but may be amelanotic; any pigmented conjunctival lesion with progression should be considered a MM until proved otherwise.
3. Can metastasize; mortality rate is higher with melanomas arising de novo or from primary acquired melanosis than those arising from nevi.
4. Treatment involves wide surgical excision; may involve enucleation or exenteration.

Squamous Cell Carcinoma (SCC)

1. Malignant transformation of conjunctival epithelial cells with invasion of underlying substantia propria (if the basement membrane remains intact, the lesion is defined as carcinoma-in-situ).
2. Usually appears as an irregularly elevated whitish gelatinous mass; the mass may exhibit leukoplakia and may extend onto corneal surface.
3. Histopathology shows hyperkeratosis, dyskeratosis, acanthosis and full-thickness dysplasia of conjunctival epithelium; there is invasion of underlying substantia propria.
4. Result of prolonged actinic exposure; may occur in preexisting pterygia and pingueculae.

5. SCC may metastasize through lymphatics and blood vessels.
6. SCC should be completely resected if at all possible; radiation and cryotherapy may be used as adjuncts; it is important not to damage Bowman's membrane during removal, since it is an effective barrier to the spread of SCC.
7. Good prognosis if removed completely before metastasis.

Sebaceous Cell Carcinoma

See Blepharitis section, above.

1. May invade conjunctiva through direct extension or pagetoid spread.
2. Should be suspected in patients with recurrent chalazia and recalcitrant or unilateral blepharitis.
3. Conjunctival biopsy if sebaceous cell carcinoma is suspected; stain specimen with oil red O.

Lymphoma

1. May be localized to the conjunctival tissue or may be systemic with conjunctival involvement.
2. Complete surgical removal in cases of localized conjunctival lymphoma; if the lymphoma is systemic, then an oncologist should direct the treatment regimen.

Basal Cell Carcinoma

1. The conjunctiva may become secondarily involved through local extension of a lid basal cell carcinoma.
2. If conjunctiva is involved, exenteration may be needed.

Ocular Cicatricial Pemphigoid (OCP)

History and Etiology   OCP is characterized by recurrent blister and bullae formation of the skin and the mucus membranes. It is an immunologically mediated disease; deposition of immunoglobulins and complements in the basement membrane of the conjunctiva has been demonstrated in some patients with OCP. In most cases the etiology of OCP is unknown; medications (e.g., idoxuridine, pilocarpine, and timolol) have been occasionally reported as causes of OCP. The disease usually affects patients older than 50 to 60 years of age, with a female predominance.

Physical Examination   Depending on the stage or progression of the disease, examine the following:

1. Conjunctiva
   a) Vesicles, hyperemia (especially during active phase)
   b) Progressive fibrosis; shrinkage; symblepharon
   c) Keratinization (due to dry eye associated with OCP)
2. Cornea
   a) SPK; keratinization (secondary to dry eye)
   b) Formation of pannus and pseudopterygium
3. Eyelids: entropion, trichiasis
4. Other lesions
   a) Oral pharynx: desquamatous gingivitis, vesiculobullous eruptions
   b) Skin: may show recurrent vesiculobullous nonscarring eruptions or localized erythematous plaques.

Workup   Not usually necessary; biopsy with immunologic studies may be necessary in questionable cases.

Differential Diagnosis

1. Stevens-Johnson syndrome
2. Chemical burn
3. Sjögren's syndrome
4. Atopic keratoconjunctivitis
5. Scleroderma (progressive systemic sclerosis)
6. Radiation injury
7. Medication-induced (epinephrine, idoxuridine, pilocarpine, timolol, and dipivefrin have been implicated)
8. Membranous conjunctivitis can lead to scarring of conjunctiva
9. Trachoma
10. Paraneoplastic pemphigus

Treatment

1. Dry eyes: artificial tears; punctal occlusion; goggles; moist chamber glasses.
2. Trichiasis: epilation; cryotherapy or electrocautery; surgical correction of accompanying lid abnormality.
3. Progressive shrinkage of conjunctival fornices: systemic corticosteroids for acute inflammation; immunosuppressives (e.g., cyclophosphamide) or dapsone may be used to prevent progressive shrinkage of conjunctiva.

4. Keratoprothesis may be necessary for patients with end-stage disease and good macular function.
5. Surgery may exacerbate conjunctival disease in OCP and should be entertained only when the disease is quiet.

Course Characterized by variable progressive shrinkage of conjunctival fornices, punctuated by periods of active inflammation.

Parinaud's Oculoglandular Syndrome

History and Etiology This is characterized by unilateral conjunctivitis with enlargement of the ipsilateral preauricular, submandibular, or cervical lymph nodes. Etiologies include cat-scratch disease, tularemia, tuberculosis, syphilis, mumps, sporotrichosis, coccidioidomycosis, and lymphogranuloma venereum.

Physical Examination

1. Conjunctival injection with or without chemosis
2. Conjunctival granulomas or follicles
3. Enlarged preauricular, submandibular, or cervical nodes
4. Mucopurulent discharge; pseudoptosis

Workup

1. Complete blood count, FTA-ABS, PPD, and serum titers for tularemia if suspected.
2. Chest x-ray for coccidioidomycosis if suspected.
3. Biopsy of the enlarged nodes may be necessary.

Differential Diagnosis Lymphoma and leukemia.

Treatment Appropriate antibiotics for infectious causes (streptomycin for tularemia, penicillin for syphilis, tetracycline for cat-scratch fever, isoniazid (INH) and rifampin for tuberculosis, and antifungals for coccidioidomycosis and sporotrichosis). An internist or specialist in infectious disease should be consulted if cat-scratch fever is not the entity. In cat-scratch fever, removal of the conjunctival granuloma can be curative.

Course Depends on the underlying etiology.

Prognosis With proper treatment, signs and symptoms of Parinaud's oculoglandular conjunctivitis will usually resolve.

Peripheral Limbal Disease

History and Etiology

1. Infections (e.g., bacterial, viral, fungal; see Ulcers section, below).
2. Immune-mediated disease (e.g., vernal keratoconjunctivitis, Mooren's ulcer, phlyctenulosis; see Conjunctivitis section, above).
3. Degenerations (e.g., arcus, band keratopathy, Terrien's, pellucid; see Degenerations section, above).
4. Masses (e.g., dermoids, pterygium, melanoma, sebaceous cell carcinoma; see Degenerations section, above; Neoplasms and Premalignant Lesions section, above).
5. Pigmentation (e.g., alkaptonuria and adrenochrome; see Pigmentation section, below).
6. Others (e.g., superior limbic keratoconjunctivitis [SLK], dry eyes; see Theodore's SLK section, below; Dry Eye section, above).
7. Associated with collagen-vascular diseases.

Peripheral Corneal Melt

Mooren's Ulcer

This is an idiopathic chronic ulceration of peripheral cornea without any associated collagen-vascular disease.

Clinical Features

1. Elderly patients
2. Exacerbations and remissions
3. Pain, decreased vision, and photophobia during exacerbations; 25% bilateral

Clinical Findings

1. Peripheral gutter-like stromal thinning; starts at about 3 or 9 o'clock position; eventually becomes circumferential and progresses centrally.
2. During exacerbations, the overlying corneal epithelium is absent with stromal infiltration, ulceration, and edema; vascularization of peripheral gutter may occur.
3. Anterior chamber reaction and glaucoma may accompany corneal pathology.
4. Spontaneous perforation occurs rarely.

Workup   A diagnosis of exclusion; laboratory studies (ESR, complete blood count, ANA, chest x-ray, liver enzymes, RF, and FTA-ABS) to exclude diseases associated with peripheral corneal ulceration.

Treatment

1. Soft contact lens to prevent lid from hitting the overhanging central corneal edge.
2. Topical steroids for unilateral cases.
3. Systemic steroids for bilateral cases.
4. Resection of limbal conjunctiva.
5. Immunosuppressive agents in unresponsive cases.
6. Tissue glue (cyanoacrylate) may be useful for impending or small perforations; can also halt the melting process.
7. Lamellar graft may be needed to reinforce areas of extreme corneal thinning or large perforation.
8. Penetrating keratoplasty if extensive stromal thinning and corneal scarring.

Differential Diagnosis

1. Peripheral corneal guttering associated with collagen-vascular diseases (RA, Wegener's granulomatosis, polyarteritis nodosa, and SLE).
2. Peripheral corneal guttering associated with scleritis; Mooren's ulcer is typically not associated with scleritis.
3. Noninflammatory peripheral corneal thinning: furrow degeneration and pellucid marginal degeneration.

Atypical African Form   Bilateral (about 75%); younger age; faster progression; spontaneous perforation more common; poorer prognosis.

Peripheral Corneal Melt Associated with Collagen-Vascular Diseases

These diseases include RA, SLE, Wegener's granulomatosis, and polyarteritis nodosa. These four entities have different systemic and ocular findings.

Rheumatoid Arthritis

1. Systemic findings: symmetrical chronic inflammation of peripheral joints; positive RF; pleural effusion; pleurisy; Raynaud's phenomenon.
2. Ocular findings: episcleritis; scleritis; associated corneal findings; keratoconjunctivitis sicca.

Systemic Lupus Erythematosus

1. Systemic findings: arthritis; malar rash and photosensitivity; glomerulonephritis; anemia; pleurisy; pleural effusion; Raynaud's phenomenon; pericarditis.
2. Ocular findings: episcleritis; scleritis; dry eye; retinal vasculitis, cotton wool spots.

Polyarteritis Nodosa

1. Systemic findings: aneurysms; fever and malaise; cutaneous ulceration and livedo reticularis; gastrointestinal hemorrhages; glomerulonephritis; pericarditis; hepatitis B antigenemia.
2. Ocular findings: scleritis; choroidal and retinal vasculitis; hypertensive retinopathy.

Wegener's Granulomatosis

1. Systemic findings: glomerulonephritis; granulomatous vasculitis of pulmonary arteries; purulent sinusitis.
2. Ocular findings: peripheral corneal melt; proptosis and orbital pseudotumor; scleritis; conjunctivitis; retinal vasculitis; papilledema.

Pigmentation

Cornea Verticillata [Vortex Keratopathy]

1. Has been termed vortex dystrophy in the past, although it is not a true corneal dystrophy; vision rarely affected.
2. Superficial gold-to-brown pigment granules in a vortex pattern centered in the inferior cornea.
3. Histologically, the granules appear in the basal cells of the corneal epithelium.
4. Associated disorders:
   a) Fabry's disease: an X-linked recessive disorder with α-galactosidase deficiency; tortuosity of conjunctival and retinal vessels may occur; female carriers may demonstrate the typical corneal findings and spoke-like peripheral cortical lenticular opacities.
   b) Disorder induced by medication: amiodarone, indomethacin, chloroquine, chlorpromazine, and quinacrine hydrochloride; vortex pattern in epithelium will usually disappear with cessation of medications.

Iron

Hudson-Stähli Line

1. In the corneal epithelium between the middle and the lower one-third of the cornea; source of iron is tears.
2. Normal variant; typically seen in elderly patients.

Stocker's Line   In corneal epithelium anterior to pterygium.

Fleischer Ring   In corneal epithelium at the base of the cone in keratoconus.

Ferry Line   In corneal epithelium anterior to a filtering bleb.

Blood Staining

1. In corneal stroma of eyes with history of hyphema and elevated IOP (e.g., trauma, neovascular glaucoma, juvenile xanthogran-uloma).
2. Treatment: lower IOP; PK if unresolving and vision is severely affected.

Siderosis   In corneal epithelium, Bowman's membrane, or stroma; a result of corneal iron foreign bodies.

Melanin

Adrenochrome

1. Located beneath the corneal epithelium, in Bowman's membrane and anterior stroma, and also in conjunctiva.
2. Due to chronic use of eyedrops containing epinephrine.

Krukenberg's Spindle   On and in the endothelium; seen in pigment dispersion syndrome and pigmentary glaucoma. Iris transillumination defects typically associated.

Melanokeratosis   In epithelium; seen in blacks; normal.

Ochronosis (Alkaptonuria)

1. In the peripheral superficial corneal stroma.
2. Pigmentation of the sclera and episclera may also be present; ear cartilage may also be pigmented.
3. An autosomal recessive disorder caused by lack of homogentisic acid oxidase; arthritis and cardiovascular disease (valvulitis) may develop.

Copper

Kayser-Fleischer Ring

1. In the peripheral Descemet's membrane; often first evident with gonioscopy and usually starts superiorly.

2. Associated with Wilson's disease.
3. Corneal deposits indistinguishable from Kayser-Fleischer ring may occur in progressive intrahepatic cholestasis; chronic active hepatitis; primary biliary cirrhosis; chalcosis.

Multiple Myeloma   Copper deposition is usually located over the central portion of Descemet's membrane; associated with hypercupremia.

Chalcosis

1. Caused by intraocular foreign body containing copper.
2. Associated findings: corneal deposits resembling Kayser-Fleischer ring; heterochromia irides; sunflower cataract; endophthalmitis (purulent endophthalmitis if the content of copper is more than 85%).

Silver

In the stroma, just anterior to the Descemet's membrane; usually due to chronic use of eyedrops containing silver (e.g., Argyrol) or chronic environmental exposure.

Gold [Corneal Chrysiasis]

1. Deposits of dust-like material in deep stroma with colors varying from yellow to violet.
2. Can result from chronic gold therapy (e.g., for RA).
3. May have accompanying dermatitis or stomatitis.

Refractive Surgery

Radial Keratotomy [RK]

1. Procedure to reduce myopia by making radial partial-thickness incisions into cornea (usually about 80% depth); results in flattening of central cornea.
2. Prospective Evaluation of Radial Keratotomy (PERK) study showed 76% of eyes attained an uncorrected visual acuity of 20/40 or better; 55% of eyes had a refractive error of 1 D or less after surgery.
3. Problems with RK include lack of predictability and fluctuations of refractive error after surgery.

Excimer Laser Surface Ablation

1. Procedure (under investigation) to reduce myopia (and possibly other forms of refractive errors) by ablating corneal tissue and flattening the cornea.
2. Excimer laser can ablate superficial corneal lesions (e.g., Reis-Bückler's dystrophy and Salzmann's degeneration) as well.

Keratomileusis

1. After removal of the anterior portion of the cornea (lenticle), keratomileusis changes the front corneal curvature by lathing the stromal side of the lenticle.
2. Can be used to correct hyperopia and myopia.
3. Few surgeons are performing keratomileusis; technology and machinery are extremely complicated.

Keratophakia

Used to correct aphakia by placing (sandwiching) a donor lenticle (which is precut from a donor corneal stroma) into the host corneal stroma.

Epikeratophakia

1. Used to correct refractive error by suturing a donor lenticle on top of the host cornea.
2. Used in aphakia and keratoconus.

Ruiz Procedure

Reduces astigmatism and myopia by making partial-thickness radial and tangential incisions.

Transverse Incisions

Used to reduce astigmatism.

Relaxing Incisions

1. Correct astigmatism after penetrating keratoplasty.
2. Partial-thickness incision made in or near the wound in the steepest meridian.
3. In cases where relaxing incisions alone did not work or if the astigmatism is high, compression sutures are placed through the wound and tied tightly along the flattest meridian.

Wedge Resection

In cases of very high astigmatism, a wedge of tissue can be removed in the flat meridian, which is then sutured.

Rejections in Corneal Transplantation

History and Etiology   Rejection of a corneal graft is an immunologically mediated response against the graft that occurs about 6 weeks or later after surgery. Predisposing factors include recipients of a relatively young age, stromal vascularization, and previous rejections.

Symptoms   Sudden onset of a red eye, pain, photophobia, or decreased vision.

Physical Examination   Corneal graft rejections may be epithelial or endothelial.

Epithelial Rejection

1. Usually occurs within months after transplantation.
2. Two forms:
   a) Elevated line of corneal epithelium representing replacement of donor epithelium with that of host.
   b) Subepithelial infiltrates, resembling those in EKC.

Endothelial Rejection

1. Khoudadoust's line (a line of keratic precipitates marching across donor endothelium) or diffuse keratic precipitates indicating diffuse endothelial cell loss.
2. Stromal and epithelial edema.
3. Anterior chamber reaction.
4. Injection of conjunctival vessels.

Differential Diagnosis

1. Primary graft failure occurs immediately postoperatively and is due to faulty donor endothelium.
2. Progressive loss of donor endothelium may lead to graft failure; may also occur with prolonged flat chamber and iris or vitreous touch.
3. Epithelial downgrowth:
   a) May resemble an endothelial rejection line.
   b) Characteristics: large (epithelial) cells in anterior chamber; faint membrane on the surface of iris, which whitens with argon laser; ocular hypertension.
   c) Paracentesis fluid contains epithelial cells.
4. Recurrence of HSV keratouveitis: often difficult to distinguish from graft rejection; in HSV, stromal edema and KP usually

involve both the donor and host cornea; in graft rejection only the donor cornea is involved.

Treatment

1. For subepithelial infiltrates or epithelial rejection:
   a) Topical 1% prednisolone or 0.1% dexamethasone, one drop every 2 hours for 2 days, then one drop every 3 hours for 3 days, then one drop every 4 hours for 4 days.
   b) Steroid ointment may be used at bedtime.
2. For endothelial rejection:
   a) Topical 1% prednisolone or 0.1% dexamethasone, one drop every hour while awake.
   b) Steroid ointment is used at bedtime.
   c) Systemic prednisone (80 mg p.o. q.d.) for at least 1 week, if stromal edema is present.
   d) Cycloplegia.
   e) If limited to a particular quadrant, subconjunctival injection of steroids may be given adjacent to the quadrant.
   g) Steroids tapered according to clinical response.

Follow up   Initial weekly visits at least; visits may be spaced further as patient responds.

Course   Resolution of corneal graft rejection may take a few weeks; if there is no clinical response after 3 weeks of intensive steroid treatment, the course of rejection is not likely to be reversed.

Prognosis   Good with prompt treatment, 80%–90% of corneal graft rejections can be reversed. Every corneal transplant patient is at the risk of rejection throughout life; the longer the patient remains free from rejection, the less likely it is to occur.

Stevens-Johnson Syndrome (Erythema Multiforme Major)

History and Etiology   A serious systemic illness characterized by mucosal ulcerations, skin lesions, fever, and ocular involvement. Precipitating factors may be infectious or drug-related. Viruses, bacteria, fungi, and *Mycoplasma pneumoniae* have been associated with Stevens-Johnson syndrome, with HSV and *M. pneumoniae* having the strongest association. Drugs that have been reported in association with Stevens-Johnson syndrome include sulfonamides, which have been implicated the most, and dilantin.

Physical Examination

1. Diagnosis based on the following criteria:
   a) Skin lesions: vesicles, bullae, epidermal necrosis, and target lesions (erythema nodosum); most often on dorsal surfaces of the extremities but can also be on the trunk in severe cases.
   b) Erosions of mucosal membranes: oral and nasal mucosa, conjunctiva, esophagus, vagina, urethra, and anus.
   c) Systemic: malaise, fever, headache, prostration.
2. Ocular findings:
   a) Acute changes: eyelid swelling, ulceration and crusting; conjunctivitis with membranes or pseudomembranes; anterior uveitis.
   b) Late changes:
      i) Conjunctiva: subconjunctival scarring, forniceal foreshortening, symblepharon formation.
      ii) Lids: trichiasis, lagophthalmos, and entropion.
      iii) Obstruction of the ducts of the lacrimal glands and also the puncta and canaliculi due to fibrosis.
      iv) Dry eye caused by the loss of conjunctival goblet cells, leading to keratinization of conjunctiva, SPK, corneal erosion, and possibly perforation.

Workup   No specific laboratory studies; immunoglobulins and complements deposited at the dermal-epidermal junction; HLA-Bw44 is associated with Stevens-Johnson syndrome.

Differential Diagnosis   See Ocular Cicatricial Pemphigoid section, above.

Treatment

1. Hydration: oral or intravenous
2. Systemic steroids (e.g., 60–80 mg of prednisone daily) and topical steroids; systemic steroid treatment is controversial.
3. Ocular lubrication; tarsorrhaphy; punctal occlusion.
4. Frequent lysis of symblepharon.
5. Surgical correction of trichiasis and lid abnormalities.
6. Buccal membrane graft.

Follow-up   Hospitalization and follow-up according to severity.

Course All patients will develop stomatitis; 63%, conjunctivitis; and 61% balanitis, vaginitis, or urethritis. The conjunctiva is the only mucous membrane that undergoes scarring. Recurrences rarely occur.

Prognosis Mortality rate between 2% and 25%.

Theodore's Superior Limbic Keratoconjunctivitis (SLK)

History and Etiology Characterized by chronic inflammation of the superior limbic conjunctiva and papillary reaction of the superior palpebral conjunctiva. Thyroid dysfunction is often associated with superior limbic keratoconjunctivitis. The etiology is unknown although it may be associated with contact lens wear.

Symptoms
1. Foreign body sensation, pain.
2. Photophobia, tearing.

Physical Examination
1. Localized inflammation of superior bulbar conjunctiva.
2. Papillary reaction of the superior tarsal conjunctiva.
3. SPK of superior cornea, limbus, and bulbar conjunctiva.
4. Thickening of superior limbus.
5. Filamentary keratitis; pseudoptosis; blepharospasm.

Workup Clinical diagnosis; thyroid function tests.

Treatment
1. Silver nitrate, 0.25% to 1.0% solution (*do not* use silver nitrate sticks), applied to the superior bulbar and palpebral conjunctiva; symptoms may return in few days to months.
2. Acetylcysteine 10% (Mucomyst) drops four to five times daily.
3. Recession or resection of superior bulbar conjunctiva.

Follow-up See patient during exacerbations; no cure for SLK; symptoms will return after any therapy.

Course Usually a bilateral condition; can undergo exacerbations and remissions; even alternating between the two eyes.

Prognosis Good; not a visually threatening disorder.

Thygeson's Superficial Punctate Keratopathy

History and Etiology   Usually affects patients under the age of 40; insidious onset characterized by exacerbations and remissions; both sexes are involved equally. Etiology is unknown.

Symptoms   Photophobia, tearing, and foreign body sensation.

Physical Examination   Small punctate epithelial lesions that often stain slightly with fluorescein, appear gray and slightly elevated, and are concentrated in the central cornea.

Workup   Laboratory studies are not necessary; a diagnosis of exclusion.

Differential Diagnosis   HSV keratitis; adenovirus keratitis; keratitis associated with measles or mumps.

Treatment   Topical corticosteroids (use least amount possible to control symptoms); soft bandage contact lens.

Follow-up   See patient during exacerbations; adjust steroids according to patient's symptoms.

Course

1. Exacerbations and remissions; exacerbation lasts about 2 weeks, and remission about 4 to 6 weeks.
2. The disease eventually burns out in several years.
3. Topical steroids may prolong the course of the disease.

Prognosis   Excellent; no permanent ocular sequelae.

Ulcers

Definition   A defect in the cornea with absence of epithelium and underlying stromal loss. Etiologies include:

1. infectious (e.g., bacterial, viral, fungal, and protozoa)
2. noninfectious—associated with collagen-vascular diseases; metaherpetic; dry eye; shield ulcer associated with VKC; hypersensitivity reaction (e.g., staphylococcal blepharitis); idiopathic (e.g., Mooren's ulcer).

Infectious Corneal Ulcers

Bacterial

Common organisms include *Staphylococcus; Pseudomonas; Moraxella; S. pneumococcus. Neisseria, Hemophilus, Corynebacterium,* and *Listeria* can penetrate intact corneal epithelium.

Predisposing Factors Contact lens wear, especially extended-wear lenses, and immunosuppression (e.g., topical steroids).

Clinical Presentation Acute onset; pain, photophobia, and decreased vision.

Clinical Features

1. Discharge: mucus discharge may indicate pseudomonas infection; purulent discharge may indicate gonococcal infection.
2. Conjunctival inflammation.
3. Epithelial defect with underlying stromal loss.
4. Stromal infiltrates and edema.
5. Anterior chamber cells and flare; hypopyon.

Workup

1. Corneal scraping for gram and giemsa stains; cultures and sensitivities.
2. Culture media should include
   a) thioglycolate (for anaerobes)
   b) blood agar (good for most bacteria)
   c) chocolate agar (good for *Neisseria* and *Hemophilus*)
   d) Sabouraud's agar (for fungus)

Treatment

1. Initially treat empirically:
   a) Fortified cefazolin (50 mg/ml, one drop every hour) with gentamicin (13.5 mg/ml) or tobramycin (9 mg/ml) every hour around the clock.
   b) If allergic to penicillin or cephalosporins, use vancomycin (50 mg/ml) eyedrops in place of fortified cefazolin.
   c) Subconjunctival injections or systemic antibiotics are indicated with concomitant corneal perforation, limbal involvement, or endophthalmitis.
2. Adjust antibiotics according to cultures and sensitivities. Slowly taper antibiotics.
3. Cycloplegia.
4. Cyanoacrylate glue, patch graft, or PK may be necessary if cornea is perforated.

Course   Depends on the organism:

1. *Pseudomonas* progresses more rapidly than *Staphylococcus* or *Moraxella*.
2. *Moraxella* more common in alcoholics and debilitated patients.

Fungal

For example: *Candida, Fusarium, Aspergillus,* and *Penicillium*.

Predisposing Factors   Trauma; chronic ocular surface disease; topical steroids.

Clinical Features   Pain and photophobia; decreasd vision; indolent onset.

Clinical Findings   Epithelium is usually not intact, but it may be; stromal infiltrates with feathery borders; satellite lesions; anterior chamber reaction; hypopyon.

Workup   Same as in bacterial corneal ulcer.

Treatment

1. Initially, natamycin 5%, one drop every hour around the clock; alternatively, amphotericin B 0.15%.
2. Topical miconazole 1%, clotrimazole 1%, and econozole 1% have been used by others; topical fluconazole may penetrate the cornea better but appears to have a more limited spectrum.
3. Oral ketoconazole may be used.
4. Flucytosine (acts synergistically with amphotericin B) in candida keratitis.
5. Adjust regimen according to culture results and clinical response.
6. Penetrating keratoplasty in cases unresponsive to medical management.
7. Steroids and lamellar keratoplasty are contraindicated.

Acanthamoeba [A. polyphaga and A. castellani]

Predisposing Factors   Trauma; contact lens wear.

Clinical Features   Pain (typically out of proportion to the clinical findings); photophobia; indolent onset with exacerbations and remissions.

Clinical Findings SPK with epithelial edema; epithelial defect (may or may not be present); stromal infiltrates (ring-shaped or perineural).

Workup

1. Gram, and giemsa stains; cultures and sensitivities.
2. Microscopic examination of corneal scraping; formalin-fixed and stained with hematoxylin and eosin or periodic acid–Schiff stain; calcofluor white.
3. Cell culture on non-nutrient agar overlaid with *E. coli.*
4. Corneal biopsy if necessary.

Differential Diagnosis Topical anesthetic abuse.

Treatment

1. Initially, Brolene and Neosporin drops every hour and Brolene ointment at night.
2. Miconazole 1%, clotrimazole 1%, and ketoconazole 1% are advocated by some.
3. Ketoconazole (200 mg p.o. b.i.d.).
4. Use of topical steroids advocated by some.
5. Penetrating keratoplasty necessary if medical regimens are ineffective, but it may recur in a corneal graft.

Prevention

1. Contact lens wearers should be warned not to make own saline or to swim with their contact lenses.
2. Heat disinfection of contact lenses.

Noninfectious Corneal Ulcers

See the following sections, above: Conjunctivitis, Dry Eye (Keratoconjunctivitis Sicca), Herpes Simplex Virus, Herpes Zoster Ophthalmicus, and Peripheral Limbal Disease.

Selected Readings

Bacteria and Gram Stains

Brinser JH. Ocular bacteriology. In: Tabbara KF, Hyndiuk RA, eds. Infections of the Eye. Little, Brown: Boston, 1986, pp. 115–50.

Blepharitis

Browning DJ, Proia AD. Ocular rosacea. Surv Ophthalmol 1986;31:145–58.
McCulley JP. Blepharoconjunctivitis. Int Ophthalmol Clin 1984;24(2):65–77.

Conjunctivitis

Ullman S, Roussel TJ, Forster RK. Gonococcal keratoconjunctivitis. Surv
Ophthalmol 1987;32:199–208.
Tabbara KF. Chlamydial conjunctivitis. In: Tabbara KF, Hyndiuk RA, eds.
Infections of the eye. Boston: Little, Brown, 1986, pp. 421–36.
Dawson CR. Inclusion conjunctivitis. In: Fraunfelder FT, Roy FH, eds.
Current ocular therapy, 3rd ed. Philadelphia: WB Saunders, 1990,
pp. 50–51.
Allansmith MR, Korb DR, Greiner JV, Henriguez AS, Simon MA, Finnemore
VM. Giant papillary conjunctivitis in contact lens wearers. Am J
Ophthalmol 1977;83:697–708.

Degenerations

Krachmer JH. Pellucid marginal corneal degeneration. Arch Ophthalmol
1978;96:1217–21.
Varley GA, Macsai MS, Krachmer JH. The results of penetrating keratoplasty
for pellucid marginal corneal degeneration. Am J Ophthalmol
1990;110:149–52.
Mannis MJ, Krachmer JH, Rodrigues MM, Pardos GJ. Polymorphic amyloid
degeneration of the cornea: a clinical and histopathologic study. Arch
Ophthalmol 1981;99:1217–23.

Dry Eye [Keratoconjunctivitis Sicca]

Lemp MA. Recent development in dry eye management. Ophthalmology
1987;94:1299–1304.
Whitcher JP. Clinical diagnosis of the dry eye. Int Clin Ophthalmol
1987;27(1):7–24.
Gilbert JM, Weiss JS, Sattler AL, Koch JM. Ocular manifestations and
impression cytology of anorexia nervosa. Ophthalmology 1990;97:
1001–7.

Dystrophies

Waring GO, Rodrigues MM, Laibson P. Corneal dystrophies: I. dystrophies of
the epithelium, Bowman's layer and stroma. Surv Ophthalmol 1978;
23:71–122.
Waring GO, Rodrigues MM, Laibson P. Corneal dystrophies: II. endothelial
dystrophies. Surv Ophthalmol 1978;23:147–68.
Krachmer JH, Schnitzer JI, Fratkin J. Cornea pseudoguttata: a clinical and
histopathologic description of endothelial cell edema. Arch Ophthalmol
1981;99:1377–81.

Episcleritis/Scleritis

Benson WE. Posterior scleritis. Surv Ophthalmol 1988;32:297–316.
Watson PG, Hayreh SS. Scleritis and episcleritis. Br J Ophthalmol 1976;60:163–91.

Eye Banking

Medical standards of Eye Bank Association of America. Revised August 8, 1989. Washington, D.C.: Eye Bank Association of America.
Wilson SE, Bourne WE. Corneal preservation. Surv Ophthalmol 1989;33:237–59.

Herpes Simplex Virus

Binder P. Herpes simplex keratitis. Surv Ophthalmol 1977;21:313–31.

Keratoconus

Krachmer JH, Feder RS, Belin MW. Keratoconus and related noninflammatory corneal thinning disorders. Surv Ophthalmol 1984;28:293–322.
Macsai MS, Varley GA, Krachmer JH. Development of keratoconus after contact lens wear: patient characteristics. Arch Ophthalmol 1990;108:534–38.

Neoplasms and Premalignant Lesions

Folberg R, Jakobiec FA, Bernardino VB, Iwamoto T. Benign conjunctival melanocytic lesions: clinical pathologic features. Ophthalmology 1989;96:436–61.
Reifler DM, Hornblass A. Squamous cell carcinoma of the eyelid. Surv Ophthalmol 1986;30:349–65.

Ocular Cicatricial Pemphigoid

Mondino BJ. Cicatricial pemphigoid and erythema multiforme. Ophthalmology 1990;97:939–52.
Anhalt GJ, Kim SC, Stanley JR, et al. Paraneoplastic pemphigus: an autoimmune mucocutaneous disease associated with neoplasia. N Engl J Med 1990;323:1729–35.

Pigmentation

Lewis RA, Falls HF, Troyer DO. Ocular manifestations of hypercupremia associated with multiple myeloma. Arch Ophthalmol 1975;93:1050–53.

Refractive Surgery

Waring GO, Lynn MJ, Fielding B, et al. Results of the prospective evaluation of radial keratotomy (PERK) study 4 years after surgery for myopia. JAMA 1990;263:1083–91.

Vrabec MP, Florakis GJ, Krachmer JH. Corrective surgery for astigmatism. Int Ophthalmol Clin 1988;28(2):145–49.

Rejections in Corneal Transplantation

Shapiro MB, Mandel MR, Krachmer JH. Rejection. In: Brightbill FS, ed. Corneal surgery: theory, technique, and tissue. St. Louis: CV Mosby, 1986, pp. 310–21.

Alldredge OC, Krachmer JH. Clinical types of corneal transplant rejection: their manifestations, frequency, preoperative correlations, and treatment. Arch Ophthalmol 1981;99:599–604.

Stevens-Johnson Syndrome [Erythema Multiforme Major]

Mondino BJ. Cicatricial pemphigoid and erythema multiforme. Ophthalmology 1990;97:939–52.

Thygeson's Superficial Punctate Keratopathy

Goldberg DB, Schanzlin DJ, Brown SI. Management of Thygeson's superficial punctate keratitis. Am J Ophthalmol 1980;89:22–24.

Ulcers

Rosenwasser GO, Holland S. Pflugfelder SC, et al. Topical anesthetic abuse. Ophthalmology 1990;97:967–72.

Cohen EJ, Buchanan HW, Laughrea PA, et al. Diagnosis and management of Acanthamoeba keratitis. Am J Ophthalmol 1985;100:389–95.

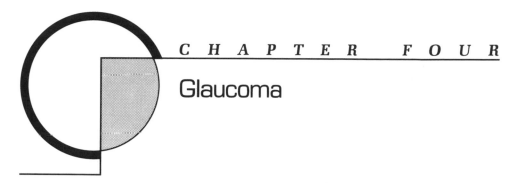

Glaucoma

Gregory L. Skuta, M.D.

Anterior Segment Anatomy and Aqueous Humor Dynamics

Definition An understanding of the mechanisms, diagnosis, and treatment of the various glaucomas is dependent on an appreciation of basic anterior segment anatomy and aqueous humor dynamics.

Anatomic and Physiologic Findings

Anterior segment anatomy, which is important in the understanding of aqueous humor dynamics, is shown in Figure 4.1.

1. Aqueous humor is derived from plasma within ciliary vasculature and produced by ciliary processes through the combination of secretion (active transport) by nonpigmented ciliary epithelium, diffusion, and ultrafiltration.

2. Blood in the capillary network of ciliary processes is derived from the major arterial circle, which is supplied by the anterior and long posterior ciliary arteries.

113

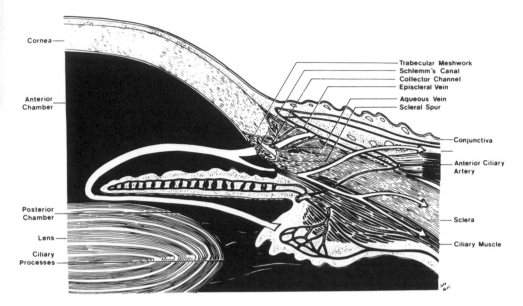

FIGURE 4.1. Cross Section of Anterior Segment Anatomy in the Primate Flow of aqueous represented by white arrow as it is formed by ciliary processes, passes around the iris into the anterior chamber, and then exits the eye by trabecular and uveoscleral routes. [From Kaufman PL. Aqueous humor outflow. In: Zandunaisky JA, Dayson H, eds. Current Topics in Eye Research. New York: Academic Press, 1984, vol. 4, pp. 97–138.]

3. Secretion (active transport) is generally independent of intraocular pressure (i.e., is pressure-independent), though it may be decreased by diminished blood flow. The enzymes adenosine triphosphatase (ATPase) and carbonic anhydrase play important roles in aqueous production.

4. Ultrafiltration is related in part to hydrostatic pressure within the capillaries of the ciliary processes and is affected by intraocular pressure, blood pressure, and plasma oncotic pressure (i.e., is pressure-dependent).

5. Aqueous humor is produced at a rate of approximately 2.0 to 2.5 μl/min; the rate is decreased during sleep by 45% ± 20%.

6. Total volume of aqueous humor is approximately 0.20 to 0.25 cc.

7. Aqueous differs in composition from plasma in the following ways:
a) Concentration of ascorbate approximately 20 times greater in aqueous than in plasma.
b) Protein concentration normally about 0.02% in aqueous compared to 7% in plasma; concentration may increase with inflammation and hypotony.
c) Aqueous contains immunoglobulin G (IgG) but not IgD, IgA, or IgM.

8. Aqueous humor passes into the posterior chamber, around the lens, and through the pupil into the anterior chamber; in the anterior chamber, it circulates in a vertical pattern in which cooler aqueous in the anterior aspect of the chamber sinks as warmer aqueous posteriorly rises.

9. Aqueous exits the eye primarily through the trabecular meshwork (80%–90% in humans) and into Schlemm's canal; from there, it passes into intrascleral collector channels, which drain into deep scleral veins, or aqueous veins, which join episcleral and conjunctival veins.

10. Most of the remainder of aqueous (10%–20%) exits by the uveoscleral route (through root of iris and ciliary muscle and into suprachoroidal space, where it leaves eye via sclera, scleral pores surrounding nerves and vessels, or vessels of optic nerve membranes).

11. Most of the resistance to aqueous outflow probably occurs at juxtacanalicular meshwork and at endothelium lining the inner wall of Schlemm's canal.

12. Uveoscleral outflow is generally relatively independent of intraocular pressure, while trabecular outflow is relatively pressure-dependent.

13. Trabecular outflow increases with cholinergics and decreases with cycloplegics, while uveoscleral outflow increases with cycloplegics and decreases with cholinergics.

14. Outflow facility (C) is estimated by the method known as tonography; normal mean value of C is 0.28 ± 0.05 μl/min/mmHg; it is usually decreased in glaucoma.

15. Intraocular pressure is determined by the rate of aqueous formation, resistance to aqueous outflow, and episcleral venous pressure as shown in the Goldmann equation:

$$P_o = F/C + P_v,$$

where

P_o = intraocular pressure (mmHg)
F = rate of aqueous formation (μl/min)
C = facility of aqueous outflow (μl/min/mmHg)
P_v = episcleral venous pressure (mmHg)

Gonioscopy

Definition Gonioscopy is a technique by which the anterior chamber angle is clinically evaluated in the diagnosis and treatment of glaucoma.

Techniques

1. The anterior chamber cannot be evaluated without special lenses owing to complete internal reflection of light coming from the angle.

2. Examination techniques include direct gonioscopy (e.g., Koeppe gonioscopy) and indirect gonioscopy (performed with mirrored gonio-lenses).

3. Direct gonioscopy is more inconvenient as it requires the patient to be in the supine position, but generally produces less distortion of the anterior chamber angle than indirect lenses.

4. Mirrored goniolenses include Goldmann one- and three-mirror lenses, Zeiss, and Posner four-mirror lenses; Goldmann lenses require use of a viscous fluid (e.g., methylcellulose), while with Zeiss and Posner lenses the patient's tears act as a fluid bridge without the need for a viscous substance.

5. Indirect lenses may make the angle appear more shallow than with direct techniques; one can improve the view by tilting the mirror toward the angle of concern or having the patient look toward the mirror being used.

6. Zeiss and Posner lenses permit compression gonioscopy, in which appositional angle closure (angle opens with compression) can be differentiated from synechial closure (angle does not open with compression).

Gonioscopic Landmarks [Fig. 4.2]

Schwalbe's Line Junction of peripheral cornea and anterior chamber angle structures.

1. Present at the termination of the corneal light wedge (where reflected beam from external corneal surface meets reflected beam on internal corneal surface).
2. May have irregular increase in pigmentation, especially in pseudoexfoliation and pigment dispersion syndromes (Sampaolesi's line).
3. Anteriorly displaced and thickened in posterior embryotoxon and Axenfeld-Rieger syndrome.

Trabecular Meshwork Band of variable pigmentation between Schwalbe's line and scleral spur.

1. Pigment usually greater posteriorly (functional meshwork) and inferiorly; pigmentation typically increased in pseudoexfoliation and pigment dispersion syndromes but may also be seen with

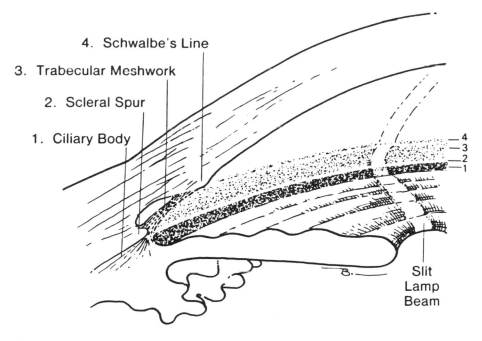

4. Schwalbe's Line

3. Trabecular Meshwork

2. Scleral Spur

1. Ciliary Body

Slit
Lamp
Beam

FIGURE 4.2. Structures in Normal Anterior Chamber Angle   [From Shields MB. Textbook of Glaucoma, 2nd ed. Baltimore: Williams and Wilkins, 1987, p. 30.]

   malignant melanoma, trauma, surgery, inflammation, and
   hyphema.
 2. May see red band (blood in Schlemm's canal) in hypotony and in
    conditions associated with increased episcleral venous pressure
    (e.g., Sturge-Weber syndrome).

Scleral Spur   White line between trabecular meshwork and ciliary
band.

 1. Represents the posterior lip of the scleral sulcus.
 2. May be crossed by iris processes: fine, lacy structures between
    which open spaces can be seen; must be differentiated from
    peripheral anterior synechiae, which are more solid and
    sheet-like and cover the angle recess.

Ciliary Body Band   Dark brown or gray band of variable width where
iris inserts.

1. Wider in myopia, more narrow in hyperopia.
2. Ciliary band is generally wider and often irregular in posttraumatic angle recession.

Angle Vessels   May see radial iris vessels, loops from the major arterial circle of ciliary body, and vertical branches of anterior ciliary arteries. Fine, branching vessels that cross scleral spur onto trabecular meshwork (as seen in iris neovascularization and Fuchs' heterochromic iridocyclitis) are not normal.

Classification Systems

1. Angle depth can be grossly estimated by the penlight method or slit lamp biomicroscopy (van Herick method).
a) Penlight method: light is shown across the anterior chamber from the temporal side; if a shadow is cast across the nasal anterior chamber (due to bowing of iris), this suggests a shallow anterior chamber.
b) Slit lamp (van Herick) method: with a thin slit beam at a 60° angle from the iris, the anterior chamber width is compared to the peripheral corneal thickness just inside the limbus; if the anterior chamber is greater than one-fourth the corneal thickness, the angle is probably deeper than Shaffer grade II (probably not occludable); if it is one-fourth the corneal thickness or less, it may be occludable (Shaffer grade II or less). Van Herick estimation of anterior chamber depth is not a substitute for gonioscopy.

2. Gonioscopy classification systems:
a) Modified Shaffer method (Fig. 4.3):

Grade IV: anterior chamber angle width 40° or greater; angle closure unlikely.
Grade III: anterior chamber angle width 20° to 40°; angle closure unlikely.
Grade II: anterior chamber angle width about 20°; angle closure possible.
Grade I: anterior chamber angle width approximately 10°; angle closure probable.
Slit: anterior chamber angle width less than 10°; angle closure likely.
Grade 0: anterior chamber angle closed.

b) Spaeth method: system that records the anterior chamber angle width in degrees, configuration of the peripheral iris, and the site of iris insertion.

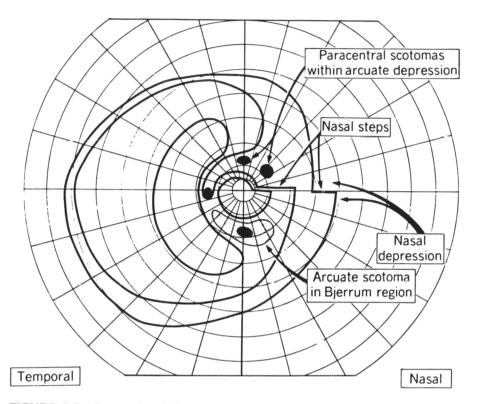

FIGURE 4.3. Composite of Glaucomatous Visual Field Defects [From Anderson DR. Perimetry: With and Without Automation, 2nd ed. St. Louis: CV Mosby, 1987, p. 157.]

c) Scheie method: system based on the degree to which angle structures can be seen; in contrast to the Shaffer system, grade IV denotes closed angle in which only Schwalbe's line is visible, while grades III, II, and I denote progressively deeper anterior chamber angles.

Principles of Perimetry in Glaucoma

Definitions

1. The normal boundaries of visual field are 60° superiorly; 75° inferiorly; 100° temporally; and 60° nasally.

2. In kinetic perimetry, a selected stimulus is moved from an "unseen" area to a "seen" area; a line that connects points at which a particular stimulus becomes visible is known as an isopter; standard Goldmann perimetry is a form of kinetic perimetry.

3. In static (threshold) perimetry, a stimulus at one location is presented at various intensities to determine the visual threshold at that point. Basic concept behind automated perimetry.

Goldmann Perimetry

1. Maximum stimulus intensity: 1000 apostilbs (apostilb, abbreviated asb, is an absolute unit of luminosity) = 1 lumen per square meter of incident surface.

2. Background illumination: 31.6 asb.

3. For a designated isopter (e.g., V-4e), Roman numeral refers to stimulus size, arabic number refers to stimulus intensity with reductions in 0.5 log-unit steps, and small letter refers to stimulus attenuation in 0.1 log-unit steps (Table 4.1).

Automated Perimetry (Humphrey and Octopus)

1. Background illumination: approximately 32 asb for Humphrey (same as Goldmann); 4 asb for Octopus.

2. Stimulus size: standard size III for Humphrey and Octopus.

3. Stimulus intensity: maximum intensity 10,000 asb for Humphrey and 1000 asb for Octopus. Thresholds in automated perimetry are reported in decibels (dB), a relative unit of measure like log units. Log units and decibels represent attenuation of light from maximum intensity. One log unit equals 10 dB (or 0.1 log unit equals 1 dB). The relationship between decibels and apostilbs for Humphrey and Octopus perimeters is shown in Table 4.2.

4. Standard programs used in glaucoma evaluation: 30-2 for Humphrey and 32 for Octopus. These establish thresholds at 76 points in the central 30°.

Visual Field Defects in Glaucoma (Fig. 4.4)

1. The first change is probably generalized constriction, followed by more focal defects.

2. Paracentral scotoma: a localized nerve fiber layer defect within 10° of fixation.

3. Seidel scotoma: an early defect extending from the blind spot.

4. Arcuate (Bjerrum) scotoma: a more extensive nerve fiber layer defect that arches from the blind spot and extends toward the nasal raphe within 10° to 20° of fixation.

TABLE 4.1

Goldmann perimetry parameters

Numeral	Stimulus Size (mm² at 30 cm)
0	$\frac{1}{16}$
I	$\frac{1}{4}$
II	1
III	4
IV	16
V	64

Number	Attenuation (log-units)	Intensity (asb)
4	0	1000
3	0.5	316
2	1.0	100
1	1.5	31.6

Letter	Attenuation (log-units)
e	0
d	0.1
c	0.2
b	0.3
a	0.4

Roman numerals refer to stimulus size. Arabic numbers refer to stimulus intensity with reductions in 0.5 log-unit steps. Small letters refer to stimulus attenuation in 0.1 log-unit steps.

TABLE 4.2

Automated perimetry parameters

Apostilb	Humphrey (dB)	Octopus (dB)
0.1	50	40
1	40	30
10	30	20
100	20	10
1000	10	0
10,000	0	—

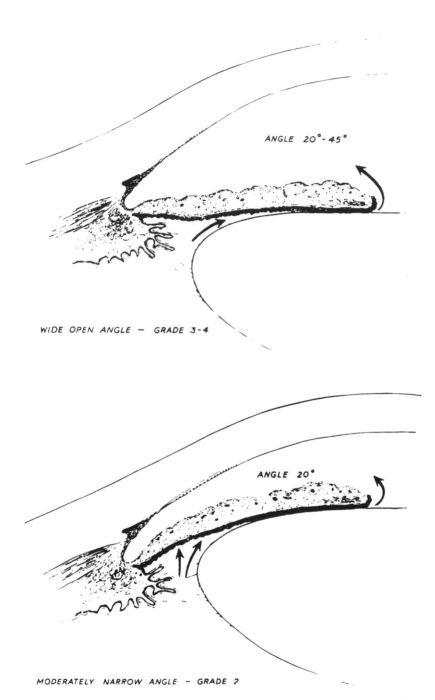

ANGLE 20°- 45°

WIDE OPEN ANGLE — GRADE 3-4

ANGLE 20°

MODERATELY NARROW ANGLE - GRADE 2

FIGURE 4.4. Shaffer Classification of Anterior Chamber Angle Configuration [From Hoskins HD, Kass MA. Becker-Shaffer's Diagnosis and Therapy of the Glaucomas, 6th ed. St. Louis: CV Mosby, 1989, pp. 108–9.]

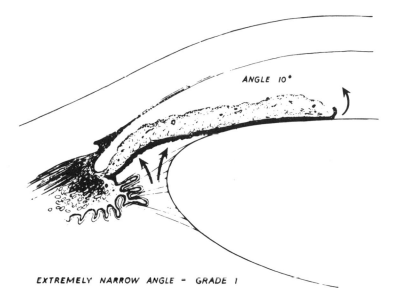

EXTREMELY NARROW ANGLE - GRADE 1

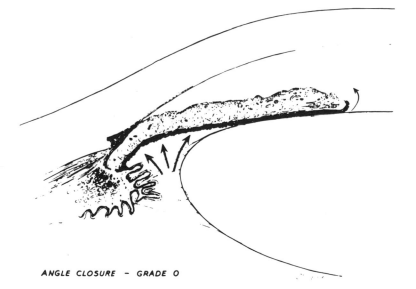

ANGLE CLOSURE - GRADE 0

5. Nasal step: a step-like defect frequently seen where nerve fibers meet along the median raphe.

6. In advanced glaucoma, may see complete double arcuate scotomas with extension to peripheral limits in all areas except temporally, resulting in central and temporal islands of vision; if the central island is lost, only the temporal island remains.

7. In glaucoma, the superior portion of the field is more commonly affected than the inferior portion.

8. Central or cecocentral scotomas are not common but have been described in glaucoma in the absence of other neurologic causes.

9. Nonglaucomatous conditions that may produce visual field defects similar to those seen in primary open angle glaucoma include optic disc drusen, anterior ischemic optic neuropathy, branch retinal artery occlusion, and optic nerve pits.

Primary Open Angle Glaucoma

Definition The most common form of glaucoma, which is clinically characterized by gonioscopically open angles, optic nerve and visual field damage, and, in most cases, increased intraocular pressure. Also known as chronic open angle glaucoma.

Epidemiology

1. Most common form of glaucoma, accounting for 60% to 70% of all adult glaucomas.
2. Second most common cause of blindness in United States and most common cause among black Americans. The relative risk of blindness from glaucoma is approximately eight times greater in blacks than whites. Optic nerve damage may occur at an earlier age in blacks and is generally more severe at the time of detection. Blacks are often more refractory to therapeutic interventions than whites.
3. At least 80,000 Americans are blind from glaucoma.
4. Approximately 2 million Americans have glaucoma, though only about half are aware of their condition.
5. Five to 10 million Americans have increased intraocular pressure; the risk of progression to glaucoma is 0.5% to 1.0% per year.
6. Risk of glaucomatous optic nerve damage increases with age and the level of intraocular pressure.
7. At the time of initial screening, one-third to one-half of patients

with primary open angle glaucoma will have normal intraocular pressure.

8. Approximately one-sixth of patients with findings consistent with primary open angle glaucoma have intraocular pressures consistently below 21 mmHg. Such patients are said to have "normal tension glaucoma" or "low tension glaucoma" (see Normal Tension (Low Tension) Glaucoma section, below).

9. In addition to race, risk factors include a family history of glaucoma, cardiovascular disease, diabetes, and myopia.

Clinical Findings

1. Increased intraocular pressure in most cases. The diurnal variation of intraocular pressure is usually 3 to 6 mmHg in normal persons; may be 30 mmHg or more in patients with primary open angle glaucoma; usually highest in early morning.

2. Glaucomatous optic nerve damage characterized by cup-to-disc ratio asymmetry of more than 0.2 between eyes, thinning of or notching to the disc rim, vertical elongation of the cup, flame-shape hemorrhage at the disc margin, or progressive generalized enlargement of the cup.

3. Focal defects or diffuse damage of the retinal nerve fiber layer may precede obvious optic nerve damage.

4. Glaucomatous abnormalities of the visual fields, including generalized constriction, nasal steps, paracentral defects, and arcuate defects (see Principles of Perimetry in Glaucoma section, above).

5. Findings are generally bilateral but may be asymmetric.

6. Adult onset.

7. Gonioscopically open angles with normal appearance.

8. No evidence of a secondary etiology.

9. An intraocular pressure rise following dilation and in the presence of an open angle is more common in patients with primary open angle glaucoma than normal individuals. This phenomenon is more likely in patients on miotic therapy.

10. Patients with primary open angle glaucoma are much more likely to develop intraocular pressure elevation when given topical corticosteroids than normal individuals.

Differential Diagnosis

1. Pseudoexfoliative glaucoma
2. Pigmentary glaucoma
3. Corticosteroid-induced glaucoma
4. Angle-recession glaucoma

5. Subacute or chronic angle closure glaucoma
6. Glaucoma associated with increased episcleral venous pressure

Management

1. Should establish a target pressure below which progressive damage is felt to be less likely.
2. Topical beta-blockers are usually the first choice for therapy, if there are no medical contraindications such as obstructive pulmonary disease, atrioventricular block, or congestive heart failure.
3. Epinephrine agents typically have minimal additional effect on intraocular pressure when added to a beta-blocker.
4. Cholinergic agents with increasing concentrations as needed are more likely to have an additive effect with beta-blockers.
5. If a beta-blocker or cholinergic (or epinephrine agent) or combination thereof is inadequate in controlling intraocular pressure, a systemic carbonic anhydrase inhibitor may be added.
6. If medical therapy is inadequate in controlling glaucoma, argon laser trabeculoplasty is an alternative. It is initially successful in controlling intraocular pressure in 85% of patients, although approximately 50% require further surgery in 3 to 5 years.
7. If the above measures are inadequate, glaucoma filtering surgery is performed. Primary filtering surgery successfully lowers intraocular pressure in 75% to 85% of patients, though some require medical therapy to achieve success.

Normal Tension (Low Tension) Glaucoma

Definition   A condition in which the intraocular pressure is consistently 21 mmHg or below in the presence of optic nerve or visual field findings that are compatible with primary open angle glaucoma.

Clinical Findings

1. Glaucomatous visual field and optic nerve abnormalities as seen in primary open angle glaucoma (see Primary Open Angle Glaucoma section, above). Some investigators believe visual field defects are more steeply sloped and closer to fixation in normal tension glaucoma than in primary open angle glaucoma.
2. Intraocular pressures are consistently ≤ 21 mmHg.
3. Flame-shaped hemorrhages of the optic nerve are believed to be more common in normal tension glaucoma than in primary open angle glaucoma.

4. Proposed mechanisms of damage include decreased perfusion of the optic nerve and unusual susceptibility of the optic nerve to intraocular-pressure-induced damage.
5. Increased incidence of migraine among patients with normal tension glaucoma is suggestive of a vasospastic component, at least in some patients.

Differential Diagnosis

1. Primary open angle glaucoma with undetected intraocular pressure elevations.
2. Secondary glaucoma associated with past intraocular pressure elevations (e.g., pigmentary glaucoma, corticosteroid-induced glaucoma, past uveitis with increased intraocular pressure).
3. Subacute angle closure glaucoma with intermittent intraocular pressure elevations.
4. Ischemic optic neuropathy: usually a history of sudden visual loss; may be induced by an episode (or episodes) of systemic hypotension related to dysrhythmia, blood loss, etc.
5. Compressive optic neuropathy (e.g., from tumor or aneurysm): often associated with decreased visual acuity or central scotoma.
6. Optic nerve anomalies (e.g., optic disc drusen or pits).
7. Past retinal vascular event (e.g., branch retinal artery occlusion).

Management

1. Careful history and ophthalmic evaluation to rule out other potential causes of optic nerve or visual field changes.
2. Diurnal intraocular pressure curve to rule out possibility of pressure elevations.
3. If clinical findings are "atypical" for glaucoma and compressive neuropathy is a possibility, consider computed tomography or magnetic resonance imaging scan.
4. To rule out other causes of optic neuropathy, evaluate carotid arteries (palpation, auscultation, and if indicated, carotid flow studies); possible laboratory studies include sedimentation rate, complete blood count, VDRL, fluorescent treponemal antibody-absorption (FTA-ABS) test, antinuclear antibody, rheumatoid factor, B12, and folate tests.
5. If no evidence of active disease (e.g., optic disc hemorrhage or evidence of progressive optic nerve or visual field damage), damage may be related to a past event (e.g., severe hypotension). Patients with such "nonprogressive disease" are usually followed without treatment.
6. In the presence of active or progressive disease, the treatment goal is usually maximal lowering of intraocular pressure by

medical therapy, argon laser trabeculoplasty, or glaucoma filtering surgery.

Pseudoexfoliation Syndrome

Definition   A condition often accompanied by a secondary open angle glaucoma and typically characterized by deposition of pseudoexfoliative material on the anterior lens surface and elsewhere in the anterior segment. Also commonly known as exfoliation syndrome.

Epidemiology

1. Typically affects elderly patients, often in their seventies.
2. Commonly described among Scandinavians but seen in numerous populations, including other Europeans, Australian aborigines, Southern Bantu tribe of South Africa, Indians, Pakistanis, and Navaho Indians.
3. In the United States, appears to be more common among women.

Clinical Findings

1. Often clinically unilateral (40%–50%) on initial presentation, though it frequently becomes bilateral.
2. Pseudoexfoliative material on anterior lens surface, typically in bull's-eye pattern. Material is also frequently seen on the pupillary border. It may also be seen on the corneal endothelium, in the anterior chamber angle, on zonules, and on ciliary processes.
3. "Moth-eaten" pattern of peripupillary iris transillumination.
4. Pupillary ruff defects are frequent in affected eyes.
5. Increased pigmentation of trabecular meshwork, though it is patchier and less homogeneous than in pigment dispersion syndrome.
6. Heavy pigment dispersion may be seen after dilation, sometimes with marked increase in intraocular pressure.
7. May be element of angle closure (in one series, peripheral anterior synechiae were noted in 14% and occludable angles in another 18%).
8. If associated with glaucoma (percentage varies depending on population studied), visual field defects and optic nerve damage similar to that with primary open angle glaucoma (POAG).
9. May be associated with spontaneous dislocation of the lens and phakodonesis.
10. Intraocular pressure response to topical corticosteroids similar to that of normal persons (much less frequent than in patients with POAG).

Differential Diagnosis

1. Pigment dispersion syndrome or pigmentary glaucoma:
   a) Krukenberg's spindle.
   b) Denser, more homogeneous pigmentation of trabecular meshwork.
   c) Peripheral radial iris transillumination defects.
   d) Young myopes (male predominance).
2. True lens exfoliation:
   a) Secondary to infrared exposure, intense heat.
   b) Characteristic scrolled appearance of lens capsule.
   c) Infrequently associated with glaucoma.

Management

1. Medical management similar to POAG, though often more resistant to medical therapy.
2. Typically excellent initial response to argon laser trabeculoplasty, though may lose effect with time.
3. Trabeculectomy has success rate similar to that for POAG.
4. With extracapsular cataract extraction, increased risk of developing zonular dialyses.

Pigment Dispersion Syndrome

Definition   A condition often accompanied by a secondary open angle glaucoma and characterized by typical anterior segment findings of pigment dispersion.

Epidemiology

1. Pigment dispersion syndrome is probably as common or more common in women than in men.
2. Pigmentary glaucoma (pigment dispersion with increase in intraocular pressure, or visual field loss, and optic disc changes) is more common in men (typically young male myope).
3. Onset usually around third decade in men, later in women.
4. May decrease in severity later in life.
5. Described but rare in blacks (presumably due to thicker, more compact iris structure).

Clinical Findings

1. Krukenberg's spindle: usually vertical deposition of pigment on central corneal endothelium.
2. Midperipheral (radial) iris transillumination defects and pigment deposition on anterior iris surface.

3. Pigment on zonules and posterior lens capsule (heaviest where zonules attach to capsule). The posterior lens capsular pigmentation is often called Scheie's line or Scheie's stripe.
4. On gonioscopy, a dense homogeneous band of trabecular pigment as well as pigment anterior to Schwalbe's line (Sampaolesi's line) is present; also seen is a concavity of the midperipheral iris, where anterior packets of zonules rub against peripheral iris pigment epithelium, resulting in dispersion of pigment.
5. Exercise and mydriasis may liberate pigment, with or without elevation in intraocular pressure.
6. Pigment may initially obstruct trabecular meshwork with eventual degeneration and sclerosis of trabeculae in some eyes.
7. Pigmentary glaucoma may initially be more difficult to control than POAG; with time, however, a smaller pupil and enlarging lens may decrease zonule-iris apposition and associated pigment dispersion.
8. Approximately 6% of patients with pigment dispersion syndrome develop retinal detachments.

Differential Diagnosis

1. Pseudoexfoliation syndrome
2. Uveitis
3. Ocular melanosis
4. Intraocular melanoma
5. POAG with excessive pigmentation

Management

1. Similar to treatment for POAG.
2. Theoretically, miotics (pilocarpine, thymoxamine) eliminate contact between zonules and iris and decrease pigment dispersion.
3. Argon laser trabeculoplasty: initially good response but may lose effect within months.
4. Response to filtering surgery generally good.

Corticosteroid-Induced Glaucoma

Definition   A secondary open angle glaucoma induced by chronic use of topical or systemic corticosteroids.

Epidemiology

1. A minority of the general population develops increased intraocular pressure with long-term corticosteroids.

2. There is a greater risk of developing increased intraocular pressure on corticosteroids in patients with POAG, their first-degree relatives, and patients with diabetes and high myopia.
3. It was once theorized that the genes which control the intraocular pressure response to corticosteroids and the inheritance of POAG are related.

Clinical Findings

1. May be caused by exogenous corticosteroids, including eyedrops and ointments, periocular injections, and systemic (oral, topical/skin, injection); may also be caused by endogenous corticosteroids (e.g., Cushing's syndrome).
2. Topical corticosteroids may be more likely to produce intraocular pressure rise than systemic administration.
3. Intraocular pressure effects of systemic and topical corticosteroids may be additive.
4. Increased intraocular pressure as early as 1 to 2 weeks after beginning treatment, or months to years later.
5. Intraocular pressure may become markedly elevated.
6. In young children, resembles primary infantile glaucoma; in most cases, resembles POAG with gonioscopically open angle, optic nerve cupping, and visual field defects.
7. Can resemble normal tension glaucoma if a history of past corticosteroid treatment and associated intraocular pressure rise with subsequent decline in intraocular pressure after discontinuation of corticosteroid.
8. In uveitis, it may be difficult to distinguish steroid-induced glaucoma from increased intraocular pressure secondary to ocular inflammation.
9. Intraocular pressure increase is related to potency, dose, frequency, route of administration, presence of other conditions, and individual responsiveness.
10. Fluorometholone and medrysone are less likely to induce intraocular pressure elevation than preparations such as prednisolone and dexamethasone; medrysone has limited corneal penetration and less of an intraocular pressure effect than fluorometholone.
11. Theories of pathogenesis include the mucopolysaccharide theory (accumulation of glycosaminoglycans in trabecular meshwork owing to stabilization of lysosomal membranes and inhibition of catabolic enzymes which depolymerize glycosaminoglycans) and the phagocytosis theory (corticosteroids inhibit phagocytosis of aqueous debris by trabecular endothelial cells).

Management

1. Diagnosis of corticosteroid-induced glaucoma confirmed by discontinuation of medication with subsequent drop in intraocular pressure.
2. Intraocular pressure usually declines in a few days to several weeks; persistent elevations reported, which may be unmasking of underlying POAG or chronic damage to outflow channels.
3. May have to treat pressure medically until it responds to discontinuation of drug.
4. If steroids are necessary, use a weaker drug, lower the concentration or dosage of the drug, or use a drug with less tendency to elevate intraocular pressure (see item 10 under "Clinical Findings," above).
5. With periocular injections, may be necessary to remove the residual drug.
6. If persistent intraocular pressure elevations are unresponsive to medical therapy, one can consider argon laser trabeculoplasty, but this may be of minimal help.
7. Glaucoma filtering surgery may be necessary in some cases.

Glaucoma and Increased Episcleral Venous Pressure

Definition   Group of conditions associated with increased episcleral venous pressure and, in some cases, a secondary glaucoma.

Clinical Findings

1. Episcleral venous pressure is normally 8 to 12 mmHg.
2. May be measured with specially designed instruments.
3. With increased episcleral venous pressure, there is prominence of conjunctival and episcleral blood vessels as well as blood in Schlemm's canal.
4. Causes of increased episcleral venous pressure are obstruction to venous outflow, arteriovenous fistulas, familial, and idiopathic.
5. Causes of obstruction to venous outflow are thyroid ophthalmopathy, superior vena cava syndrome, retrobulbar tumors and orbital pseudotumor, cavernous sinus thrombosis, and radiation.
6. Conditions associated with arteriovenous fistulas are carotid cavernous fistulas, dural shunt syndrome, orbital varices, and Sturge-Weber syndrome.

Differential Diagnosis

Obstruction to Venous Outflow

Thyroid ophthalmopathy: orbital congestion and proptosis; contracture of extraocular muscles

Superior vena cava syndrome: obstruction of venous return from head caused by lesions of the upper thorax (e.g., mediastinal tumors, aortic aneurysms, mediastinitis, thrombophlebitis, constrictive pericarditis, and intrathoracic goiter); results in increased episcleral venous pressure with exophthalmos, edema and cyanosis of face and neck, and dilated veins of head, neck, and upper extremities.

Arteriovenous Fistulas

Carotid cavernous fistula: fistula between internal carotid and cavernous sinus venous complex; typically after severe head injury; pulsating exophthalmos, bruit over globe, conjunctival chemosis, engorgement of epibulbar veins, restriction of motility, and evidence of ocular ischemia.

Dural shunt syndrome (dural sinus fistula): fistula between meningeal branch of internal or external carotid and cavernous sinus of adjacent dural vein; minimal proptosis; no pulsation or bruit.

Orbital varices (orbital arteriovenous shunts): intermittent exophthalmos with increased episcleral venous pressure noted after stooping or Valsalva maneuver; secondary glaucoma not common but reported.

Sturge-Weber syndrome (encephalotrigeminal angiomatosis): Portwine stain hemangioma involving the skin in trigeminal distribution; glaucoma present in half of cases with involvement of ophthalmic and maxillary divisions of cranial nerve V; glaucoma due to developmental anomaly of anterior chamber angle or increased episcleral venous pressure or both.

Familial Increased Episcleral Venous Pressure

- Unilateral or bilateral
- No associated history of trauma
- No clear etiology

Idiopathic Increased Episcleral Venous Pressure

- Typically in elderly but may be seen in young adults.
- Usually unilateral.
- Cause of increased episcleral venous pressure unknown.
- Associated glaucoma may be severe.

Management

1. Eliminate cause of increased episcleral venous pressure, if possible; repair of arteriovenous fistulas may normalize intraocular pressure, though complications include anterior segment, optic nerve, and cerebral ischemia.
2. Aqueous suppressants (beta-blockers, carbonic anhydrase inhibitors) are the most effective form of medical therapy.
3. Argon laser trabeculoplasty has a minimal role in treatment.
4. With glaucoma filtering surgery, an increased risk of uveal effusion and suprachoroidal hemorrhage exists (consider prophylactic sclerotomies).

Uveitis-Associated Glaucoma

Definition   Secondary glaucoma associated with ocular inflammation from a variety of causes. The glaucoma may be associated with an open angle, angle closure, or a combination of the two.

Clinical Findings

1. Typical findings associated with uveitis are conjunctival injection and ciliary flush; keratic precipitates of cornea; anterior chamber cells, flare, and fibrin; iris nodules; posterior synechiae; peripheral anterior synechiae; cataract formation; vitreous cells and debris; and chorioretinitis.
2. Gonioscopically, there may be normal-appearing angle, peripheral anterior synechiae, and prominent or abnormal vessels.
3. Intraocular pressure elevation, if present, may be secondary to the following:
   a) Swelling/dysfunction of trabecular sheets and/or endothelial cells
   b) Accumulation of inflammatory material within the trabeculum
   c) Angle closure secondary to iris bombé caused by dense posterior synechiae
   d) Development of peripheral anterior synechiae unrelated to pupillary block

e) Release of prostaglandins and breakdown of blood-aqueous barrier with subsequent increase in aqueous proteins

f) Anterior segment neovascularization

g) Corticosteroid therapy

Differential Diagnosis

1. *Acute anterior uveitis:* nonspecific iridocyclitis which is often idiopathic; most common cause of intraocular pressure elevation with uveitis.
2. *Fuchs' heterochromic iridocyclitis:* mild anterior uveitis with heterochromia, posterior subcapsular cataract, and secondary glaucoma; usually unilateral; uveitis mild with minimal cell and flare response; fine stellate keratic precipitates; stromal atrophy of iris; fine vessels in angle may bleed during intraocular surgery.
3. *Glaucomatocyclitic crisis (Posner-Schlossman syndrome):* mild anterior uveitis with marked intraocular pressure elevation; usually unilateral; episodic with episodes lasting hours to weeks; recurrence variable, monthly to yearly; may be more common in patients with underlying primary open angle glaucoma; minimal anterior chamber cells or flare with few fine nonpigmented keratic precipitates; pressure elevations usually not associated with optic nerve damage.
4. *Sarcoidosis:* 38% with ocular involvement (e.g., anterior uveitis, chorioretinitis, retinal periphlebitis); of these, approximately 15% have acute iridocyclitis, 50% have chronic granulomatous iridocyclitis, and 10% have glaucoma.
5. *Trabeculitis:* bilateral, often recurrent; gonioscopically, there are gray or slightly yellow precipitates on meshwork with irregular peripheral anterior synechiae; often respond dramatically to topical corticosteroids.
6. *Other uveitic disorders associated with glaucoma:* infectious diseases (e.g., syphilis, herpes simplex, herpes zoster, rubella, mumps, toxoplasmosis, toxocariasis, cytomegalovirus, tuberculosis), joint diseases (juvenile rheumatoid arthritis, ankylosing spondylitis, Reiter's syndrome, psoriatic arthritis); gastrointestinal diseases (ulcerative colitis, Crohn's disease, Whipple's disease); Behçet's disease; Vogt-Koyanagi-Harada syndrome; sympathetic ophthalmia; pars planitis; lens-induced uveitis; scleritis and episcleritis; and interstitial keratitis.

Management

1. Control of inflammation with topical, periocular, or systemic corticosteroids and cycloplegic agents; nonsteroidal anti-

inflammatory agents and immunosuppressive agents sometimes used.

2. Glaucoma management includes aqueous suppressants (beta-blockers and carbonic anhydrase inhibitors); in general, miotics should be avoided as they may increase inflammation.
3. If pupillary block results from posterior synechiae, laser iridotomy is necessary.
4. Argon laser trabeculoplasty is generally not effective but may occasionally be useful in eyes with "burnt out" inflammatory disease.
5. Glaucoma filtering surgery appropriate in glaucoma uncontrolled by medical therapy; increased risk of surgical failure; postoperative antimetabolite therapy (e.g., 5-fluorouracil or mitomycin) should therefore be considered.
6. If uncontrolled by filtering surgery, further modalities include placement of an aqueous shunting device (e.g., Molteno implant) or cyclodestructive procedure.

Lens-Induced Glaucoma

Definition   A group of secondary glaucomas related to increasing lens size (phacomorphic), lens dislocation, release of abnormal proteins by cataractous lenses (phacolytic), release of lens material after trauma or surgery (lens particle glaucoma), or inflammation related to immune sensitization to lens material (phacoanaphylaxis).

Clinical Findings

1. In phacomorphic glaucoma, increasing lens thickness with age results in progressive closure of anterior chamber angle through anterior displacement of lens-iris diaphragm and increased pupillary block.
2. Anterior lens dislocation into the pupillary space or anterior chamber (e.g., microspherophakia) may produce pupillary block.
3. In phacolytic glaucoma, an advanced (usually mature) cataract leaks lens proteins through an intact lens capsule; produces aqueous cells and intense flare with obstruction of the trabecular meshwork by protein-laden macrophages; often there are white particles on anterior lens surface and in the aqueous.
4. In lens particle glaucoma, release of lens material after ocular surgery or trauma results in inflammation and secondary obstruction of the trabecular meshwork.

5. In phacoanaphylaxis, an intense inflammatory reaction secondary to immune sensitization of the patient to his or her own lens protein occurs; rare condition but may occur after trauma or extracapsular cataract extraction in which lens material remains in eye.

Management

1. In phacomorphic glaucoma, lens extraction results in deepening of the anterior chamber angle; if lens removal is not an option, one could attempt to relieve any element of pupillary block with laser iridotomy.
2. In glaucoma associated with lens dislocation and pupillary block, treatment generally consists of laser iridotomy; pupillary dilation with cycloplegic and sympathomimetic agents is another option to pull lens posteriorly (cholinergics may exacerbate block, especially in microspherophakia); lens removal may be necessary in a few cases.
3. In phacolytic glaucoma, lens extraction generally results in resolution of glaucoma; intracapsular cataract extraction has been traditionally recommended, though extracapsular extraction with placement of a posterior chamber intraocular lens has also been reported to be successful.
4. In lens particle glaucoma, medical treatment is indicated initially though removal of liberated lens material or the lens itself is often necessary.
5. In phacoanaphylaxis, treat inflammation and secondary glaucoma; removal of residual lens material may be necessary.

Angle Closure Glaucoma

Primary Angle Closure Glaucoma

Definition   An acute glaucoma typically characterized by the abrupt onset of ocular pain and injection secondary to the development of pupillary block and closure of the anterior chamber angle.

Epidemiology

1. Less common than primary open angle glaucoma though incidence not clearly established.
2. May have a hereditary influence.
3. Among whites, appears to be more common in women than men.
4. Less common among American blacks and Indians.

5. Among Eskimos, relatively high prevalence: an estimated 2% to 3% of persons over age 40.

Clinical Findings

1. Eyes with small anterior segments are predisposed to pupillary block and primary angle closure glaucoma.
2. Thickening of the lens and reduction in pupil size with age may also increase the likelihood of angle closure.
3. Attacks are often precipitated by exposure to dim light, emotional upset, or pharmacologic dilation.
4. Typically present with sudden onset of pain, decreased vision, halos, ocular injection; autonomic stimulation often produces nausea, vomiting, bradycardia, and diaphoresis.
5. Marked conjuctival injection and ciliary flush.
6. Corneal epithelial edema; sometimes stromal edema and folds in Descemet's membrane.
7. Shallow anterior chamber centrally but more shallow peripherally with iris bombé configuration; anterior chamber inflammation common.
8. Pupil in mid-dilated (3.5–6 mm diameter) position (at which point vector forces result in maximal conditions for pupillary block); may be irregular and sluggish or nonreactive.
9. May have sector atrophy of the iris (usually greater superiorly) and pigment dispersion.
10. Glaucomflecken of lens (anterior lens opacities).
11. Intraocular pressure usually highly elevated (usually > 40 mmHg and often > 50 mmHg).
12. Anterior chamber angle gonioscopically closed, though may be possible to open with compression if no permanent peripheral anterior synechiae; gonioscopy of fellow eye generally exhibits narrow angle.
13. Optic nerve may appear normal; in acute attack, can see hyperemia and edema of nerve; following attack, can see optic nerve pallor with or without cupping.
14. Visual fields most often show generalized constriction, though nerve fiber bundle defects may develop.

Differential Diagnosis

1. *Neovascular glaucoma:* see section on this topic, below.
2. *Uveitic (inflammatory) glaucoma:* see Uveitis-Associated Glaucoma section, above.
3. *Glaucomatocyclitic crisis:* see Uveitis-Associated Glaucoma section, above.
4. *Ciliary block glaucoma:* see section on this topic, below.

5. *Suprachoroidal hemorrhage:* see Differential Diagnosis in Ciliary Block Glaucoma section, below.
6. *Iridocorneal endothelial syndrome:* see section on this topic, below.
7. *Lens-induced glaucoma:* see section on this topic, above.
8. *Aphakic and pseudophakic pupillary block.*
9. *Angle closure after scleral buckling surgery:* secondary to inflammation, uveal congestion with anterior rotation of the ciliary processes, and mechanical anterior displacement of the lens-iris diaphragm; generally responds to topical corticosteroids but occasionally requires peripheral iridoplasty, drainage of suprachoroidal fluid, or adjustment of scleral buckle.
10. *Angle closure after panretinal photocoagulation and central retinal vein occlusion:* secondary to ciliary body congestion; generally responds to topical corticosteroids, cycloplegics, and aqueous suppressants; occasionally requires peripheral iridoplasty.
11. *Nanophthalmos:* condition characterized by small hyperopic eyes with a high lens-to-eye volume ratio and thickened sclera; treatment of narrow anterior chamber angles may require laser iridotomy and sometimes peripheral iridoplasty; increased risk of massive uveal effusions in association with intraocular surgery (prophylactic sclerotomies recommended).
12. *Angle closure due to tumors and cysts:* intraocular tumors (e.g., malignant melanoma of choroid and ciliary body) may produce anterior displacement of the lens-iris diaphragm and angle closure; similarly, epithelial cysts of the iris and ciliary body may produce anterior shift of the iris; for cysts causing significant angle closure, treatment options include puncture with argon or neodymium:yttrium-argon-garnet (Nd:YAG) laser.
13. *Epithelial and fibrovascular ingrowth:* may occur after trauma or due to inadequate postoperative wound apposition; can produce severe secondary angle closure glaucoma.

Management
1. Topical beta-blocker (and, possibly, topical apraclonidine).
2. One to four drops of 1% to 2% pilocarpine over 30 minutes (additional pilocarpine is unlikely to be beneficial and may induce further ocular congestion and inflammation); thymoxamine, an α-adrenergic antagonist, may also be useful in the induction of miosis, though it is not commercially available in the United States. However, Dapiprazole, a similar agent, is now commercially available.
3. Oral acetazolamide (250–500 mg) and oral osmotic agents (glycerin or isosorbide, 1–2 g/kg); if patient is unable to tolerate

oral agents, may administer intravenous acetazolamide and mannitol.

4. Topical corticosteroids may help reduce ocular inflammation associated with the attack.
5. If the attack is not broken by medical therapy, consider corneal compression with tonometer tip, cotton-tipped applicator, muscle hook, or four-mirror goniolens to push aqueous into peripheral anterior chamber.
6. Definitive treatment surgical: argon or Nd:YAG laser iridotomy.
7. In some cases a peripheral iridoplasty is useful.
8. If unable to complete laser iridotomy, consider surgical peripheral iridectomy.
9. Residual glaucoma after iridotomy may require chronic medical therapy; argon laser trabeculoplasty or glaucoma filtering surgery may be necessary in medically uncontrolled eyes.
10. As the risk of an angle closure attack is increased in the fellow eye (50%–75% over 5–10 yrs), prophylactic laser iridotomy should also be performed in this eye.

Other Angle Closure Glaucomas

Subacute Angle Closure Glaucoma

1. Intermittent episodes of blurred vision and ocular discomfort; may be relieved by light-induced or sleep-induced miosis.
2. Repeated episodes may result in development of permanent peripheral anterior synechiae.
3. Initial treatment consists of laser iridotomy; if intraocular pressure remains increased after laser iridotomy, long-term medical therapy or further surgical treatment may be required.

Chronic Angle Closure Glaucoma

1. Also known as "creeping angle closure glaucoma"; most common type of angle closure among blacks; generally asymptomatic.
2. Appositional angle closure with or without presence of permanent peripheral anterior synechiae; if peripheral anterior synechiae are present, they tend to begin superiorly.
3. May be induced or worsened by chronic cholinergic therapy.
4. Treatment consists of laser iridotomy, though permanent trabecular damage or peripheral anterior synechiae may require long-term medical therapy or filtering surgery or both for intraocular pressure control. Argon laser trabeculoplasty is an option if enough open angle remains.

Plateau Iris Configuration and Syndrome

1. "Plateau iris configuration": relatively flat iris insertion with abrupt posterior turn near iris insertion; often has an element of pupillary block, which responds to laser iridotomy.
2. "Plateau iris syndrome": even in presence of laser iridotomy, angle closure may be present as peripheral iris bunches up to occlude angle; may require chronic miotic therapy or peripheral laser iridoplasty.

Ciliary Block Glaucoma

See section on this topic, below.

Neovascular Glaucoma

Definition A secondary glaucoma characterized by anterior segment neovascularization with eventual closure of the anterior chamber angle and elevated intraocular pressure.

Epidemiology

1. Generally associated with underlying retinal ischemia.
2. Predisposing disorders:
   a) Diabetic retinopathy (most common cause)
   b) Ischemic central retinal vein occlusion (second most common cause)
   c) Other retinal disorders (central retinal artery occlusion, branch retinal vein occlusion, chronic retinal detachment, retinoblastoma, retinopathy of prematurity, sickle cell retinopathy)
   d) Carotid artery obstructive disease (probably third most common cause)
   e) Uveitis
   f) Carotid-cavernous fistula
3. Iris neovascularization is strongly correlated with the degree of retinal ischemia. Signs of ischemia include extensive retinal capillary nonperfusion on fluorescein angiography, decreased vision, 10 or more cotton-wool spots, significant relative afferent pupillary defect, reduced b/a wave ratio ($<$ 1.2) on electroretinography.

Clinical Findings

1. In iris neovascularization without glaucoma, the first sign is increased permeability of blood vessels at the pupil margin by fluorescein angiography.

2. Clinically, dilated tufts of vessels first appear at pupil margin, which progress toward the iris root. For differentiation of new versus engorged vessels, see Table 4.3.
3. In "open angle" glaucoma, more extensive iris or angle neovascularization is found; a fibrovascular membrane covers the angle and anterior iris surface; may see anterior chamber inflammation and hyphema.
4. In secondary "angle closure" glaucoma, which is typically severe, contracture of the membrane leads to progressive synechial angle closure, flattening of the iris stroma, ectropion uvea, and pupillary dilation.
5. Anterior segment neovascularization is believed to result from forward diffusion of angiogenic factors released by hypoxic retinal tissue.

Differential Diagnosis

1. *Fuchs' heterochromic iridocyclitis:* fine iris and angle vessels; may develop hyphema with surgical manipulation of the eye; eye generally white and quiet.
2. *Uveitic (inflammatory) glaucoma:* may be difficult to differentiate vascular engorgement from neovascularization. See Table 4.3 and Uveitis-Associated Glaucoma section, above.
3. *Acute angle closure glaucoma:* see Angle Closure Glaucoma section, above. Gonioscopy of the fellow eye may be helpful since a narrow angle is generally present.

Management

1. Aqueous suppressants (beta-blockers and carbonic anhydrase inhibitors).
2. Cholinergics are rarely helpful and should be avoided in the

TABLE 4.3

Differentiation of neovascularization from engorged vessels

Characteristic	New Vessels	Engorged Vessels
Size	Irregular	Uniform
Course	Irregular	Radial
Branching	Frequent	None within iris
Location	Iris surface	Iris stroma

presence of active neovascularization (increase inflammation and cause further breakdown of blood-aqueous barrier).

3. Topical corticosteroids and cycloplegic agents.
4. Panretinal photocoagulation to treat underlying ischemic process and eliminate or reduce anterior segment neovascularization. (Panretinal cryoablation is an alternative when medium precludes panretinal photocoagulation.)
5. Goniophotocoagulation with argon laser (0.2 s duration, 50–100 μm spot size, and 100–200 mW power) may be an adjunct in some cases but does not eliminate need for retinal ablation.
6. Surgical management includes trabeculectomy with careful intraoperative hemostasis (postoperative 5-fluorouracil or intraoperative mitomycin may increase success rate), placement of aqueous shunting device (e.g., Molteno implant), or cyclodestructive procedure (e.g., cyclocryotherapy, Nd:YAG transscleral cyclophotocoagulation).

Iridocorneal Endothelial (ICE) Syndrome

Definition A unilateral condition characterized by corneal endothelial abnormalities, progressive formation of peripheral anterior synechiae, and iris defects. Corneal edema and secondary glaucoma are common. Clinical variants include progressive essential iris atrophy, Chandler's syndrome, and iris-nevus (Cogan-Reese) syndrome.

Epidemiology

1. Typically affects patients in early to middle adulthood.
2. Whites more commonly affected.
3. Reported female-to-male ratios vary from 2:1 to 5:1.
4. Family history negative.

Clinical Findings

1. Spectrum of findings including corneal endothelial abnormalities, corneal edema, progressive peripheral anterior synechiae (usually to or beyond Schwalbe's line), secondary glaucoma (in one series, 77% required treatment of increased intraocular pressure and 44% required filtering surgery), breaks in iris stroma and pigment epithelium, and iris nodules.
2. Almost always unilateral, though rare bilateral cases reported.
3. In progressive (essential) iris atrophy, iris changes predominate: pupil displacement toward heaviest peripheral anterior synechiae; frequent ectropion iridis toward direction of

displacement; stromal thinning and stretch holes on side opposite pupillary distortion.

4. In Chandler's syndrome, corneal changes predominate: "fine hammered silver appearance" of corneal endothelium; corneal edema may occur with normal or only slightly elevated intraocular pressure; iris atrophy mild without hole formation; pupil round or slightly oval.

5. In Cogan-Reese (iris-nevus) syndrome, fine pedunculated nodules on iris surface with matted appearance of stroma and loss of normal iris crypts or a velvety whorl-like iris surface with loss of iris crypts.

6. Specular microscopy: affected eyes show endothelial cell pleomorphism, loss of cellular mosaic, and intracellular blackout areas; fellow eyes generally normal though may show some cellular pleomorphism.

7. Clinical findings explained by membrane theory: endothelialization of anterior chamber angle with ectopic corneal endothelium and abnormal Descemet's membrane extending across trabecular meshwork onto anterior iris surface.

Differential Diagnosis

1. *Fuchs' corneal endothelial dystrophy:* usually bilateral; lacks iris atrophy and peripheral anterior synechiae.

2. *Posterior polymorphous dystrophy:* usually bilateral and familial; posterior corneal changes often vesicular.

3. *Axenfeld-Rieger syndrome:* congenital, bilateral, familial; may be associated with maxillary hypoplasia and other systemic manifestations.

4. *Aniridia:* bilateral, familial.

5. *Iridoschisis:* tends to occur in elderly; usually bilateral.

6. *Neurofibromatosis:* bilateral; nodules flatter than ICE syndrome and more like ordinary nevi.

7. *Melanoma:* usually solitary but may be multiple.

Management

1. Medical and/or surgical control of glaucoma and corneal edema.

2. In medical treatment of glaucoma, aqueous suppressants are the most effective.

3. In one series, filtering surgery successfully controlled intraocular pressure in 69% of patients but was only 42% successful in controlling corneal edema.

4. In another series, a 1-year success rate of 64% was achieved for the first trabeculectomy; 39% at 3 years.

Ciliary Block Glaucoma

Definition   A relatively rare form of angle closure glaucoma in which aqueous is misdirected into the vitreous cavity in predisposed eyes, resulting in shallowing of the anterior chamber angle and angle closure. Also known as malignant glaucoma, direct lens block, aqueous misdirection syndrome, and cilio-vitreo-lenticular block.

Clinical Findings

1. Most commonly seen after intraocular surgery (e.g., surgical peripheral iridectomy, glaucoma filtering surgery, cataract extraction) in eyes with chronic or acute angle closure glaucoma.
2. The anterior chamber is shallow or flat even in the presence of a patent iridectomy; unlike the appearance in pupillary block, the anterior chamber in ciliary block is usually uniformly shallow.
3. Elevated intraocular pressure, often 40 mmHg or higher.
4. More likely to occur in phakic eyes with small anterior segments, which predispose to misdirection of aqueous into the vitreous cavity, anterior displacement of the lens-iris diaphragm, and the clinical findings as described above.
5. Aphakic or pseudophakic eyes, iridovitreal synechiae, a dense or thickened vitreous face, or adherence of the vitreous to the ciliary body may predispose to posterior misdirection of aqueous.
6. Usually worsened by cholinergic agents and can be induced by miotic therapy.

Differential Diagnosis

1. *Pupillary block and acute angle closure glaucoma:* typically there is iris bombé, shallow anterior chamber peripherally, and deeper chamber centrally; responds to laser iridotomy or surgical iridectomy.
2. *Suprachoroidal hemorrhage:* often associated with sudden onset of pain, shallow or flat anterior chamber, and, frequently, elevated intraocular pressure; dark choroidal elevations are usually seen on fundus examination.
3. *Wound leaks or serous choroidal detachment:* may cause a shallow anterior chamber, though the intraocular pressure is usually low.

Management

1. Discontinuation of any miotic agents.
2. Administration of topical cycloplegic (e.g., atropine 1% q.i.d.) and sympathomimetic agent (e.g., phenylephrine 2.5%–10% q.i.d.) to

decrease ciliary body tone, increase tension on zonules, and produce retrodisplacement of lens.

3. Aqueous suppressants (beta-blockers and carbonic anhydrase inhibitors) to reduce the amount of aqueous being directed posteriorly and to lower intraocular pressure.

4. Hyperosmotic agents to shrink the vitreous and help re-establish normal aqueous flow.

5. Topical corticosteroids to reduce inflammation and any associated uveal congestion.

6. Within 4 to 5 days, intensive medical therapy may result in resolution of ciliary block in approximately 50% of cases; after an appropriate response, therapy can be tapered, though most eyes will require continuation of atropine indefinitely.

7. Prior to or in conjunction with initiation of medical therapy, laser iridotomy may be performed in the absence of a patent iridotomy or iridectomy to treat or rule out any possible element of pupillary block.

8. Argon laser treatment of ciliary processes through patent iridectomy has also been described in the treatment of phakic eyes.

9. If unresponsive to above, a vitrectomy (standard pars plana vitrectomy preferable to needle aspiration of vitreous) and anterior chamber reformation (with air, balanced salt solution, or sodium hyaluronate) is indicated.

10. In eyes unresponsive to vitrectomy, lens extraction may become necessary.

11. In aphakic or pseudophakic ciliary block, photodisruption of the anterior vitreous face and the posterior capsule with the Nd:YAG laser may result in resolution of the ciliary block.

Primary Infantile Glaucoma

Definition A developmental defect in the trabecular meshwork and anterior chamber angle of a neonate or infant, which is clinically characterized by increased intraocular pressure, corneal enlargement and edema, and optic nerve cupping. Also known as primary congenital glaucoma and trabeculodysgenesis. If the child is over age 3, it is called juvenile glaucoma.

Epidemiology

1. One out of 10,000 births.
2. Bilateral in 65% to 80%.
3. Male-to-female preponderance of 3:2 in the United States.

4. Inheritance: autosomal recessive with variable penetrance versus multifactorial.

Clinical Findings

1. Classic triad on presentation: epiphora, blepharospasm, and photophobia.
2. Enlarged corneal diameter and globe, corneal edema, and breaks in Descemet's membrane.
3. The normal neonatal cornea is 10 to 10.5 mm in horizontal diameter, increasing by 0.5 to 1.0 mm in the first year; enlargement greater than 12 mm is usually due to increased intraocular pressure; breaks in Descemet's membrane (Haab's striae) are usually horizontal centrally and parallel to limbus peripherally.
4. Increased intraocular pressure; when patient is under anesthesia, check the intraocular pressure as soon as light anesthesia is induced since halothane may lower intraocular pressure.
5. On gonioscopy, one usually finds an anterior iris insertion and may see translucency of the trabecular surface.
6. Optic nerve cupping may occur rapidly and early but may reverse with intraocular pressure control.
7. Increased intraocular pressure was once felt to be secondary to a membrane (Barkan's membrane) obstructing flow through the trabecular meshwork. More likely explanations are compressed trabecular tissue (which may visually simulate a membrane); a failure of usual atrophy, resorption, or cleavage of angle tissues; or failure of the ciliary body and iris to slide posteriorly.

Differential Diagnosis

1. *Nasolacrimal duct obstruction:* not usually associated with photophobia; no corneal haze or enlargement.
2. *Megalocornea:* abnormal corneal enlargement (>13 mm) with normal intraocular pressure, absence of breaks in Descemet's membrane, and no optic nerve cupping.
3. *Obstetrical trauma:* breaks in Descemet's membrane are often vertical; usually unilateral (more commonly left eye because of typical left occiput anterior presentation of infant's head).
4. *Maternal rubella syndrome:* often also associated with deafness, cardiac abnormalities, mental retardation, and cataracts.
5. *Congenital hereditary endothelial dystrophy (CHED):* autosomal recessive condition characterized by bilateral corneal edema with marked stromal thickening; corneal diameters and intraocular pressures are normal.

6. *Lowe's oculocerebrorenal syndrome:* X-linked recessive disease characterized by renal tubular acidosis, cataracts, and glaucoma.
7. *Other metabolic diseases:* corneal clouding (without enlargement) due to mucopolysaccharidoses, cystinosis, and corneal lipidosis.
8. *Axial myopia:* often there is a tilted optic nerve head, myopic crescents, and choroidal mottling.
9. *Secondary infantile glaucomas:* include Axenfeld-Rieger syndrome (see section on this topic, below), Sturge-Weber syndrome (see Glaucoma and Increased Episcleral Venous Pressure section, above), and neurofibromatosis.

Management

1. The definitive treatment is surgical.
2. Goniotomy is the most widely used procedure, though it may not be possible in the presence of a cloudy cornea; complications include iridodialysis, cyclodialysis, hyphema, and peripheral anterior synechiae.
3. Trabeculotomy is appropriate when a hazy cornea precludes goniotomy and is the primary choice for some surgeons; complications include hyphema, Descemet's tears, iridodialysis, and cyclodialysis.
4. Reassess glaucoma status 3 to 6 weeks after surgical intervention.
5. Overall success rate of 80% with goniotomy and trabeculotomy, though reoperations are often necessary (10%–35%).
6. Prognosis better if presentation at 1 to 12 months; worse if presentation in first month or after 12 months.
7. Even with successful control of intraocular pressure, visual loss may result from amblyopia, corneal scarring, refractive error, and permanent optic nerve damage.

Axenfeld-Rieger Syndrome

Definition   A secondary developmental condition typically exhibiting bilateral abnormalities of the cornea, anterior chamber angle, or iris. Frequently complicated by secondary glaucoma. Also known as anterior chamber cleavage syndrome, mesodermal dysgenesis of the cornea and iris, and primary dysgenesis mesodermalis of the iris.

Epidemiology

1. Bilateral developmental disorder usually diagnosed by childhood.
2. Frequent positive family history of the condition (autosomal dominant inheritance), though sporadic cases are common.
3. No sex predilection.

Clinical Findings

1. Posterior embryotoxon: anterior displacement of Schwalbe's line; anatomic variation in 8% to 15% of normal eyes; as an isolated finding, there is no increased risk of associated glaucoma.
2. Axenfeld's anomaly: prominent anterior Schwalbe's line with thin to broad tissue strands from peripheral iris to Schwalbe's line.
3. Rieger's anomaly: peripheral anterior segment abnormalities with iris changes, including stromal thinning and atrophy, corectopia, and ectropion uvea.
4. Rieger's syndrome: ocular anomalies plus nonocular defects, including microdontia, hypodontia, maxillary hypoplasia, and anomalies of pituitary gland.
5. Corneal abnormalities (other than above) include small or enlarged corneas.
6. Secondary glaucoma develops in approximately 60% of patients, usually between early childhood and adulthood; it is believed to result from maldevelopment of the trabecular meshwork and Schlemm's canal as part of more general maldevelopment of structures derived from neural crest cells.
7. Rare ocular associations include strabismus, limbal dermoids, cataracts, choroidal hypoplasia, retinal detachment, macular degeneration, optic nerve hypoplasia, and chorioretinal colobomas.

Differential Diagnosis

1. *Iridocorneal endothelial syndrome:* usually unilateral, nonfamilial, and progressive, with predilection for women in young adulthood.
2. *Posterior polymorphous dystrophy:* generally with associated blisters or vesicles of posterior cornea.
3. *Iridoschisis:* separation of anterior iris stroma from deeper layers; usually occurs in the elderly.
4. *Peter's anomaly:* generally bilateral (80%) autosomal recessive or sporadic disorder characterized by central corneal opacities with abnormal Descemet's membrane, iris strands to the margins of the corneal defect, and anterior polar cataracts; secondary glaucoma in 50% of cases; other associations are microphthalmos, keratolenticular adhesions, blue sclera, and aniridia.

Management

1. Secondary glaucoma is often difficult to control.
2. Medical therapy consists of aqueous suppressants (beta-blockers

and, if necessary, carbonic anhydrase inhibitors); in some cases, cyclotonia from pilocarpine is believed to produce trabecular collapse.
3. Argon laser trabeculoplasty is ineffective.
4. Goniotomy and trabeculotomy have limited success in infants; trabeculectomy shows success rates consistent with surgery in this age group.

Hypotony

Definition   Abnormally low intraocular pressure (<6 mmHg).

Epidemiology   Most commonly seen after ocular surgery or ocular trauma; may also be associated with systemic and vascular disease.

Clinical Findings

1. Abnormally low intraocular pressure (usually <6 mmHg).
2. May find associated shallow anterior chamber, iridocyclitis, ciliochoroidal detachment, retinal detachment, or cyclodialysis cleft.
3. Complications of hypotony include breakdown of blood-aqueous barrier, iridocyclitis, macular and disc edema, and corneal stromal thickening and folds in Descemet's membrane.

Differential Diagnosis

1. Hypotony following ocular surgery (e.g., glaucoma surgery, cataract surgery)
   a) Wound leak: detected by careful Seidel testing.
   b) Iridocyclitis.
   c) Overfiltration after glaucoma filtering surgery.
   d) Ciliochoroidal detachment: often found in association with early postoperative hypotony after glaucoma filtering surgery; due to the accumulation of serous fluid in the suprachoroidal space.
   e) Retinal detachment.
   f) Inadvertent cyclodialysis cleft: seen clinically as separation of the iris or ciliary body from the sclera; allows direct communication between anterior chamber and suprachoroidal space and, thus, increased uveoscleral outflow.
   g) Perforation of sclera with retrobulbar needle or bridle suture.

2. Hypotony following ocular trauma
   a) Scleral rupture
   b) Iridocyclitis
   c) Retinal detachment
   d) Cyclodialysis cleft
   e) Ciliochoroidal detachment
3. Bilateral hypotony
   a) Osmotic dehydration secondary to diabetes or uremia
   b) Myotonic dystrophy
4. Other causes
   a) Vascular occlusion (e.g., carotid obstructive disease)
   b) Prephthisis bulbi

Management

1. Treatment of underlying problem (e.g., iridocyclitis, retinal detachment, scleral rupture, wound leak, if possible).
2. Treatment of cyclodialysis cleft: dilation of pupil to increase likelihood of spontaneous closure; if unsuccessful, treatment of cleft with argon laser, diathermy, or direct suturing.

Medical Therapy of Glaucoma

Definition   Initial therapy for glaucoma generally consists of administration of topical and, later, systemic medications. Four general classes of drugs used are beta-blockers, epinephrine agents, cholinergic agents, and carbonic anhydrase inhibitors.

β-Adrenergic Inhibitors

Clinical Information

1. Timolol (Timoptic), levobunolol (Betagan), and metipranolol (Optipranolol) are nonselective beta-blockers which act on β_1 and β_2 receptors; similar in potency.
2. Betaxolol (Betoptic) is a selective beta-blocker with primary action on β_1 (cardiac) receptors; minimal effect on β_2 (pulmonary) receptors; probably slightly less potent than nonselective agents.
3. Beta-blockers are the most widely used class of drugs for glaucoma therapy; usually first choice for treatment unless contraindication exists.
4. Mechanism of action: lower intraocular pressure by reducing aqueous production by 30% to 40%.

5. Generally administered twice daily, though once daily treatment may be appropriate in some patients.

Side Effects

1. Ocular
   a) Dry eyes
   b) Decreased corneal sensation
   c) Superficial punctate keratopathy
   d) Dilated pupil with concomitant treatment with epinephrine agent
2. Systemic
   a) Exacerbation of obstructive pulmonary disease (much less likely with selective beta-blocker).
   b) Decreased pulse rate and myocardial contractility; exacerbation of atrioventricular block and congestive heart failure.
   c) Central nervous system effects: depression, confusion, loss of libido.
   d) May mask symptoms of hypoglycemia in diabetic patients.

Adrenergic Agonists

Clinical Information

1. Epinephrine available in hydrochloride, borate, and bitartrate forms.
2. Dipivefrin (Propine) 0.1% solution is a lipophilic prodrug with 17-fold greater corneal penetration than epinephrine; converted to epinephrine by esterases in cornea; intraocular pressure effects similar to 1% to 2% epinephrine, though decreased external and systemic side effects when compared to epinephrine.
3. Mechanism of action: epinephrine may initially increase aqueous production; the ultimate effect of lowering intraocular pressure is due to increased trabecular (and probably uveoscleral) outflow.
4. Generally administered twice daily.
5. Less effective than topical beta-blockers in initial glaucoma therapy.
6. Minimal additive effect with beta-blockers, though appears to be greater effect with betaxolol (selective beta-blocker) than with nonselective beta-blockers.

Side Effects

1. Ocular
   a) Hyperemia and irritation
   b) Allergic blepharoconjunctivitis

    c) Follicular hypertrophy
    d) Adrenochrome deposits
    e) Ocular cicatricial pemphigoid
    f) Macular edema in aphakic eyes
    g) Pupillary dilation, especially when used in combination with topical beta-blocker
2. Systemic
    a) Palpitations with tachycardia and dysrhythmias
    b) Premature ventricular contractions
    c) Increased blood pressure
    d) Anxiety and tremor

Cholinergic Agents

Clinical Information

1. First agents used in glaucoma therapy (1870s).
2. Direct parasympathomimetic agents: mimic acetylcholine effects on motor endplates; include pilocarpine and carbachol.
3. Indirect parasympathomimetic agents: inhibit acetylcholinesterase to produce local accumulation of acetylcholine; include echothiophate, physostigmine, demecarium, diisopropyl fluorophosphate. (Carbachol has some indirect effects.)
4. Mechanism of action: contraction of ciliary musculature with subsequent traction on scleral spur and altered configuration of trabecular meshwork or Schlemm's canal or both, to produce increased facility of aqueous outflow.
5. Sustained delivery systems: ointment (pilopine gel) and membrane-controlled delivery system (Ocusert).
6. Pilocarpine (0.5%–10%) generally administered four times a day; carbachol (0.75%–3.0%) administered three times a day; echothiophate (phospholine iodide) (0.03%–0.25%) administered twice a day.
7. Cholinergics provide significant additional intraocular pressure effect in combination with epinephrine, beta-blockers, and carbonic anhydrase inhibitors.

Side Effects

1. Ocular
    a) Ciliary muscle spasm with associated brow ache, induced myopia, and anterior movement of lens-iris diaphragm (can produce angle closure).
    b) Miosis and decreased dark adaptation.
    c) Vascular congestion and breakdown of blood-aqueous barrier

(cholinesterase inhibitors should be stopped at least 2 weeks before surgical procedures if possible).
d) Posterior synechiae, especially with cholinesterase inhibitors.
e) Retinal detachment (evidence circumstantial) due to vitreoretinal traction caused by contraction of ciliary musculature.
f) Cataractogenesis, especially with cholinesterase inhibitors; initially fine anterior subcapsular vacuoles; cholinesterase inhibitors, therefore, used primarily in aphakia and pseudophakia.
g) Iris cysts near pupil margin (most commonly in children on cholinesterase inhibitor for accommodative esotropia); treat with phenylephrine.
h) Atypical band keratopathy in past due to preservative phenylmercuric nitrate.
i) Allergic conjunctivitis and dermatitis.
j) Ocular cicatricial pemphigoid (pseudopemphigoid) and stenosis of lacrimal canaliculi.
2. Systemic
a) In high concentrations, include nausea, vomiting, diarrhea, bradycardia, salivation, diaphoresis.
b) Indirect agents deplete plasma cholinesterase (pseudocholinesterase), which hydrolyses succinylcholine and local anesthetics with ester linkage group (procaine, tetracaine); if succinylcholine used as muscle relaxant during induction of general anesthesia, may develop prolonged respiratory paralysis; with local anesthetics, toxicity may occur. Depletion of pseudocholinesterase begins within 2 weeks; peaks in 5 to 7 weeks; requires several weeks for recovery. Antidotes for systemic toxicity: intravenous atropine, 1 to 2 mg or more as needed; intravenous pralidoxime chloride (Protopam), a cholinesterase reactivator, 25 mg/kg.

Carbonic Anhydrase Inhibitors (CAI)

Clinical Information

1. Administered systemically (orally or intravenously).
2. Acetazolamide (Diamox) and methazolamide (Neptazane) most widely used; dichlorphenamide and ethoxzolamide also available.
3. Mechanism of action: reduce intraocular pressure by inhibition of carbonic anhydrase (within the ciliary body necessary in aqueous production) and induction of metabolic acidosis; aqueous humor formation suppressed by 40% to 60%.
4. Of all patients 30% to 50% fail to tolerate long-term treatment

with carbonic anhydrase inhibitors (CAI) due to systemic side effects.

5. CAI effect additive to secretory inhibition of beta-blockers.
6. Topical CAI currently being developed and studied in clinical trials; previous efforts limited by needs for high degree of inhibition of carbonic anhydrase and adequate corneal penetration to achieve intraocular pressure effect.

Side Effects

1. Ocular: transient myopia possibly due to ciliary body swelling.
2. Systemic
   a) Paresthesias.
   b) Gastrointestinal: nausea, diarrhea, weight loss, loss of appetite.
   c) Central nervous system: malaise, fatigue, depression, confusion, loss of libido.
   d) Ureteral colic/nephrourolithiasis: related to decreased urinary citrate, which normally improves calcium solubility; theoretically less chance of stone formation with methazolamide than acetazolamide since former causes less reduction in urinary citrate.
   e) Skin rash.
   f) Hematologic reactions, including aplastic anemia.
   g) Teratogenicity in laboratory animals.
   h) Avoid use during pregnancy in humans: sacrococcygeal teratoma and multiple congenital anomalies have been described.
   i) Potassium loss: minimal with CAI alone; greater if combined with thiazides.
   j) Sickle cell disease: acidosis produces hypoxia and more sickling; less acidosis with methazolamide.
   k) Chronic obstructive pulmonary disease: patients with compensatory metabolic alkalosis may develop respiratory and metabolic acidosis.
   l) Renal insufficiency: acetazolamide excreted unmetabolized; methazolamide excreted 25% unchanged.
   m) Cirrhosis: may prevent ammonia secretion.

Hyperosmotic Agents
Clinical Information

1. Mechanism of action: increases osmotic pressure of plasma relative to aqueous/vitreous; may also alter intraocular pressure by affecting osmoreceptors in hypothalamus.

2. More effective with low molecular weight and when confined to extracellular space (i.e., poor ocular penetration).
3. Intravenous administration generally has more rapid and greater effect than oral administration.
4. Usual dose: 1 to 2 g/kg.
5. Mannitol: agent of choice for intravenous use; usually used as 20% solution; penetrates eye poorly (extracellular); less irritation than urea if extravasates.
6. Urea: for intravenous use but now seldom used; penetrates eye fairly well; may get rebound elevation in pressure; if it extravasates, sloughing and phlebitis occur.
7. Glycerin: for oral use; available as 50% or 75% solution; penetrates eye poorly (extracellular); may cause nausea and vomiting; metabolized (caloric).
8. Isosorbide: also for oral use; available as 45% or 50% solution; less nausea and vomiting than glycerin; excreted unmetabolized in urine (better for diabetic patients).
9. Effects of osmotic agents may last 6 to 8 hours; may be repeated if necessary.

Systemic Side Effects

1. Nausea and vomiting
2. Diuresis
3. Shrinkage of cerebral cortex: headache; traction on meningeal vessels; subarachnoid/subdural hemorrhage
4. Pulmonary edema; congestive heart failure

Glaucoma Laser Surgery

Definition   Procedures using the argon or neodymium:yttrium-argon-garnet (Nd:YAG) laser to create openings in the iris (laser iridotomy), directly treat the trabecular meshwork to lower intraocular pressure (laser trabeculoplasty), or cause contracture of the peripheral iris (laser iridoplasty or gonioplasty).

Laser Iridotomy

1. Indicated for treatment of conditions associated with pupillary block, most commonly acute and chronic angle closure glaucoma.
2. May be performed with argon blue-green or Nd:YAG lasers.
3. Guidelines for treatment:
    a) Administer 2% to 4% pilocarpine for two to three doses to place iris on stretch.

b) Administer topical anesthetic and use Abraham (or similar) contact lens.

c) Treat outer one-third of superior iris, preferably superonasally (to avoid potential macular injury); also avoid treatment directly at 12 o'clock position as accumulation of air bubbles may prevent completion of treatment; when penetration achieved, one generally sees a burst of pigment and can usually visualize the anterior lens capsule.

d) Parameters for treatment with argon laser: 50 to 100 μm spot size, 500 to 2000 mW power, and 0.05 to 0.2 seconds duration; settings may vary depending on iris pigmentation and thickness of iris stroma.

e) Parameters for treatment with Nd:YAG laser: approximately 70 μm spot size, 3 to 10 mJ power, 1 to 3 pulses per burst.

4. Complications:

a) Corneal epithelial or endothelial burns with argon laser; may see "shattered glass" endothelial injury with Nd:YAG.

b) Focal nonprogressive lenticular opacities.

c) Transient elevation of intraocular pressure (8 mmHg or more in 30%–35% of argon and Nd:YAG iridotomies in one study); may be blunted by preoperative and postoperative administration of apraclonidine (Iopidine), an α-adrenergic agonist that reduces aqueous flow; postoperative monitoring for 1 to 2 hours after treatment is necessary.

d) Transient postoperative inflammation (may cause development of posterior synechiae, more commonly after argon laser iridotomy).

e) Bleeding with Nd:YAG laser (due to lack of thermal coagulative effects seen with argon laser); should avoid iris vessels; bleeding usually transient and can be decreased by gentle pressure with Abraham lens, though occasional hyphema may occur.

f) Closure of iridotomy secondary to proliferation of iris pigment epithelium; occurs in up to 30% of patients after argon laser iridotomy; easily reopened with light retreatment; rare (<1%) after Nd:YAG iridotomy.

Argon Laser Trabeculoplasty

1. Indicated for open angle glaucoma uncontrolled by maximum tolerated medical therapy.

2. Most effective in primary open angle glaucoma, pseudoexfoliative glaucoma, and pigmentary glaucoma; generally ineffective in uveitic glaucomas and developmental and juvenile glaucomas.

3. An initial clinically significant intraocular pressure reduction

occurs in 70% to 90% of patients; the effect is usually maximal by 4 to 6 weeks; the typical intraocular pressure reduction is 6 to 9 mmHg; 5-year success rate is approximately 50%.

4. Treatment may be repeated though intraocular pressure effect generally less than with initial treatment; the likelihood of a sustained postoperative intraocular pressure rise is greater with retreatment.

5. Believed to increase aqueous outflow and lower intraocular pressure by tightening trabecular beams or stimulating cellular activity in the trabecular meshwork or both.

6. Guidelines for treatment with argon blue-green laser:
   a) Apply topical anesthetic and use Goldmann-type gonioscopy lens.
   b) Treat at midportion of trabecular meshwork at junction of pigmented and nonpigmented meshwork.
   c) Treatment endpoint: blanching of tissue or small bubble formation.
   d) May treat 180° or 360°; generally 20 to 25 applications per quadrant for total of 80 to 100 over 360°.
   e) Typical treatment parameters: 50 μm spot size, 0.1 second duration, and 500 to 1500 mW power.
   f) Treat postoperatively with topical corticosteroid for 4 to 7 days.

7. Complications:
   a) Transient postoperative intraocular pressure rise (according to one study, >5 mmHg in 34% of patients and >10 mmHg in 12%); may be reduced by preoperative and postoperative administration of apraclonidine; postoperative monitoring of intraocular pressure is necessary for 1 to 2 hours.
   b) Peripheral anterior synechiae (more common with more posteriorly placed burns).
   c) Transient mild postoperative anterior uveitis.
   d) Corneal epithelial burns.
   e) Microscopic hemorrhages (rare).

Argon Laser Iridoplasty (Gonioplasty) Argon laser iridoplasty may be indicated to eliminate appositional closure or widen the angle in such conditions as plateau iris syndrome, nanophthalmos, and angle closure following scleral buckling surgery or panretinal photocoagulation. It may also be used in conjunction with argon laser trabeculoplasty in areas where the angle is narrow or prominent iris rolls are present.

1. Guidelines for treatment:
   a) Topical anesthetic applied and Abraham or goniolens used.
   b) Ten to 15 applications per quadrant placed to contract iris and open angle; should avoid confluent burns to decrease likelihood of developing iris atrophy.
   c) Typical treatment parameters (relatively long burns of low intensity): 200 to 500 μm spot size, 0.2 to 0.5 seconds duration, and 200 to 500 mW power.
2. Complications
   a) Iris atrophy (see above)
   b) Transient mild iritis
   c) Transient postoperative intraocular pressure rise
   d) Corneal endothelial burns

Selected Readings

Anterior Segment Anatomy and Aqueous Humor Dynamics

Glaucoma, lens, and anterior segment trauma. Basic and clinical science course, section 8. San Francisco: American Academy of Ophthalmology, 1989, pp. 24–26.

Kaufman PL. Aqueous humor dynamics. In: Tasman W, Jaeger EA, eds. Duane's clinical ophthalmology. Philadelphia: JB Lippincott, 1985, vol. 3, pp. 1–24.

Shields MB. Aqueous humor dynamics. I. Anatomy and Physiology. In: Textbook of glaucoma, 3rd ed. Baltimore: Williams and Wilkins, 1992, chap. 2, pp. 5–36.

Gonioscopy

Palmberg P. Gonioscopy. In: Ritch R, Shields MB, Krupin T, eds. The glaucomas. St. Louis: CV Mosby, 1989, vol. 1, chap. 18, pp. 345–59.

Glaucoma, lens, and anterior segment trauma. Basic and clinical science course, section 8. San Francisco: American Academy of Ophthalmology, 1989, pp. 32–37.

Principles of Perimetry in Glaucoma

Anderson DR. Perimetry: with and without automation, 2nd ed. St. Louis: CV Mosby, 1987.

Drance SM, Anderson DR, eds. Automatic perimetry in glaucoma. A practical guide. Orlando, Florida: Grune and Stratton, 1985.

Primary Open Angle Glaucoma

Primary open angle glaucoma. Preferred practice pattern. San Francisco:
    American Academy of Ophthalmology, 1989, pp. 1–31.
Glaucomas suspect. Preferred practice pattern. San Francisco: American
    Academy of Ophthalmology, 1989, pp.1–8.
Hoskins HD Jr, Kass MA. Primary open-angle glaucoma. In: Becker-Shaffer's
    Diagnosis and therapy of the glaucomas, 6th ed. St. Louis: CV Mosby,
    1989, chap. 18, pp. 277–307.

Normal Tension (Low Tension) Glaucoma

Werner EB. Low-tension glaucoma. In: Ritch R, Shields MB, Krupin T, eds.
    The glaucomas. St. Louis: CV Mosby, 1989; vol. 2, chap. 44, pp. 797–812.
Levene RZ. Low tension glaucoma: a critical review and new material. Surv
    Ophthalmol 1980;24:621–64.

Pseudoexfoliation Syndrome

Skuta GL. Pseudoexfoliation syndrome, pigment dispersion syndrome, and
    the associated glaucomas. In: Tasman W, Jaeger EA, eds. Duane's
    clinical ophthalmology. Philadelphia: JB Lippincott, 1989, vol. 3, chap.
    54B, pp. 1–10.
Layden WE. Exfoliation syndrome. In: Ritch R, Shields MB, Krupin T, eds.
    The glaucomas. St. Louis: CV Mosby, 1989; vol. 2, chap. 56, pp. 997–
    1015.

Pigment Dispersion Syndrome

Skuta GL. Pseudoexfoliation syndrome, pigment dispersion syndrome, and
    the associated glaucomas. In: Tasman W, Jaeger EA, eds. Duane's
    clinical ophthalmology. Philadelphia: JB Lippincott, 1989; vol. 3, chap.
    54B, pp. 10–17.
Richardson TM. Pigmentary glaucoma. In: Ritch R, Shields MB, Krupin T,
    eds. The glaucomas. St. Louis: CV Mosby, 1989; vol. 2, chap. 55, pp.
    981–95.

Corticosteroid-Induced Glaucoma

Kass MA, Johnson T. Corticosteroid-induced glaucoma. In: Ritch R, Shields
    MB, Krupin T, eds. The glaucomas. St. Louis: CV Mosby, 1989; vol. 2,
    chap. 64, pp. 1161–68.
Shields MB. Steroid-induced glaucoma. In: Textbook of glaucoma, 3rd ed.
    Baltimore: Williams and Wilkins, 1992; chap. 20, pp. 374–80.

Glaucoma and Increased Episcleral Venous Pressure

Weinreb RN, Jeng S, Goldstick BJ. Glaucoma secondary to elevated episcleral
    venous pressure. In: Ritch R, Shields MB, Krupin T, eds. The glaucomas.
    St. Louis: CV Mosby, 1989; vol. 2, chap. 62, pp. 1127–40.

Shields MB. Glaucomas associated with elevated episcleral venous pressure. In: Textbook of glaucoma, 3rd ed. Baltimore: Williams and Wilkins, 1992; chap. 17, pp. 329–335.

Uveitis-Associated Glaucoma

Alward WLM. Uveitic glaucoma. In: Tasman W, Jaeger EA, eds. Duane's clinical ophthalmology. Philadelphia: JB Lippincott, 1989; vol. 3, chap. 54D, pp. 1–11.
Krupin T, Feitl ME. Glaucoma associated with uveitis. In: Ritch R, Shields MB, Krupin T, eds. The glaucomas. St. Louis: CV Mosby, 1989; vol. 2, chap. 67, pp. 1205–23.

Lens-Induced Glaucoma

Richter C, Epstein DL. Lens-induced open-angle glaucoma. In: Ritch R, Shields MB, Krupin T, eds. The glaucomas. St. Louis: CV Mosby, 1989; vol. 2, chap. 57, pp. 1017–26.
Liebmann JM, Ritch R. Glaucoma secondary to lens intumescence and dislocation. In: Ritch R, Shields MB, Krupin T, eds. The glaucomas. St. Louis: CV Mosby, 1989; vol. 2, chap. 58, pp. 1027–45.
Gressel MG. Lens-induced glaucoma. In: Tasman W, Jaeger EA, eds. Duane's clinical ophthalmology. Philadelphia: JB Lippincott, 1989; vol. 3, chap. 54A, pp. 1–9.

Angle Closure Glaucoma

Lowe RF, Ritch R. Angle-closure glaucoma. In: Ritch R, Shields MB, Krupin T, eds. The glaucomas. St. Louis: CV Mosby, 1989; vol. 2, section III, chap. 46–48, pp. 825–64.
Hoskins HD Jr, Kass MA. Angle-closure glaucoma with pupillary block. In: Becker-Shaffer's Diagnosis and Therapy of the glaucomas, 6th ed. St. Louis: CV Mosby, 1989; chap. 16, pp. 208–37.
Skuta GL. The primary and secondary angle closure glaucomas. In: Podos SM, Yanoff M, eds. Textbook of ophthalmology. New York: Gower, in press.
Simmons RJ, Belcher CD III, Dallow RL. Primary angle-closure glaucoma. In: Tasman W, Jaeger EA, eds. Duane's clinical ophthalmology. Philadelphia: JB Lippincott, 1985; vol. 3, chap. 53, pp. 1–32.

Neovascular Glaucoma

Wand M. Neovascular glaucoma. In: Ritch R, Shields MB, Krupin T, eds. The glaucomas. St. Louis: CV Mosby, 1989; vol. 2, chap. 60, pp. 1063–1110.
Deuker DK. Neovascular glaucoma. In: Epstein DL. Chandler and Grant's Glaucoma, 3rd ed. Philadelphia: Lea and Febiger, 1986; chap. 24, pp. 378–90.

Iridocorneal Endothelial (ICE) Syndrome

Shields MB. Progressive essential iris atrophy, Chandler's syndrome, and the iris-nevus (Cogan-Reese) syndrome: a spectrum of disease. Surv Ophthalmol 1979;24:3–20.

Shields MB, Bourgeois JE. Glaucomas associated with primary disorders of the corneal endothelium. In: Ritch R, Shields MB, Krupin T, eds. The glaucomas. St. Louis: CV Mosby, 1989; vol 2., chap. 54, pp. 963–77.

Ciliary Block Glaucoma

Luntz MH, Rosenblatt M. Malignant glaucoma. Surv Ophthalmol 1987;32:73–93.

Simmons RJ, Thomas JV, Yaqub MK. Malignant glaucoma. In: Ritch R, Shields MB, Krupin T, eds. The glaucomas. St. Louis: CV Mosby, 1989; vol. 2, chap. 70, pp. 1251–63.

Primary Infantile Glaucoma

DeLuise VP, Anderson DR. Primary infantile glaucoma (congenital glaucoma). Surv Ophthalmol 1983;28:1–19.

Hoskins HD Jr, Kass MA. Developmental and childhood glaucoma. In: Becker-Shaffer's Diagnosis and therapy of the glaucomas, 6th ed. St. Louis: CV Mosby, 1989; chap. 21, pp. 355–81.

Axenfeld-Rieger Syndrome

Shields MB, Buckley E, Klintworth GK, Thresher R. Axenfeld-Rieger syndrome. A spectrum of developmental disorders. Surv Ophthalmol 1985;29:387–409.

Shields MB. Axenfeld-Rieger syndrome: a theory of mechanism and distinctions from the iridocorneal endothelial syndrome. Trans Am Ophthalmol Soc 1983;81:736–84.

Hypotony

Pederson JE. Hypotony. In: Tasman W, Jaeger EA, eds. Duane's clinical ophthalmology. Philadelphia: JB Lippincott, 1984; vol. 3, chap. 58, pp. 1–8.

Pederson JE. Ocular hypotony. In: Ritch R, Shields MB, Krupin T, eds. The glaucomas. St. Louis: CV Mosby, 1989; vol. 1, chap. 13, pp. 281–90.

Medical Therapy of Glaucoma

Hoskins HD Jr, Kass MA. Adrenergic antagonists. In: Becker-Shaffer's Diagnosis and therapy of the glaucomas, 6th ed. St. Louis: CV Mosby, 1989; chap. 25, pp. 453–69.

Shields MB. Adrenergic inhibitors. In: Textbook of glaucoma, 3rd ed. Baltimore: Williams and Wilkins, 1992; chap. 27, pp. 480–499.

Hoskins HD Jr, Kass MA. Adrenergic agonists. In: Becker-Shaffer's
Diagnosis and therapy of the glaucomas, 6th ed. St. Louis: CV Mosby,
1989; chap. 24, pp. 435–52.

Shields MB. Adrenergic stimulators. In: Textbook of glaucoma, 3rd ed.
Baltimore: Williams and Wilkins, 1992; chap. 26, pp. 462–79.

Hoskins HD Jr, Kass MA. Cholinergic drugs. In: Becker-Shaffer's Diagnosis
and therapy of the glaucomas, 6th ed. St. Louis: CV Mosby, 1989; chap.
23, pp. 420–34.

Shields MB. Cholinergic stimulators. In: Textbook of glaucoma, 3rd ed.
Baltimore: Williams and Wilkins, 1992; chap. 25, 446–61.

Friedland BR, Maren TH: Carbonic anhydrase inhibitors. In: Ritch R,
Shields MB, Krupin T, eds. The glaucomas. St. Louis: CV Mosby, 1989;
vol. 1, chap. 26, pp. 539–49.

Hoskins HD Jr, Kass MA. Carbonic anhydrase inhibitors. In: Becker-Shaffer's
Diagnosis and therapy of the glaucomas, 6th ed. St. Louis: CV Mosby,
1989; chap. 26, pp. 470–84.

Feitl ME, Krupin T. Hyperosmotic agents. In: Ritch R, Shields MB, Krupin T,
eds. The glaucomas. St. Louis: CV Mosby, 1989; vol. 1, chap. 27, pp.
551–55.

Hoskins HD Jr, Kass MA. Hyperosmotic agents. In: Becker-Shaffer's
Diagnosis and therapy of the glaucomas, 6th ed. St. Louis: CV Mosby,
1989; chap. 27, pp. 485–91.

Glaucoma Laser Surgery

Higginbotham EJ, Shahbazi MF. Laser therapy in glaucoma: an overview and
update. Int Ophthalmol Clin 1990;30(3):187–97.

Shields MB. Surgery of the anterior chamber angle. In: Textbook of
glaucoma, 3rd ed. Baltimore: Williams and Wilkins, 1992; chap. 34, pp.
538–60.

Shields MB. Surgery of the iris. In: Textbook of glaucoma, 3rd ed. Baltimore:
Williams and Wilkins, 1992; chap. 35, pp. 561–76.

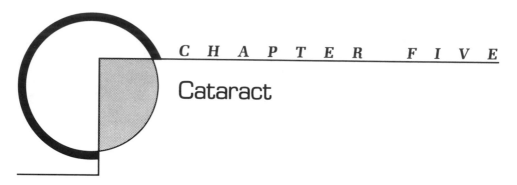

Cataract

Thomas A. Farrell, M.D.

General Considerations

A cataract is any opacification of the crystalline lens. However, the term is reserved primarily for lenticular opacities that disturb or interfere with visual acuity. Epidemiologic studies find that 10% of Americans have cataracts, and more than 50% of the population over age 65 are affected (Liebowitz et al. 1980; National Advisory Eye Council 1987).

Etiology

1. Age: 70% of Americans age 75 or greater have lens opacities.
2. Systemic diseases: diabetes mellitus (snowflakes), hypocalcemia (white spots), myotonic dystrophy (Christmas tree), Wilson's disease (sunflower).
3. Medications: corticosteroids, dose-dependent; miotics; thorazine (anterior subcapsular).
4. Trauma (mechanical, radiation).
5. Ocular inflammation or tumors.

For a complete list of all ocular and systemic associations with cataract, consult the chapter on cataracts in *Pathobiology of Ocular Disease* (Klintworth and Garner 1982).

Symptoms

1. Painless loss of vision, either distance or near, involving predominantly central vision.
2. Glare: loss of visual performance caused by light scattering within the eye, which degrades the contrast of the retinal image. Manifests as a significant degradation of vision in bright sunlight or a disturbance of vision by oncoming car headlights at night.
3. Monocular diplopia.
4. Polyopia: multiple images, most often experienced at night (e.g., automobile tail-lights are described as multiple streamers, streaks, or bubbles).

Physical Findings

Refraction

1. Retinoscopy reflex aberrations include a dull red reflex, dark spoke opacities in the peripheral reflex, or central and paracentral black "granular" opacities.
2. Myopic shift in refractive error.

Slit Lamp Biomicroscopy Lens opacifications are classified according to the zone of lens involvement (Figs. 5.1–5.4) (Chylack 1985).

FIGURE 5.1. Anatomy of the Adult Crystalline Lens

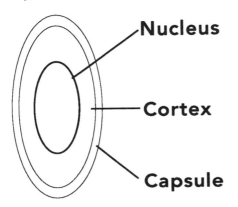

Nucleus

Cortex

Capsule

FIGURE 5.2. Nuclear Sclerotic Cataract

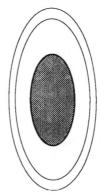

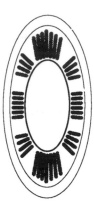

FIGURE 5.3. Cortical Cataract

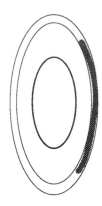

FIGURE 5.4. Posterior Subcapsular Cataract

Nuclear sclerosis: progressive compression and hardening of the lens nucleus is accompanied by gradual darkening of the chromophores in the nucleus, from yellow to green-brown to red-brown (Fig. 5.2). The sclerosis of the nucleus produces the myopic shift in the refraction, and the color changes cause a late decrease in hue discrimination.

Cortical cataract: spokes of interfibrillar protein-deficient fluid accumulations form in the cortical zone of the lens. These spokes are made up of younger, newer lens fibers that encircle the nucleus and radiate from the lens equator into the anterior and posterior cortex (Fig. 5.3). Cortical spokes can take on a significant amount of fluid so that the lens anteroposterior dimensions increase in size (intumescent cataract).

Posterior supcapsular cataract: crystalline, granular opacities found in the posterior subcapsular zone form a coalescence of vacuoles and flakes (Fig. 5.4). These opacities are in the youngest fibers that have migrated posteriorly from the lens epithelium.

Mature cataract: a mature cataract is one with a total opacification of the lens, causing the cortex to be completely white. A mature cataract with liquefied cortex that floats the sclerotic nucleus, usually by gravity to the bottom of the capsule, is known as a morgagnian cataract.

Additional Evaluations   A complete ocular examination including refraction, tonometry, pupillary responses, biomicroscopy of the anterior segment, and dilated fundus examination is essential to begin evaluations for cataract.

Macular function assessment: pinhole visual acuity is an easy, inexpensive, well-tested method of assessing macular function if performed with patience. An improved acuity with the pinhole is most likely due to the presence of refractive changes induced by the lens opacities, while poorer acuity suggests macular dysfunction. Methods using potential acuity meters, laser interferometry, and contrast sensitivity tests are not standardized to date, and their reliability has not been established (American Academy of Ophthalmology 1990).

Glare testing: various devices for glare testing are available but are also not standardized. A simple, quick and inexpensive method of glare assessment can be made by having the patient read the standard Snellen acuity chart through a 1-inch viewing aperture in a white 5-by-8-inch card held at 33 cm. A 75 to 100 watt standard reading light illuminates the card face. Visual acuity is tested with the light off and again with it on. Patients with 20/40 to 20/50 acuity and posterior subcapsular cataracts typically have 20/100 or poorer vision with this test.

Echography: B scan ultrasonography should be performed any time a cataract prevents visualization of the posterior retina, to rule out other causes for the reduced acuity that would change the method of surgical intervention or treatment, such as retinal detachment or tumor mass.

Differential Diagnosis Visually significant cataracts are usually obvious, and few ophthalmic disorders mimic them. confusion can exist when the root cause for the loss of vision is not recognized in the presence of lenticular opacities.

Other Causes of Painless Visual Loss

- Macular degeneration
- Diabetic macular edema
- Anterior ischemic optic neuropathy
- Retinal detachment
- Myopic degeneration
- Posterior uveitis (cystoid macular edema in pars planitis)

Other Causes of Glare

- Posterior uveitis
- Retinal ischemia

Cataract Management

Medical Management

There are no established effective medical therapies for cataracts to date (Chylack 1985). Aldose reductase inhibitors may prove beneficial in diabetic cataracts. Discontinuation of known cataractogenic medications (e.g., corticosteroids) can prevent progression. Myopic shifts may be corrected with spectacles.

Surgical Management

Indications for surgery are as follows:

1. Subjective: loss of patient's ability to function in usual capacity.
2. Objective: vision loss in the presence of cataractous lens changes consistent with the patient's visual acuity.
3. Educational: patient's decision that potential benefits of surgery outweigh the cost, demands, and possible complications. This requires appropriate instruction of the risks and benefits of surgery.
4. Other indications: sight-threatening lens-incited diseases (phacomorphic or phacolytic glaucoma) or the need to adequately visualize the fundus to provide treatment and assessments of other potentially serious ocular conditions (e.g., adequately clear medium for photocoagulation of retinal proliferative vascular disease).

Preoperative Assessment

General Medical Evaluation The patient should be in the best state of health possible. Collaborate with the patient's primary physician to ensure the best medical management of chronic obstructive pulmonary disease, arteriosclerotic cardiovascular disease, bleeding disorders, or diabetes mellitus.

Current Medications The surgeon must review all patient medications as some may change the timing, technique, or possible outcome of surgery (e.g., aspirin or coumadin). It is best to have the patient's primary physician manage the temporary discontinuation of the medications (especially coumadin) prior to surgery. In general, aspirin-like medications should be stopped 7 to 10 days before surgery. Note that multiple medications, both prescription and over-the-counter formulations, have components that can prolong the bleeding time, prothrombin time (PT), or partial thromboplastin time (PTT). See Table 5.1.

TABLE 5.1

Medications that may cause increased bleeding during eye surgery:

Acetylsalicylic acid	Excedrin	Naprosyn
Advil	4-Way Cold Tablets	Naproxen
Alka-Seltzer	Feldene	Nuprin
Anacin	Fenoprofen	Orudis
Anaprox	Fiorinal	Panwarfin
Ansaid	Flurbiprofen	Pepto-Bismol
Ascriptin	Heparin	Persantine
Aspirin	Ibuprofen	Phenylbutazone
Bufferin	Indocin	Piroxicam
Butazolidin	Indomethacin	Ponstel
Clinoril	Ketoprofen	Rufen
CoAdvil	Measurin	Sulindac
Coumadin	Meclofenamate	Tolectin
Diclofenac	Meclomen	Tolmetin
Diflunisal	Medipren	Trendar
Dipyridamole	Mefenamic	Triaminicin
Disalcid	Midol	Ursinus
Dolobid	Momentum	Vanquish
Ecotrin	Motrin	Voltaren
Empirin	Nalfon	Warfarin

Medications that do not have to be stopped and may be continued as needed:

Acetaminophen	Darvon	Propoxyphene
Allerest	Datril	Trental
Anacin-3	Excedrin PM	Trilisate
Darvocet	Panadol	Tylenol

Mental Status   Patient must be able to comprehend the nature of the surgery and be able to participate in postoperative care. If not, suitable arrangements must be made in advance with the patient's family, friends, or community service agencies.

Ophthalmologic Management

1. External eye should be free of concurrent lid, external, or ocular infections. Deep-set eyes or prominent brows may interfere with ease of surgery.

2. Intraocular pressure control should be optimal.
3. Anterior segment assessment including the following:
   a) Cornea: especially status of the endothelium. Low cell counts may alter type of cataract surgery, and consideration of a corneal transplant at the time of surgery if edema is present.
   b) Anterior chamber depth.
   c) Anterior chamber angle gonioscopy if considering an anterior chamber angle intraocular lens.
   d) Pupillary dilation: avoid dilating the patient the day before surgery as this may result in less mydriasis on the day of surgery.
   e) Lens position.
4. Posterior segment evaluation including the macula and the peripheral retina. Any retinal breaks should be prophylactically treated if appropriate.
5. Special tests:
   a) Keratometry (K): check calibration; repeat measurements for unusually high or low values (i.e., < 40 or > 46 diopters [D]); average K values should be within 1 D of each other.
   b) Biometry: intraocular lens calculation. Many formulas are available to calculate the power of the intraocular lens (IOL) to be used in surgery. Parameters required include the A constant for the IOL, axial length, and keratometry. Formulas should also be modified based on an individual surgeon's past results. Check calibration; repeat measurement if eye is unusually short or long (i.e., < 21 or > 25 mm); compare axial length of both eyes—they should be within 0.2 mm or less of each other. Select IOL power appropriate for patient's needs and refraction of fellow eye (to avoid problems with aniseikonia postoperatively). Err on the side of a little myopia.

Informed Consent   The nature of the surgery, all its potential risks, complications, and likelihood of success must be discussed with the patient (best with a third party present who is a friend or relative of the patient). It is incumbent upon the operating surgeon to obtain the consent personally. Patients remember instructions best when given both verbally and in writing.

Prophylactic Preoperative Antibiotics   There is no consensus on this issue (American Academy of Ophthalmology 1989). The operating surgeon should use antibiotics in a judicious, consistent, and appropriate manner during the perioperative period in keeping with her or his views. Antimicrobials do not supplant proper aseptic surgical technique.

Optical Correction of Aphakia

Intraocular Lens Implantation

This is the current standard of care for visual correction after the cataract has been removed.

Posterior Chamber IOL   This implant constitutes 96% of cataract operations. An adequate posterior capsule of the lens is required to insert a posterior chamber lens. Multiple designs of the basic optical disc (optic) with flexible arms (haptics) for support are used and include lenses made of one piece of polymethylmethacrylate (PMMA), investigational foldable lenses, and innovative multifocal designs (Duffey et al. 1990).

Multifocal IOLs typically combine refractive and diffractive optics to produce simultaneous focusing of both distant and near objects. Only one image is perceived at a time. With the increase in depth of field comes a decrease in contrast, which is one of the significant drawbacks with this type of IOL.

A posterior chamber intraocular lens with a biconvex or planoconvex optic design has been shown to be associated with capsular opacification in 7% of cases after 5 years, as opposed to other lens optic designs for which posterior capsular opacification was 40% or more after 5 years (Born and Ryan 1990).

Anterior Chamber IOL   A backup lens used when implanting a posterior chamber IOL is not feasible because there is a large posterior capsule tear or primary intracapsular extraction has been performed. One anterior chamber lens design has been shown to have fewer complications (hyphema, uveitis, and glaucoma): the multiflex design, one piece of PMMA with flexible haptics providing four-point anterior chamber angle support. Anterior chamber IOLs are not recommended for patients with glaucoma. Posterior chamber IOLs sutured in place (either to the iris or haptic fixation to the ciliary sulcus with transcleral fixation) are under investigation as an alternative to the anterior chamber IOL (Lubniewski et al. 1990).

IOL Advantages

1. No distorting magnification
2. No significant additional optical correction necessary for functional vision

3. Full field of vision
4. Cosmetically very acceptable

IOL Disadvantages

1. Additional surgical manipulation to insert
2. Dislocation, decentration, and inflammation
3. Corneal endothelial damage over time
4. Secondary hemorrhages and glaucoma

Aphakic Contact Lens

This lens is used when no IOL can be implanted and there is good vision in the fellow eye. A contact lens will reduce the difference in image size between the two eyes (assuming the fellow eye is phakic) to a tolerable 8%. Some ocular conditions preclude success with a contact lens (e.g., dry eyes). Many elderly patients have problems managing the care and handling of contact lenses.

Advantages

1. Minimized image magnification
2. Can reduce or correct irregular astigmatism
3. Full field of vision

Disadvantages

1. Variable visual acuity
2. Cost; lens replacement for loss, damage and deposits, and frequent follow-up office visits
3. Manipulation; cleaning, inserting, and storing

Spectacles

Aphakic spectacles are still prescribed in cases where no intraocular lens implantation is feasible and contact lens wear is not possible. This is an uncommon occurrence today. Precise optical fitting, vertex distance, and pantoscopic tilt are critical to ensure successful aphakic spectacle wear.

Advantages   They are safe.

Disadvantages

1. Image magnification (20 + %)
2. Cosmetically unattractive

3. Serious spherical aberrations (image jump, ring scotoma) affecting ability to ambulate and operate a motor vehicle

---

Cataract Surgery

Methods

1. Intracapsular extraction: < 10%
2. Extracapsular extraction: > 90%
   a) Planned extracapsular extraction > 65% (Leaming 1990)
   b) Phacoemulsification: > 35% (Leaming 1990)

Anesthesia

Perioperative Sedation   Many patients tolerate local anesthesia without the addition of any sedation. Midazolam HCl, 0.5 to 1.0 ml intravenously just before injecting the local anesthetic, acts as a sedative and amnesiac and is short acting. Other options are

1. meperidine HCl (50 mg i.m.), alone or with
2. hydroxyzine HCl (50 mg i.m.), and
3. diazepam (2–5 mg i.m. or i.v.).

Beware that all these drugs can produce respiratory depression and hypotension.

Local Anesthetic Agents   One common mix includes lidocaine 2%, with or without epinephrine, mixed in equal amounts with bupivicaine 0.75% with hyaluronidase (150 National Formulary [NF] units) to promote tissue absorption.

1. Advantages over a general anesthetic include less systemic stress, less postoperative pain, less postoperative nausea, and earlier ambulation.
2. Disadvantages include less control of the patient, possible retrobulbar hemorrhage preventing the operation, perforation of the globe, optic nerve damage from the needle, or severe respiratory depression from intrasheath injection, and cardiac or respiratory depression from systemic absorption.

Techniques
1. Facial block can be achieved by one of four methods:
   a) Nadbath: infiltration of the area just posterior and inferior to the auditory meatus (behind the ear) where the facial nerve exits the stylomastoid foramen.

    b)   O'Brien, infiltration of the nerve just anterior to the tragus of the ear.

    c)   Atkinson, infiltration of the facial nerve branches in the area halfway from the tragus to the lateral canthus.

    d)   VanLint, infiltration of facial nerve branches just lateral to the lateral canthus.

2. Retrobulbar block: the traditional method has the patient looking up and in while the retrobulbar needle is introduced into the muscle cone from below and lateral to the globe. The needle pierces the orbital septum at the junction of the middle and lateral one-third of the inferior orbital rim. Anesthetic mix of 3 to 5 ml is all that is needed to provide prompt anesthesia, pupil dilation, and akinesia.

    a)   Advantages are excellent and rapid-onset anesthesia and akinesia.

    b)   Disadvantages are globe perforation and optic nerve penetration (especially with long and sharp disposable needles), and retrobulbar hemorrhage.

    c)   In a modified retrobulbar technique, the patient looks straight ahead while a 1.5-inch or shorter retrobulbar needle is directed into the muscle cone. In this way, one avoids placing the optic nerve in the path of the retrobulbar needle, which is safer; however, there is a slower onset of anesthesia and akinesia.

3. Peribulbar block: This technique is gaining wider acceptance and involves the injection of larger volumes of anesthetic outside the muscle cone, posterior to the orbital septum (Weiss and Deichman 1989). It is a safer technique in that it avoids the risk of optic nerve injury but requires more time to take as well as a greater risk of systemic side effects, and the akinesia may not be as effective as a retrobulbar block.

Surgical Techniques

All cataract surgeons use fairly standard techniques that are comfortable, easy, and may even be unique to them in performing their surgery, so their outcomes are optimized and consistent. The following is a relatively generic cataract extraction procedure. Cataract surgery in the United States is currently done under the operating microscope.

    Bridle suture: not required unless the eye is deep-set.

    Peritomy: incisions are more accurately placed and wound closure is simpler with a conjunctival flap; also perilimbal hemostasis is easier.

Incision: grooved, step, or scleral tunnel types all should enter the anterior chamber in the same place, anterior to the trabecular meshwork. The incision must be large enough to admit instruments into the eye without stripping Descemet's membrane and be adequate for nucleus expression in planned extracapsular extraction. Posterior sutures minimize astigmatism, and step or beveled incisions theoretically promote better wound healing by virtue of their greater surface area.

Capsulotomy: for extracapsular extractions, an adequate anterior capsule opening must be fashioned with scissors, with cystotome, or by controlled tearing (capsulorhexis). Many elect to use viscoelastic substances to optimize anterior chamber depth control, protect the corneal endothelium, and enhance pupillary dilation. Viscoelastics or balanced salt solution may also be used for loosening the nucleus in preparation for phacoemulsification or expression.

Lens material removal: after either manual expression or phacoemulsification of the nucleus, the residual lens remnants (mainly cortical fibers) may be aspirated with manual or automated systems, with their respective advantages and shortcomings. Manual systems have the benefit of not requiring expensive backup or skilled ancillary staff and are easily repaired with items universally available. Automated units are generally faster and part of phacoemulsification units.

Wound closure: multiple single mattress sutures, double cross-stitch sutures, or running sutures are the surgeon's choice. Individual mattress sutures may be removed to control postoperative with-the-rule astigmatism earlier than running or cross-stitch suture closure techniques.

Postoperative Management

1. Prior to discharge, the patient's vital signs should be stable, he or she should have mild eye pain if any, and be able to take liquids by mouth. The follow-up appointment should be confirmed.
2. Postoperative medications usually include an antibiotic-steroid combination, which is continued for several weeks at the discretion of the surgeon.
3. Restrictions on activity depend on the size of the incision and also should be individualized to the particular patient.
4. Follow-up appointments should generally occur at 1 day, 1 week, 3 weeks, and 6 weeks postoperatively, but also should be tailored

to the particular setting (American Academy of Ophthalmology 1989).

Special Surgical Situations
Subluxated and Dislocated Lens

Etiology

1. Trauma.
2. Marfan's syndrome, lens usually dislocates superiorly and temporally (autosomal dominant, cardiac disease, tall stature).
3. Homocystinuria, lens usually dislocates inferiorly and nasally (autosomal recessive, mental retardation, tall stature, risk of embolism with general anesthetic).
4. Weill-Marchesani syndrome (autosomal recessive, short stature, small lenses).
5. Spherophakia.

Signs Iridodonesis, phacodonesis, appearance of zonules, high astigmatism, or high myopia.

Surgical Management

Indications

1. Visual loss uncorrectable with either phakic or aphakic correction
2. Pupillary block
3. Phacolytic glaucoma

Procedures

1. Extracapsular extraction if subluxation is minimal and adequate zonules. Caveat: systemic conditions with subluxated lens have deficient zonules.
2. Preferred method is lensectomy via pars plana (Reese and Weingeist 1987) unless nucleus is very sclerotic, then a combined approach is helpful. If the lens capsule is intact and the eye is quiet, the lens can be observed.
3. Intracapsular extraction.

Complications

1. Retinal detachment
2. Vitreous loss

Cataracts in Children

Etiology   Most common associations:

1. Down syndrome
2. Hereditary
3. Persistent hyperplastic primary vitreous
4. Convulsive disorders or central nervous system impairment (includes hyperglycemia, hypoglycemia, hypocalcemia, and galactosemia)
5. Prematurity
6. Rubella (retained fetal nuclei)

Intervention

1. Visually significant bilateral cataracts in the neonate should be treated surgically within weeks of discovery.
2. Amblyopia is the major concern, and delay in cataract removal or in visual rehabilitation may forsake an eye to 20/200 vision in spite of a successful operation.
3. Monocular cataract surgery also demands aggressive intervention to restore vision, and serious dedication and understanding of the parents in the treatment of the amblyopia (Drummond et al. 1989).

Surgery   Extracapsular extraction and limited anterior vitrectomy using a fairly large bore aspirating or cutting instrument.

Complications

1. Opacification of the posterior capsule
2. Glaucoma
3. Retinal detachment

Optical Correction

Bilateral Aphakia

1. Aphakic spectacles
2. Contact lenses

Monocular Aphakia

1. Contact lens
2. Investigational: intraocular lens, refractive surgery

Complications of Cataract Surgery

Operative Complications

Retrobulbar Hemorrhage   This may cause enough pressure on the globe to compress the central retinal artery! A retrobulbar hemorrhage can be recognized by progressive proptosis, reduced retropulsion, spreading ecchymosis, and lids that cannot be retracted from the globe. Treat by tamponade if the intraocular pressure has not occluded the central retinal artery; other measures include

1. lateral canthotomy and
2. paracentesis if the IOP is elevated or if the artery is pulsating or collapsed on ophthalmoscopy.

Expulsive Hemorrhage   A suprachoroidal hemorrhage of sufficient volume to expel intraocular contents.

1. Signs of a suprachoroidal hemorrhage
   a) Shallowing of the anterior chamber with sudden increase in the intraocular pressure
   b) Gaping of the wound with iris prolapse that will not reposit
   c) Dark-colored mounds in the pupil reflex
2. Treatment
   a) Immediate closure of the eye with 8-0 or heavier sutures (a good reason to use a temporary closure suture that is of stouter caliber than 10-0 nylon)
   b) Assess the intraocular pressure: if it is very high, perform posterior sclerotomies; if it is moderately elevated, control medically with hyperosmotic agents, carbonic anhydrase inhibitors, and topical beta-blockers until a controlled pars plana vitrectomy, lens remnant removal, and drainage of liquified suprachoroidal blood can be performed.
3. Prevention of this event is possible by observing the following:
   a) Ensure a normal blood pressure at surgery
   b) Lower intraocular pressure before entering the eye
   c) Minimize amount of retrobulbar anesthesia
   d) Elevate head of bed when operating

Vitreous Loss   Usually occurs at the time of nucleus expression during planned extracapsular extraction or with a rupture in the posterior capsule during cortex removal (Osher and Cionni 1990).

1. Treatment: meticulous cleaning of the vitreous from the wound and anterior vitrectomy.

2. Sequelae of vitreous loss:
   a) Wound leak and filtering blebs
   b) Chronic inflammation with cystoid macular edema
   c) Epithelial downgrowth and secondary glaucoma
   d) Retinal detachment
   e) Corneal decompensation and bullous keratopathy
   f) Distorted pupil
3. Prevention may be achieved by checking the following if positive vitreous pressure is noted:
   a) Check lid speculum position and traction sutures
   b) Loosen the nucleus
   c) Consider intravenous mannitol
   d) Consider iridectomy
   e) Vitreous tap: enter eye 4 mm from the limbus with a 23 gage needle; remove 0.25 cc of liquid vitreous.

Capsule Tear Implantation of a posterior chamber lens may be possible if there is adequate zonule integrity and capsule to guide the lens into the capsule bag or, with aid of a glide, to direct the lens into the ciliary sulcus (Osher and Cionni 1990).

Descemet's Membrane Detachment Usually happens at a wound site that is too small to admit the injuring surgical instrument. Treatment is as follows:

1. Unscroll with the aid of viscoelastic material and inject air into the anterior chamber to hold in place.
2. Suture in place if air is not effective or a large tear.

Dislocation of the Nucleus into the Vitreous This complication is more common for inexperienced phacoemulsification surgeons but also is possible in extracapsular extractions. Treatment is as follows:

1. Close the eye.
2. Vitrectomy and lens remnant extraction via the pars plana at an appropriate time.

Postoperative Complications

Endophthalmitis

Usually occurs early in the first week after surgery, but may be delayed longer depending on the etiologic agent. Bacterial cases present early and fungal later.

1. Signs and symptoms of pain, loss of vision, chemosis, hypopyon uveitis, and vitritis obscuring the details of the posterior retina are typical.
2. Treatment starts with a vitreous tap (or a limited vitrectomy if possible) for diagnostic cultures and intravitreal broad spectrum antibiotics such as gentamicin, cefazolin, and vancomycin. Additional high-dose antibiotics are given intravenously, subconjunctivally, and topically. The initial antibiotics are selected for optimal broad spectrum activity until gram stains and cultures isolate the causative agent, then specific antibiotics are used.
3. Fungal endophthalmitis presents serious challenges as antifungal agents are less effective in penetrating the eye, and the indolent presentation of the infection delays the diagnosis.
4. Corticosteroids are an important adjunct therapy to minimize the effects of the inflammation accompanying endophthalmitis.

Corneal Edema

1. Early corneal edema relates to trauma of surgical manipulation, from lens expression to IOL insertion, and postoperative ocular hypertension.
2. Treatment: topical corticosteroids and intraocular pressure control.
3. Bullous keratopathy is usually a late sign of endothelial damage from cataract surgery and often requires penetrating keratoplasty.

Wound Healing Problems

Leaks Treated with patching and carbonic anhydrase inhibitors or topical beta-blockers (e.g., timolol) initially, or surgical repair if serious (loss or shallowing of anterior chamber).

Iris Prolapse Repaired if seen early but later may be left alone if asymptomatic, small, and covered adequately by conjunctiva.

Astigmatism Commonly with-the-rule astigmatism is present in the early postoperative healing period. Selective suture cutting can help reduce this astigmatism, but late wound shifting can induce significant against-the-rule astigmatism. Caveat: do not rush to cut sutures before 6 weeks if there is less than 2 D of with-the-rule astigmatism. Keratorefractive surgery may be required for disabling astigmatism later.

Glaucoma

Reduce the pressure with topical beta-blockers and carbonic anhydrase inhibitors and treat the root cause if secondary to any of the following:

1. Pupillary block.
2. Inflammation.
3. Hyphema.
4. Corticosteroids.
5. Retained lens material.
6. Viscoelastic material.
7. Endophthalmitis.
8. Epithelial downgrowth (presents as a white line on the corneal endothelial surface). One can diagnose with an argon laser to the iris. It will whiten if a membrane is present. Treatment may include a total iridectomy or cyclectomy.
9. Aqueous misdirection.

Uveitis

A certain amount of postoperative intraocular inflammation is to be expected, but an uncommon sterile or noninfectious endophthalmitis can occur after

1. intraocular lens implantation,
2. injection of unsuspected toxic material into the anterior chamber.
3. retained lens material reaction.

Treatment requires differentiating the sterile severe uveitis from an infectious endophthalmitis. This is a diagnosis of exclusion.

Retinal Detachment

Occurs in less than 2% of eyes following extracapsular cataract surgery and typically presents in the first 6 months after surgery (Coonan et al. 1985; Kraff and Sanders 1990). Those at risk (who should be followed carefully during the first postoperative year) are patients with

1. retinal detachment of the fellow eye,
2. axial myopia,
3. lattice degeneration, or
4. intraoperative vitreous loss.

Cystoid Macular Edema [CME]

Clinically symptomatic CME is present in up to 2% of the patients following extracapsular cataract surgery and usually manifests as visual loss 2 to 6 months after surgery. Those at greatest risk for developing CME have had

1. surgical complications, especially vitreous loss with persistent vitreous adherence to the cataract wound, or
2. chronic postoperative inflammation.

Treatment includes corticosteroids, nonsteroidal anti-inflammatory drugs, acetazolamide, neodymium:yttrium-argon-garnet (Nd:YAG) laser severing adherent anterior segment vitreous bands, and vitrectomy in long-standing (> 6 mo) cases.

Posterior Capsule Opacification

A common sequela of extracapsular surgery that occurs in approximately 40% to 50% of patients within 5 years of the cataract surgery. A posterior chamber lens with a convex posterior surface appears to significantly reduce the incidence of posterior capsule opacification (Born and Ryan 1990).

1. Treatment is to open the capsule with a knife-needle or the Nd:YAG laser. The laser is preferred as the risks of anesthetic complications and the introduction of bacteria into the eye are eliminated.
2. Complications of Nd:YAG capsulotomy:
   a) Ocular hypertension in the immediate postlaser period that can be effectively prevented in most cases with apraclonidine drops before and after treatment.
2. Pitting of the lens.
3. Retinal detachment.

Selected Readings

American Academy of Ophthalmology. Cataract in the otherwise healthy eye. Preferred practice pattern. San Francisco: American Academy of Ophthalmology, 1989.

American Academy of Ophthalmology. Contrast sensitivity and glare testing in the evaluation of anterior segment disease. Ophthalmology 1990;97:1233–37.

Born CP, Ryan DK. Effect of intraocular lens optic design on posterior capsule opacification. J Cataract Refract Surg 1990;16:188–92.

Chylack LT. The crystalline lens and cataract. In: Pavan-Langston D, ed. Manual of ocular diagnosis and therapy. Boston: Little, Brown, 1985, Chap. 6.

Coonan P, Fung WE, Webster RD Jr, et al. The incidence of retinal detachment following extracapsular cataract extraction: a ten year study. Ophthalmology 1985;92:1096–1101.

Drummond GT, Scott WE, Keech RV. Management of monocular congenital cataracts. Arch Ophthalmol 1989;107:45–51.

Duffey RJ, Zabel RW, Linstrom RL. Multifocal intraocular lenses. J Cataract Refract Surg 1990;16:423–29.

Klintworth GK, Garner A. The causes, types, and morphology of cataracts. In: Garner A. Klintworth GK, eds. Pathobiology of ocular disease, part B. New York: Marcel Dekker, 1982, pp. 1223–72.

Kraff MC, Sanders DR. Incidence of retinal detachment following posterior chamber intraocular lens surgery. J Cataract Refract Surg 1990;15:447–80.

Leaming DV. Practice styles and preferences of ASCRS members—1989 survey. J Cataract Refract Surg 1990;16:624–32.

Liebowitz HM, Kreuger DE, Maunder LR, et al. The Framingham Eye Study monograph: an ophthalmological and epidemiological study of cataract, glaucoma, diabetic retinopathy, macular degeneration, and visual acuity in a general population of 2,631 adults, 1973–1975. Surv Ophthalmol (Suppl) 1980;24:335–610.

Lubniewski AJ, Holland EJ, VanMeter WS, Gussler D, Parelman J, Smith ME. Histologic study of eyes with transclerally sutured posterior chamber intraocular lenses. Am J Ophthalmol 1990;110:237–43.

National Advisory Eye Council. Vision research; a national plan: 1983–1987. Bethesda, Maryland: US DHHS. PHS Publ (NIH) No. 87-2755, 1987.

Osher RH, Cionni RJ. The torn posterior capsule: its intraoperative behavior, surgical management, and long-term consequences. J Cataract Refract Surg 1990;15:490–94.

Weiss JL, Deichman CB. A comparison of retrobulbar and periocular anesthesia for cataract surgery. Arch Ophthalmol 1989;107:96–98.

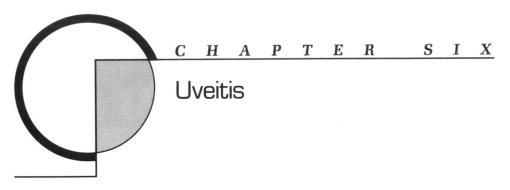

Uveitis

Michael J. Weiss, M.D., Ph.D.
Diane Kraus, M.D.

Basics of Uveitis

Uveitis History

The evaluation of a patient with uveitis should include the following information:

1. Age, sex, and race of patient.
2. History of present illness: eye symptoms, unilateral or bilateral disease, onset time and course, response to any previous treatment, and any associated systemic findings.
3. Past ocular history.
4. Past medical history: check for history of
   a) sarcoid, tuberculosis (rule out granulomatous uveitis),
   b) intestinal disease (e.g., Whipple's disease, ulcerative colitis), regional enteritis; (rule out recurrent iridocyclitis),
   c) ankylosing spondylitis, juvenile rheumatoid arthritis, HLA-B27 positivity (rule out iridocyclitis),
   d) multiple sclerosis (rule out intermediate uveitis),

   e) collagen vascular disease (rule out retinal vasculitis),
   f) urethritis (rule out Reiter's syndrome), and
   g) immunosuppressive disease (rule out endogenous
       opportunistic infection).
5. Travel history
   a) San Joaquin Valley (rule out coccidiomycoses).
   b) Ohio-Mississippi-Missouri Valley (rule out histoplasmosis).
   c) Central and South America (rule out cysticercosis, amebiasis,
       onchocerciasis).
   d) West Africa (rule out onchocerciasis).
   e) Mid Atlantic, New England area (rule out Lyme disease).
6. Sexual history: ?sexually active, ?sexual orientation, ?number of
   sexual contacts, ?history of venereal disease (rule out ocular
   syphilis, cytomegalovirus [CMV] retinitis).
7. Dietary history: Did mother of patient ingest undercooked meat
   (e.g., steak tartar) during her pregnancy? (rule out toxoplasmosis).
8. Pet history: ?exposure to cats or dogs (rule out toxoplasmosis and
   toxocariasis).
9. Drug history: ?intravenous drug use (rule out opportunistic
   infection such as fungal endophthalmitis, CMV retinitis).

Criteria Used for the Classification of Uveitis

Onset and Duration of the Disease

Acute uveitis is defined as inflammatory activity that, with appropriate intervention, lasts less than 3 months (usually between 2 and 6 wks). The inflammatory activity may recur (acute-recurrent), but between episodes, the patient is inflammation-free. In contrast, chronic uveitis is characterized by inflammatory activity that persists beyond 3 months despite appropriate intervention. Periodic exacerbation of the baseline chronic inflammatory activity may also occur (chronic-recurrent). Both acute and chronic uveitis may have a sudden or insidious onset.

Severity of Inflammatory Activity

Anterior segment inflammation should be graded as shown in Tables 6.1 and 6.2. A grading system of vitreous inflammatory activity utilizing photographic standards for vitritis has also been proposed. In addition to these grading systems, the International Uveitis Study Group has suggested that severity of disease be graded according to the extent of visual damage. Severe inflammation is defined as a greater than 50% visual loss as assessed by visual acuity or electroretinogram (ERG), whereas mild inflammation would be less than a 50% loss.

TABLE 6.1

Grading of aqueous cells

Cells/Slit Beam Field	Grade
1–2	Rare
3–5	Trace
5–10	1+
10–20	2+
20–50	3+
Over 50	4+

Light intensity and magnification should be maximal. The slit beam should be 1 mm long and 1 mm wide.

Anatomic Region of Involvement

Iritis: inflammatory activity confined to the anterior chamber.

Iridocyclitis: iritis plus cells in the retrolental space signifying ciliary body involvement.

Intermediate uveitis: characterized by inflammatory findings predominantly at the pars plana and far retinal periphery.

Posterior uveitis: characterized by inflammatory findings located posterior to the vitreous base. Depending on the primary site of involvement, posterior uveitis may be subclassified focal, multifocal, or diffuse choroiditis, chorioretinitis, retinochoroiditis, or neurouveitis.

Panuveitis: inflammatory findings involving the entire uveal tract.

TABLE 6.2

Grading of aqueous flare

Amount of Flare	Grade
Faint (barely seen)	1+
Moderate (iris details clearly seen)	2+
Marked (iris details hazily seen)	3+
Intense (plastic aqueous with fibrin)	4+

Light intensity and magnification should be maximal. The slit beam should be 1 mm long and 1 mm wide.

Response to Steroid Therapy

Should be categorized as resistant or responsive. If responsive, control by maintenance dosing of steroids.

Signs

External

1. Lid swelling, conjunctival chemosis (rule out endophthalmitis).
2. Lacrimal gland enlargement, conjunctival follicles (rule out sarcoid).
3. Perilimbal flush (rule out cyclitis).
4. Episcleritis, scleritis (rule out intraocular inflammation).

Cornea

1. Keratitis (rule out herpes simplex or herpes zoster uveitis).
2. Stromal vascularization.
3. Keratic precipitates:
   a) Usually located in the inferior corneal region.
   b) Fine (nongranulomatous) keratic precipitates are composed of lymphocytes and polymorphonuclear leukocytes.
   c) Mutton-fat (granulomatous) keratic precipitates are composed of lymphocytes and macrophages.

Anterior Segment

1. Cells and flare: chronic flare without cells is not an indication of active uveitis and should not be treated.
2. Hypopyon (rule out Behçet's disease, endophthalmitis, HLA-B27-related uveitis).
3. Iris nodules:
   a) Koeppe: located at pupillary margin; may be seen in granulomatous and nongranulomatous inflammation.
   b) Bussaca: located in mid-iris stroma; seen only in granulomatous inflammation.
4. Anterior and posterior synechiae.
5. Cataract formation (usually posterior subcapsular).
6. Iris atrophy (rule out Fuchs' heterochromic iridocyclitis, viral uveitis).
7. Rubeosis irides.
8. Intraocular pressure may be high or low.

Vitreous

1. Vitreous cells, opacities.
2. Snowballs (rule out sarcoid).
3. Snowbanking (rule out pars planitis).
4. Posterior vitreous separation.
5. Posterior keratic precipitates: line the posterior hyaloid.

Fundus

1. Cystoid macular edema.
2. Vascular alterations: sheathing of arteries and veins, vessel narrowing, retinal hemorrhages, exudates, cotton-wool spots.
3. Chorioretinal lesions.
4. Optic disc hyperemia, papillitis, granuloma, or atrophy.
5. Retinal or subretinal neovascularization.

Syndromes That May Masquerade as Anterior Uveitis

Rhegmatogenous retinal detachment: a mild anterior uveitis may accompany a retinal detachment.

Intraocular foreign body: may have iris heterochromia and anterior segment inflammation simulating Fuchs' heterochromic iridocyclitis.

Intraocular neoplasm: for example, retinoblastoma (may present with a pseudohypopyon due to tumor cells in the anterior chamber), malignant melanoma (may demonstrate flare and cells in the anterior chamber), and leukemia (early on may present with cells in the anterior chamber).

Juvenile xanthogranuloma: occurs in children under 15 years of age. Characterized by yellowish-gray iris tumors associated with spontaneous hyphemas and anterior segment inflammation. Diagnosis can be established by anterior chamber paracentesis, iris biopsy, and skin examination.

Ocular toxoplasmosis: a cause of posterior uveitis that may result in a spillover of cells in the anterior chamber.

Syndromes That May Masquerade as Posterior Uveitis

Histiocytic lymphoma: rare cause of chronic vitritis most commonly affecting patients in their sixties (age range 30–80). The disease has no sex predilection and is usually bilateral. Presents as a chronic anterior uveitis or vitritis or multifocal chorioretinitis, or combination thereof, usually unresponsive or exacerbated by steroid treatment. Diagnosis is established by anterior chamber or vitreous tap with cell marker studies.

In cases of suspected intraocular lymphoma, a workup for a systemic or central nervous system (CNS) lymphoma should also be initiated including head computed tomographic (CT) scan, lumbar puncture, chest x-ray, bone marrow biopsy, lymphangiogram, liver-spleen scan, complete blood count with differential, and serum protein electrophoresis.

Rhegmatogenous retinal detachment: pigmented anterior vitreous cells may be present (tobacco dust).

Retinitis pigmentosa: may present with vitreous cells and cystoid macular edema in addition to the classic bone spicule pigmentary changes, narrowed retinal vessels, and pale optic nerve.

Intraocular foreign body: may present with a persistent vitritis. Diagnosis can be established by ophthalmoscopy, ultrasound, or CT scanning of the globe.

Retinoblastoma: may present with vitreous cells due to diffusion of cells from the tumor mass into the vitreous.

Amyloidosis: presents with vitreal veils and membranes but without vitreal cells. The diagnosis of ocular amyloidosis can be established by a vitreous biopsy and systemic amyloidosis by a rectal mucosal biopsy. Patients with suspected amyloidosis should also undergo a systemic workup to identify any underlying immunoglobulin disorder.

Malignant melanoma: may present with vitreous cells and a secondary retinal detachment. Diagnosis is established by visualization of the tumor by ophthalmoscopy or ultrasonography.

Leukemia: may present with a retinopathy and less commonly vitritis. The retinopathy includes venous dilation and tortuosity, vascular sheathing, cotton-wool spots, hemorrhages, and grayish white nodular leukemic infiltration of the retina. Optic nerve head swelling and acute loss of vision may occur due to leukemic infiltration of the optic nerve.

A Basic Nonspecific Workup on All Patients Who Present with Anterior or Posterior Uveitis

1. Uveitis history and complete ocular examination.
2. Laboratory studies including complete blood count, erythrocyte sedimentation rate (ESR), VDRL, fluorescent treponemal antibody-absorption (FTA-ABS) test, chest x-ray, and purified protein derivative (PPD) skin test with anergy panel.
3. Further studies should be tailored to the pertinent uveitis history and findings on ocular examination (see specific disease entities).

Guidelines for the Nonspecific Treatment of Anterior and Posterior Uveitis

1. For anterior segment inflammation, begin with topical prednisolone acetate 1% every 1 to 6 hours with frequency dependent on the severity of the inflammatory reaction. If topical steroids prove inadequate, anterior subtenon injections of methylprednisolone (40–80 mg) can be administered to augment the anti-inflammatory effect. Prior to administering periocular steroids, it is advisable to use topical steroids for 6 weeks to ascertain if a patient is a steroid responder. If topical and periocular steroids prove inadequate, oral steroids (e.g., prednisone, 1–1.5 mg/kg/d) should be given. All patients on oral steroids should concomitantly be started on Zantac (150 mg p.o. b.i.d.), and a careful history and physical should be performed to rule out

1. diabetes mellitus (check fasting blood sugar),
2. hypertension (check blood pressure),
3. tuberculosis (check PPD, chest x-ray),
4. peptic ulcer disease, and
5. pregnancy.

2. Topical steroids have no place in the management of posterior segment inflammation. Posterior subtenon injections of methylprednisolone (40–80 mg) or prednisone (1–1.5 mg/kg/d p.o.) or both should be used to suppress the inflammatory response. Patients are generally kept on prednisone (1–1.5 mg/kg/d) until control of the inflammatory reaction is achieved (usually 10–14 d). Steroids are then gradually tapered until the minimum dose necessary for control of the inflammatory reaction is reached.

3. In patients who cannot tolerate the side effects of high-dose steroids or whose uveitis is unresponsive to steroids, consider the use of cyclosporin A. Cytotoxic drugs are reserved as a last resort if both steroids and cyclosporin A fail to control the inflammatory reaction.

4. Pupil management for anterior segment inflammation: cycloplegics to prevent posterior synechiae formation.

Arthritis-Related Anterior Uveitis Syndromes

Ankylosing Spondylitis

Acute recurrent anterior uveitis occurs in approximately 25% of patients with ankylosing spondylitis. Ankylosing spondylitis classically occurs in young men (age range 20–40 yrs), but women may have a milder form. Initial presenting systemic symptoms are low-back pain and stiffness, usually worse in the morning. It may present as a peripheral arthritis in children. The most commonly involved joint is the sacroiliac, but ankylosis of the spine may ultimately occur. Other features include aortic valve incompetence and heart conduction abnormalities. There is no correlation between the ocular inflammatory activity and severity of the joint disease.

Symptoms Eye pain, photophobia, and blurred vision.

Signs

1. *External:* ocular redness.
2. *Anterior segment:* nongranulomatous anterior uveitis. The uveitis is usually unilateral but tends to affect both eyes at different times. Posterior synechiae commonly develop.
3. *Vitreous:* anterior vitreous cells are present.
4. *Fundus:* macular edema may develop.

Workup History of low back pain or stiffness. Perform the following laboratory tests:

1. ESR.
2. Sacroiliac joint x-ray.
3. HLA antigen testing: a high association (85%–95%) is found between ankylosing spondylitis and HLA-B27 positivity. Since HLA-B27 may also be present in other types of anterior uveitis, HLA testing only helps to confirm the diagnosis of ankylosing spondylitis. HLA testing, therefore, need not be routinely performed when sacroiliac x-rays are positive.

Differential Diagnosis

1. Ulcerative colitis, regional enteritis, Reiter's syndrome or psoriatic arthritis.
2. Sarcoid uveitis: usually granulomatous inflammation, which commonly involves the posterior segment.
3. Idiopathic anterior uveitis: not associated with any clinical syndrome.

Treatment

1. Prednisolone acetate 1% topically. In severe cases, periocular steroids.
2. Cycloplegia.

3. Macular edema, if present, is treated by controlling the anterior segment inflammation.
4. Rheumatology referral for management of the systemic disease.

Course and Prognosis   The uveitis is acute and recurrent. It generally responds favorably to topical steroids and cycloplegics. Common complications:

1. Anterior and posterior synechia formation.
2. Secondary glaucoma due to the anterior segment inflammation or the development of synechiae. Less commonly, cataract formation and chronic cystoid macular edema develop. Although the prognosis for maintaining good vision is generally favorable, it depends on the frequency, severity, and duration of attacks.

Reiter's Syndrome

Reiter's syndrome is a chronic disease that typically affects young caucasian men (age range 20–40 yrs) and is characterized by nonspecific urethritis, conjunctivitis, polyarthritis, and mucocutaneous lesions. The full constellation of findings may take months or years to occur.

Reiter's syndrome usually follows a nonspecific urethritis. Both Chlamydia and Ureaplasma urealyticum have been isolated from urethral discharge. Less commonly, Reiter's syndrome may occur following an attack of dysentery caused by gram-negative bacteria.

Signs   Ocular involvement tends to be bilateral and symmetric.

1. *External:* a papillary or follicular mucopurulent conjunctivitis (most common eye finding) may be present with or without a nontender preauricular node.
2. *Anterior segment:* punctate keratopathy or anterior peripheral stromal infiltrates, nongranulomatous iridocyclitis with white keratic precipitates and mild to moderate flare and cell.
3. *Vitreous:* anterior vitreous cells.

Workup

1. Diagnosis is generally made on the basis of clinical criteria.
2. Check for history of arthritis, nonspecific urethritis, dysentery, and skin lesions.
3. Cultures of urethral discharge.
4. X-rays of the lower extremities and sacroiliac joints: 98% will have some rheumatologic findings.

5. Laboratory tests: no specific test will diagnose Reiter's syndrome. ESR is usually mildly elevated. HLA-B27 is positive in 65% to 75% of patients.
6. Referral to a rheumatologist and urologist for management of systemic features of the disease.

Differential Diagnosis

1. Other arthritis-related diseases with eye manifestations are ankylosing spondylitis, juvenile rheumatoid arthritis, psoriatic arthritis, and inflammatory bowel disease.
2. Beçhet's disease: in contrast to Reiter's syndrome, the oral and genital ulcers of Beçhet's disease are painful. Posterior segment involvement is a major feature.

Treatment

1. Conjunctivitis is self-limiting and requires no treatment.
2. Iridocyclitis: topical prednisolone acetate 1% and cycloplegia.
3. If chlamydia is isolated from urethral secretions, treat with tetracycline.

Course and Prognosis The course of Reiter's syndrome is characterized by remissions and recurrences. The iritis is usually acute in character but may eventually become chronic. Although the eye manifestations generally respond favorably to treatment, potential complications include the development of posterior synechiae and, rarely, secondary glaucoma. The prognosis for retention of functional vision is excellent.

Psoriasis

Psoriasis is an idiopathic skin disease characterized by erythematous plaques most commonly involving elbows and knees. Approximately 1% to 6% of patients with psoriasis also have associated arthritis, which predominantly affects the distal peripheral joints of the hands and feet. Of patients with psoriasis 30% demonstrate ocular findings, usually in association with arthritis.

Symptoms Pain, redness, photophobia.

Signs

1. *External:* conjunctivitis (most common finding) or, less commonly, episcleritis, scleritis, and dry eye.

2. *Anterior segment:* epithelial and anterior stromal infiltrates, nongranulomatous iridocyclitis with keratic precipitates, flare and cells, posterior synechiae.
3. *Vitreous:* vitreous cells may be present.

Workup   Diagnosis established on the basis of clinical presentation.

Differential Diagnosis

1. Ankylosing spondylitis
2. Reiter's syndrome
3. Crohn's disease and ulcerative colitis

Treatment   Topical prednisolone acetate 1% and cycloplegia. Oral corticosteroids for vitreous and retinal involvement.

Prognosis   The iritis is usually mild and responds to topical steroids. The prognosis for maintenance of vision is excellent.

Juvenile Rheumatoid Arthritis (JRA)

JRA is a rheumatoid-factor-negative inflammatory arthritis of at least 3 months' duration, which develops before age 16. Girls are slightly more commonly affected than boys, but girls carry a much higher risk of developing uveitis. The peak incidence of JRA occurs between ages 2 and 4, whereas the average age at the time of diagnosis of uveitis is 6. Three subgroups of JRA (systemic onset or Still's disease, polyarticular onset, and pauciarticular onset) are identified by the extent of joint involvement that occurs *during the first 3 months.* The incidence of uveitis is rare in systemic onset JRA and in the polyarticular subgroup ranges between 7% and 14%. The pauciarticular subgroup (four or fewer joints affected) carries the highest risk for the development of uveitis, with an incidence ranging between 78% and 91%. There is no correlation between the activity of the arthritis and the ocular inflammation.

Symptoms   Usually asymptomatic and detected on a routine eye examination.

Signs   Uveitis is usually bilateral.

1. *External:* quiet eye.
2. *Anterior segment:* chronic nongranulomatous iritis (1–2 + flare and cells), posterior synechia, and cataract.
3. *Vitreous:* cells in the anterior vitreous (especially with severe iritis).

Workup For patients with previously diagnosed JRA, assess the risk of developing uveitis:

1. Check history regarding the extent of joint involvement during the first 3 months of the disease. Patients who initially present with pauciarticular JRA may subsequently evolve into the polyarticular form but still have the incidence of developing uveitis associated with the pauciarticular subgroup.
2. Antinuclear antibody (ANA): between 70% and 90% of patients with JRA and uveitis are positive compared to 30% of patients without eye involvement.

Referral to a pediatric rheumatologist (a knee x-ray should be checked if JRA is suspected because this is the most commonly involved joint).

Differential Diagnosis

1. *Pediatric sarcoid:* patients less than 5 years of age present with arthritis, skin lesions, and only one-third have pulmonary symptoms. ANA is always negative, and uveitis is usually granulomatous. Chest x-ray, gallium scanning, skin testing for anergy, and testing for angiotensin-converting enzyme levels will help differentiate.
2. *Pars planitis:* bilateral nongranulomatous anterior segment inflammation, with snowbanking, absence of posterior synechiae formation, and no associated systemic illness.
3. *Ocular toxocariasis:* primarily posterior segment findings with spillover into the anterior chamber.
4. *Juvenile spondylitis:* may present with a lower limb arthritis with normal sacroiliac joints, making it difficult to distinguish from JRA. Distinguishing features include a *unilateral* anterior uveitis and a high prevalence of HLA-B27, and it typically affects *boys* at 10 years of age.

Treatment

Cycloplegia A short-acting mydriatic (tropicamide 1%) to prevent posterior synechiae formation. In mild cases, one drop at bedtime may be adequate.

Control of inflammatory response Topical steroids (prednisolone acetate 1% up to every hour initially, with gradual tapering thereafter); anterior subtenon injections of methylprednisolone or rarely systemic steroids may be necessary.

Management of secondary complications

1. Glaucoma: initially *nonmiotic* medical management including sympathomimetics, beta-blockers, and carbonic anhydrase inhibitors. If medical management fails, glaucoma surgery should be considered. Although the surgical treatment of choice is controversial, trabeculodialysis appears to offer better results than conventional filtration surgery.
2. Cataract: intraocular inflammation should be under maximum control prior to surgery. Lensectomy vitrectomy through an incision at the limbus or pars plana is the treatment of choice. The implantation of an intraocular lens (IOL) is contraindicated in children with chronic uveitis.
3. Band keratopathy can be managed by EDTA chelation.

Course and Prognosis   Most patients develop the chronic form of JRA iridocyclitis. Early detection and treatment are the keys to successful management. Once secondary complications develop, the prognosis is poor, with vision often in the 20/200 range.

Follow-up   See Table 6.3.

Beçhet's Disease

Beçhet's is an idiopathic, recurrent, multisystem inflammatory disorder (occlusive vasculitis) that has a worldwide distribution but is especially common in the Far East and in Mediterranean countries. The disease is more common in men than women (ratio of 2:1). Frequently unilateral during the early phases of eye involvement, the disease eventually becomes bilateral in 90% of patients. Peak onset is between ages 20 and 40. The diagnosis is made on the basis of clinical symptoms,

TABLE 6.3

Follow-up for JRA uveitis

Risk Factor	Recommended Screening Frequency
Systemic onset	Annual
Polyarticular onset	Every 6 mo
Pauciarticular onset	Every 3 mo
Positive ANA	Every 2 mo

From Kanski JJ. Juvenile arthritis and uveitis. Surv Ophthalmol 1990;34(4):253–267.

TABLE 6.4

Diagnostic criteria for Beçhet's disease

Major criteria

Recurrent aphthous ulcers of oral mucous membranes

Skin lesions (e.g., erythema nodosum)

Ocular inflammation

Genital ulcers usually in the scrotum or vulva

Minor criteria

Arthritis, most commonly affecting the knee joint

Ileocecal intestinal ulcers

Epididymitis

Vascular occlusive disease (e.g., obliterative thrombophlebitis)

Neurologic symptoms (neuro-Beçhet's) such as meningoencephalitis, brain-stem syndromes with cranial nerve palsies, and confusional state

which are classified by major and minor criteria (Table 6.4). Although oral ulcers are the most frequent initial symptom, ocular lesions are the most common reason for patients to seek medical attention. Of patients with Beçhet's disease 75% have ocular involvement.

Definitions Related to Diagnosis of Beçhet's Disease

Complete type: four major symptoms occurring during the clinical course.

Incomplete type: three major symptoms occurring during the clinical course or typical ocular involvement along with one other major criteria or three minor criteria.

Beçhet's suspect: two major criteria occurring during the clinical course.

Possible Beçhet: one major criteria.

Ocular Examination

1. *External:* rarely subconjunctival hemorrhage, conjunctivitis, episcleritis, filamentary keratitis, ocular muscle paralysis (neuro-Beçhet's).
2. *Anterior segment:* nongranulomatous iridocyclitis with fine keratic precipitates, flare and cells, transient hypopyon, posterior synechiae, iris atrophy, and peripheral anterior synechiae.
3. *Vitreous:* vitritis (consistent finding).

4. *Fundus:* edema of the optic nerve, localized patches of retinal edema, most often in the macular area, venous dilation, venous sheathing, yellowish-white exudates, and retinal hemorrhages. Repeated episodes may lead to branch or central retinal vein or artery occlusions, macular hole formation, optic atrophy, and retinal neovascularization.

Workup   Diagnosis usually based on clinical criteria (Table 6.4).

1. History: check ancestry, country of origin.
2. HLA-B5 and HLA-B51 (a subset of B5) are associated with Beçhet's disease in Japanese patients.
3. Beçhetine test: an indurated erythematous lesion occurs in 40% of patients secondary to needle prick or intradermal injection of saline.
4. Fluorescein angiogram: may reveal areas of marked capillary dropout and dye leakage from small and large retinal veins and peripapillary capillaries.

Differential Diagnosis

1. Sarcoid
2. Viral retinitis
3. Retinal vasculitis secondary to collagen vascular disease
4. HLA-B27 iridocyclitis

Therapy   The anterior uveitis generally responds to topical steroids and cycloplegics. Subtenon injections of steroids can augment the anti-inflammatory effect if needed. For posterior segment disease, a variety of agents have been employed:

1. Oral corticosteroids: prednisone, 1 to 2 mg/kg for 5 to 7 days during the acute attack, with a variable tapering schedule. Initially most cases will respond favorably; however, a state of resistance eventually develops leading to an increase in severity and number of recurrences.
2. Cytotoxic agents: chlorambucil is felt by some to be the cytotoxic agent of choice; azathioprine has also been shown to be effective.
3. Colchicine.
4. Cyclosporin: exacerbation of the ocular disease occurs upon cessation of the drug or reducing the dose below a certain critical level, necessitating use of the drug for years.

Course and Prognosis   The course is characterized by exacerbations and remissions of varying duration and frequency. Between episodes of active inflammation, the disease is totally quiescent. Although treatment appears to decrease the frequency and duration of attacks, the long-term prognosis for vision is poor. Since the main cause of vision loss is related to fundus changes, patients with only anterior segment involvement have a far superior visual prognosis. Complications of anterior segment involvement include glaucoma and cataracts. Complications of repeated posterior segment inflammation include macular degeneration secondary to subretinal neovascularization, retinal detachment, and phthisis bulbi.

Endophthalmitis

Exogenous Endophthalmitis

Acute Onset Exogenous Endophthalmitis

Bacterial endophthalmitis within 1 week following cataract surgery is the most frequent clinical setting, with an incidence reported between 0.05% and 0.3%. Gram-positive aerobic bacteria (e.g., *Staphylococcus epidermidis* (most common), *S. aureus, Streptococcal* sp., *Pneumococci*) account for approximately 90% of cases, 7% of cases are caused by gram-negative bacteria (e.g., *Proteus, Pseudomonas, Hemophilus influenza, Klebsiella, Escherichia coli, Enterobacter*), and 3% are of fungal etiology (e.g., *Candida, Aspergillus*). Infectious endophthalmitis following surgery should be suspected in any case where the intraocular reaction appears inappropriate to the surgery performed. The onset time of endophthalmitis is generally related to the virulence of the organism. Endophthalmitis caused by gram-positive organisms typically occurs within 7 days of surgery, and gram-negative cases within the first 4 days.

Symptoms   Eye pain, ocular redness, and decreasing vision.

Signs   May have any or all of the following findings:

1. *External:* ptosis, exophthalmos, lid swelling, restricted ocular motility, and conjunctival chemosis.
2. *Afferent pupil* defect may be present.
3. *Anterior segment:* corneal ring or abscess, corneal edema, cells and flare, hypopyon, fibrin, air bubble (anaerobic organism).
4. *Vitreous:* mild to severe vitritis, leading to a decrease or loss of the red reflex.
5. *Fundus:* retinal periphlebitis (early finding), superficial retinal hemorrhages, optic nerve head edema.

Workup

1. Complete eye examination. Rule out predisposing factors such as wound separation and vitreous wick.
2. Ultrasonogram to evaluate the posterior segment when a vitritis precludes ophthalmoscopy. The most common findings are anterior vitreous echoes and thickening of the retinochoroidal layer.
3. Anterior chamber paracentesis to sample the aqueous and a diagnostic vitrectomy to sample the vitreous. Both aqueous and vitreous samples are submitted for gram stain, giemsa stain, and cultured on the following:
   a) Solid media: blood, Mackonkey, Sabouraud's, and prereduced anaerobic blood agar.
   b) Liquid media: thioglycolate and cooked meat medium.
      Of note, cultures must be held for 2 weeks before excluding anaerobic infection.
4. Complete blood count with differential.

Differential Diagnosis

1. *Phacoantigenic endophthalmitis:* look for the presence of residual lens material.
2. *Sterile endophthalmitis:* diagnosis of exclusion.
3. *Fungal endophthalmitis:* usually has a delayed onset.
4. *Endogenous endophthalmitis:* no history of recent ocular surgery. Usually occurs in immunosuppressed patients.

Treatment   Begin as soon as the diagnosis is considered possible.

1. After sampling of the aqueous and vitreous, all cases should receive an intravitreal injection of vancomycin (1 mg/0.1 cc) and gentamicin (0.1 mg/0.1 cc). If clinical suspicion is high for anaerobic infection, substitute clindamycin (1 mg/0.1 cc) for vancomycin.
2. All cases receive subconjunctival antibiotics (e.g., gentamicin, 20–40 mg plus vancomycin, 50 mg). Subconjunctival injections may be administered daily for 3 to 4 days.
3. All cases receive systemic antibiotics for 7 to 10 days (e.g., cefazolin, 500–1000 mg i.v. q. 6 h plus gentamicin, 1.75 mg/kg i.v. load, followed by 1 mg/kg q. 8 h) (check renal function).
4. All cases receive topical fortified antibiotics (e.g., cefazolin, 50 mg/ml, alternating every 30 min with gentamicin, 15 mg/ml).
5. All cases receive topical cycloplegics (e.g., homatropine 5% t.i.d.).

Topical prednisolone acetate 1%, six times a day, should be started 24 hours after initiating antibiotic therapy.
6. Severe cases of endophthalmitis (e.g., those with hypopyons greater than 15%, vitreous opacification obliterating the red reflex, or corneal ring infiltrate) should have a therapeutic pars plana vitrectomy as part of the initial management.
7. In cases with a moderate to severe vitritis, oral steroids (e.g., prednisone 60–80 mg/d for 7 d followed by a rapid taper) can be started 24 hours following initiation of antibiotic therapy. The use of intravitreal steroids is controversial, but as an alternative to oral steroids, intravitreal dexamethasone (400 μg/0.1 ml) can be given at the time of initial vitrectomy (if a fungal etiology has been excluded).

Follow-up   In the hospital, patients should be examined at least twice daily. The antibiotic regimen should be modified as necessary depending on the clinical response to treatment and antibiotic sensitivities of isolated organisms. Repeat intravitreal antibiotic injections at 48 to 96 hours after the initial injection can be considered if the clinical response to treatment is inadequate.

Following discharge, patients should be followed closely until the ocular status is deemed stable.

Course and Prognosis   Posterior segment complications include hypotony (due to cyclitic membrane formation detaching the ciliary body), retinal detachment, and macular edema. Anterior segment complications include glaucoma secondary to anterior and posterior synechia formation and corneal decompensation. The virulence of the infecting organism is the major factor that determines the visual outcome (S. epidermidis has the best visual prognosis whereas streptococci species and gram-negative organisms carry the worst visual prognosis).

Delayed Onset Exogenous Endophthalmitis

Propionibacterium Acnes Endophthalmitis P. acnes (gram-positive non-spore-forming anaerobic bacillus) endophthalmitis presents as a low-grade chronic iridocyclitis and should be suspected in any patient with chronic uveitis following successful cataract surgery. The uveitis usually occurs 2 to 10 months after surgery but has been reported to occur years later. Many of the cases initially respond to steroids but upon tapering the inflammation returns.

Symptoms   Decreased vision and ocular pain.

Signs

1. *External:* usually quiet eye or mildly injected.
2. *Anterior segment:* chronic iridocyclitis with moderate flare and cells, granulomatous keratic precipitates, hypopyon, and a whitish plaque on the posterior capsule or IOL surface.
3. *Vitreous:* mild anterior vitritis.
4. *Fundus:* normal.

Workup Diagnostic paracentesis and vitrectomy for smear and culture (as in acute onset endophthalmitis) with emphasis on isolating anaerobes.

Differential Diagnosis

1. Sterile endophthalmitis: presents in the early postoperative period; the vitreous is usually uninvolved and resolves with steroids alone.
2. Retinal detachment masquerading as a low-grade uveitis.
3. Phacoantigenic uveitis: usually present within 2 weeks of surgery. Residual lens material may be found in the anterior chamber.
4. Fungal endophthalmitis.

Treatment Following the diagnostic workup, inject intravitreal clindamycin or a cephalosporin. If inflammation persists and cultures are positive for *P. acnes*, the lens implant and capsular bag should be removed. If the anterior hyaloid face is broken during capsule removal, an anterior vitrectomy should also be performed. There are reports of successful resolution of the inflammation with only a combination of topical periocular and systemic antibiotics.

Exogenous Fungal Endophthalmitis Fungal endophthalmitis following intraocular surgery presents within 1 week to 3 months, typically within 2 to 3 weeks. The most commonly involved fungi are *Candida* and *Aspergillus.*

Symptoms Pain, redness, and varying degrees of decreased vision.

Signs

1. *External:* ocular redness.
2. *Anterior segment:* moderate to severe flare and cells, often followed within several days by the development of a hypopyon. The aqueous gradually becomes more turbid, and stringy gelatinous strands develop in the anterior chamber. A secondary posterior corneal abscess may also develop.

3. *Vitreous:* grayish-white infiltrates may develop in the anterior vitreous associated with increasing vitritis. The vitreous "abscess" may eventually bulge forward into the anterior chamber in a horn-like fashion.

Workup See Acute Onset Endophthalmitis, above.

Differential Diagnosis See *P. acnes* endophthalmitis, above.

Treatment

1. Initially treat as an acute bacterial exogenous endophthalmitis *without* the use of steroids.
2. If the smear or cultures are positive for fungi or if there is a high clinical index of suspicion for fungal endophthalmitis, inject 5 to 10 μg of intravitreal amphotericin B. This injection can be repeated in cases of persistent infection. In cases of treatment failure or infection with *P. lilacinus,* consider the use of intravitreal miconazole, 25 to 50 μg.
3. All clinically involved tissue should be excised. If there is vitreous involvement, a pars plana vitrectomy should be performed. The lens implant need not be removed unless there is significant fungal involvement in the region of the lens, or in cases of failure to eradicate the infection.
4. If there is corneal or anterior segment involvement, begin the following:
   a) Topical natamycin 5%, amphotericin B 0.15%, or miconazole 1% every hour.
   b) Subconjunctival amphotericin B (0.5–1.0 mg) or miconazole (5–10 mg).
5. If vitreous cultures are positive for fungi, begin ketoconazole (400 mg p.o.) daily, or flucytosine (37.5 mg/kg p.o.) every 6 hours. Consultation with an infectious disease specialist is desirable.

Follow-up See Acute Onset Endophthalmitis, above.

Nonsurgical Traumatic Endophthalmitis

The incidence of endophthalmitis following penetrating trauma is estimated between 2.4% and 7.4%. Most cases are caused by aerobic gram-positive organisms, but infections by anaerobes, gram-negative organisms, fungi, or mixed flora are more common following trauma than after surgery. The most commonly isolated organism is *Bacillus* species followed by *S. epidermidis.*

Symptoms and Signs   See Acute Onset Exogenous Endophthalmitis, above.

Workup   See Acute Onset Exogenous Endophthalmitis, above. An orbital CT scan or ultrasound or both should be performed to rule out an intraocular foreign body.

Differential Diagnosis

1. Phacoantigenic endophthalmitis.
2. Sterile inflammatory reaction secondary to a retained foreign body or blood in the vitreous.

Treatment   Primary repair of penetrating injury. If the diagnosis of endophthalmitis is suspected or confirmed during initial primary repair, the aqueous and vitreous should be sampled for smear and culture and a pars plana vitrectomy performed as part of the initial management. Intravitreal injection of gentamicin, 0.1 mg/0.1 ml (or amikacin, 400 μg/0.1 ml, which is possibly preferable to gentamicin due to the emergence of gentamicin-resistant gram-negative organisms as well as the problem of macular infarction associated with the use of intravitreal gentamicin), and vancomycin, 1 mg/0.1 ml (or clindamycin, 1 mg/0.1 ml). Depending on the clinical response, intravitreal injections may be repeated 48 and 96 hours after the initial injection. Vancomycin provides better gram-positive coverage whereas clindamycin delivers superior coverage against anaerobic bacteria. Both antibiotics cover *Bacillus* and *Staphylococcus* species.

Following primary repair all patients with penetrating intraocular trauma should be started prophylactically on topical, subconjunctival, and systemic antibiotics (the use of prophylactic intravitreal antibiotics is controversial).

Topical: fortified gentamicin (15 mg/ml) alternating with fortified cefazolin (50 mg/ml) every 30 minutes.

Subconjunctival: gentamicin (40 mg) and either vancomycin (25–50 mg) or clindamycin (34 mg). Subconjunctival injections may be repeated every 12 to 24 hours.

Systemic: Gentamicin (1.75 mg/kg i.v. loading dose, followed by 1 mg/kg q. 8 h) and either clindamycin (150–900 mg/kg i.v. q. 8 h) or vancomycin (1 g i.v. q. 12 h) (check renal function).

In cases with moderate to severe vitritis, the use of steroids can be considered if a fungal etiologic agent has been excluded.

Follow-up   See Acute Onset Exogenous Endophthalmitis, above.

Prognosis The visual prognosis with posttraumatic endophthalmitis is worse than for postoperative endophthalmitis. Factors that affect the final visual outcome include severity of trauma, virulence of the infecting organism, interval between onset of endophthalmitis and treatment, and the presence of retinal breaks or detachment at the time of initial injury.

Endogenous Endophthalmitis

Fungal

Candida is the most common cause of endogenous fungal endophthalmitis followed in frequency by *Aspergillus.* The disease may affect one or both eyes. Risk factors include:

1. Intravenous drug use,
2. Debilitated patients requiring indwelling catheters for long-term antibiotic or hyperalimentation therapy,
3. Gastrointestinal surgery in chronically ill patients, and
4. Immunocompromised hosts (e.g., secondary to treatment with immunosuppressive agents, AIDS).

Symptoms Blurred vision, floaters, red eye, and ocular pain. May be asymptomatic in the early stages.

Signs

1. *External:* conjunctival hyperemia.
2. *Anterior segment:* mild to moderate flare and cells, keratic precipitates, hypopyon.
3. *Vitreous:* cells and round yellow-white vitreous opacities (puff balls).
4. *Fundus:* initially multifocal creamy-white deep retinal or choroidal lesions with indistinct margins. Left untreated, these lesions gradually enlarge and break into the vitreous cavity, giving rise to characteristic puff balls. Occasionally may have associated retinal hemorrhages with or without pale centers.

Workup

1. Check for history of risk factors.
2. Culture blood, urine, and tips of all indwelling catheters.
3. If there is significant vitreous involvement, a diagnostic vitrectomy for smear and culture should be performed.
4. Complete blood count and chemistry panel.

Differential Diagnosis

1. CMV retinitis: associated with more hemorrhages and only a relatively mild vitritis.
2. Ocular toxoplasmosis: focal area of retinitis is usually adjacent to an old healed *Toxoplasma* chorioretinal scar. Although a dense vitritis may develop, puff balls are not found.
3. Cotton-wool spots: not associated with a vitritis.
4. Pars planitis: may be confused with *Candida* endophthalmitis due to the presence of snowballs resembling Candida puff balls.
5. Other causes (e.g., *Aspergillis, Cryptococcus neoformans,* Coccidioides immitis, and *Blastomycosis*).
6. Endogenous bacterial endophthalmitis.

Treatment

1. If retinal or choroidal involvement is present with only minimal or no vitreous involvement, treatment should involve only systemic antifungals.
2. If the diagnosis of endogenous fungal endophthalmitis is highly suspected or confirmed by blood cultures or vitreous biopsy and the vitreous is more than minimally involved, a therapeutic vitrectomy should be performed, followed by intravitreal administration of 5 to 10 μg of amphotericin B.
3. In patients with endogenous fungal endophthalmitis with vitreous involvement but *without evidence of disseminated infection* (e.g., no other site of infection, negative blood, and urine cultures), a systemic antifungal agent may not be necessary.
4. Systemic antifungal agents should be used in all cases of fungal endophthalmitis *with evidence of disseminated infection.* An infectious disease specialist should be consulted to determine the optimal systemic agent. Choices include amphotericin B, flucytosine, or ketoconazole.
5. Topical cycloplegia (e.g., homatropine 5% t.i.d.).

Course and Complications Without appropriate intervention, the intraocular inflammation progressively worsens, leading to complications including vitreoretinal traction, retinal detachment, cyclitic membrane formation, and ultimately phthisis bulbi. The prognosis for salvaging useful vision is improved if treatment is begun prior to significant vitreous involvement.

Follow-up While in the hospital, patients should be examined at least once daily. If systemic antifungals are being administered, renal function should be carefully monitored and doses varied accordingly.

Bacterial

Endogenous bacterial endophthalmitis (EBE) is caused by bacteria that reach the eye by way of the bloodstream. Bilateral involvement occurs in 25% of cases, and is generally but not always present simultaneously. A wide spectrum of bacteria may cause EBE with *Bacillus cereus*, the most frequently reported organism (especially in intravenous drug users). Other reported organisms include *Streptococci* species, *Pneumococcus*, *S. aureus*, *Neisseria meningitis*, *Hemophilus influenza*, enteric gram-negative bacilli, *Nocardia asteroides*, and *Actinomyces*.

Symptoms Decreased vision.

Signs See Acute Onset Exogenous Endophthalmitis, above. Clinical involvement can be classified as anterior or posterior focal, anterior or posterior diffuse, and panophthalmitis.

Workup

1. Check for predisposing risk factors (e.g., underlying systemic disease (such as diabetes), intravenous drug use, immunocompromised host, and recent surgery or trauma.
2. Ultrasonogram if posterior segment not visible.
3. Culture blood, urine, and all indwelling catheters. Cerebrospinal fluid should also be sampled if meningitis is suspected. Cultures from nonocular sites are reliable indicators of the causative organism.
4. If the causative organism cannot be established from nonocular sources, both aqueous and vitreous samples should be obtained for smear and culture.
5. Infectious disease consultation.

Differential Diagnosis

1. Noninfectious uveitis (e.g., sarcoid, pars planitis, vernal keratoconjunctivitis, Beçhet's).
2. Infectious uveitis (e.g., toxoplasmosis, toxocariasis, tuberculosis, and syphilis).
3. Neoplasms (e.g., histiocytic lymphoma and retinoblastoma).
4. Endogenous fungal endophthalmitis.
5. Cotton-wool spots, Roth spots: are not associated with vitreous cells and are smaller (less than 1 disc diameter) than septic foci.

Treatment

1. After all cultures have been taken, broad spectrum intravenous antibiotics are used at doses recommended for severe infection for at least 2 weeks. The initial choice of antibiotics reflects the likely source of the infection and may be modified once the causative organism is identified.
2. Periocular antibiotics may be used especially in the uninvolved eye to help prevent bilateral involvement.
3. In cases classified as posterior diffuse endophthalmitis or panophthalmitis, consideration should be given to performing a pars plana vitrectomy with intravitreal injection of gentamicin (0.1 mg/0.1 ml) and vancomycin (1 mg/0.1 ml). Similar consideration should be given in posterior focal EBE if there are signs of progressive worsening after 1 to 2 days of intravenous antibiotics.
4. Topical steroids and cycloplegia with dosages varying depending on the degree of anterior segment involvement.

Prognosis   Early recognition of EBE and treatment is essential for a favorable visual outcome. With appropriate intervention, 40% of affected eyes retain useful vision. The virulence of the infecting organism is inversely related to the visual prognosis. Focal and anterior diffuse presentations have a more favorable visual outcome than do posterior diffuse and panophthalmitis.

Fuchs' Heterochromic Iridocyclitis

Fuchs' heterochromic iridocyclitis is a chronic anterior iridocyclitis of unknown etiology. Most commonly occurs in the third and fourth decades of life, affects all races, occurs equally in men and women, and is usually unilateral.

Symptoms   The most common complaint is blurred vision or floaters, but the condition may be asymptomatic. Rarely photophobia and ciliary spasm-type pain may occur.

Ocular Examination

1. *External*: quiet eye, rarely mild injection.
2. *Anterior segment*:
   a) Heterochromia: usually the hypochromic eye is involved. Heterochromia may be absent in brown-eyed patients.

b) Keratic precipitates (KP): nonpigmented, small or medium size, round or star-shaped that may involve the entire posterior surface. Fine cotton-wisp-like filaments are generally found connecting the KPs.

c) Flare and cells: usually not more than 1 to 2+.

d) Iris: due to stromal atrophy the involved iris may demonstrate a dull surface with hazily defined crypts and collarettes. The iris may also appear "moth-eaten" due to a defective pigment epithelial layer. Koeppe nodules may be present. Posterior synechiae are generally *absent*.

e) Lens: posterior subcapsular cataract.

f) Angle structures: gonioscopy may reveal neovascularization, peripheral anterior synechiae, and membranes.

g) Vitreous: cells and strands in the anterior vitreous.

h) Fundus: usually normal but may demonstrate peripheral inactive chorioretinal scars (resembling toxoplasmosis) or venous sheathing.

Workup

1. Diagnosis generally based on characteristic clinical findings.
2. In atypical cases check PPD, chest x-ray, VDRL, and FTA-ABS.
3. Consider iris angiogram, which may reveal localized ischemia, filling delays, and fluorescein leakage (from neovascular vessels).

Differential Diagnosis

1. *Posner-Schlossman syndrome:* episodic acute elevation of intraocular pressure compared to chronic elevation in Fuchs'.
2. *Pars planitis:* heterochromia and characteristic KPs are not seen.
3. *Toxoplasmosis:* will always present with an *active* chorioretinal lesion.
4. *Metallic intraocular foreign body:* may present with iris heterochromia but history of ocular trauma is generally present and entry site may be visible on examination.

Treatment   No known effective treatment.

1. Topical steroids may be used to decrease the density of KPs if central KPs are responsible for decreased vision.
2. Although generally ineffective, a trial with topical steroids may be attempted to control intraocular inflammation.
3. Cycloplegia is unnecessary since posterior synechia do not develop.

Course and Prognosis   Two main complications include cataract formation (50%) and secondary open angle glaucoma (15%–30%). Less common complications include corneal edema and cystoid macular edema. The prognosis for good vision depends on the success encountered in managing these complications. The use of an intraocular lens implant in cataract surgery is controversial. Surgical complications following cataract surgery include hyphema, glaucoma (which commonly becomes refractory to medical management), and progressive vitreous opacification.

Follow-up   Every 3 to 4 months to screen for glaucoma.

Intermediate Uveitis (Pars Planitis, Chronic Cyclitis)

Intermediate uveitis represents an anatomic classification of ocular inflammation rather than a distinct clinical entity. This disease characteristically affects healthy individuals of both sexes, typically teenagers and young adults (20 to 30 yrs). Of these patients 70% to 80% have bilateral involvement. It may occasionally be a manifestation of demyelinating disease.

Symptoms   Floaters, blurred vision, and loss of accommodation.

Ocular Examination

1. *External:* quiet eye.
2. *Anterior segment:* mild nongranulomatous iritis (KPs and posterior synechiae are generally absent). In children, there may be moderate-to-severe anterior chamber reaction KPs, band keratopathy, and the formation of posterior synechiae.
3. *Vitreous:* vitreous cells, debris, and snowballs are usually present, most prominent in the anterior and inferior vitreous cavity. As the disease progresses, a gelatinous fibroglial mass (snowbank) may be noted over the pars plana, which may extend posteriorly over the ora serrata and peripheral retina. A snowbank is not required for the diagnosis of intermediate uveitis but is a necessary clinical finding for the subgroup diagnosis of pars planitis.
4. *Fundus:* perivasculitis (venules > arterioles) most common in the retinal periphery, cystoid macular edema (most common cause of decreased vision), infrequently neovascularization of the

peripheral retina or optic nerve head with or without vitreous hemorrhage.

Workup   Diagnosis is made on the basis of the clinical findings.

1. Since steroids are the mainstay of treatment, a chest-x-ray, PPD, and VDRL-FTA should be obtained.
2. Fluorescein angiogram for cystoid macular edema.
3. Demyelinating disease workup if indicated.
4. Lyme titer.

Differential Diagnosis

1. *Sarcoidosis* can resemble intermediate uveitis because of snowballs and periphlebitis. However, in sarcoid the anterior segment involvement is usually more significant, typically presenting as a granulomatous uveitis. See Sarcoidosis section, below.
2. *Toxocariasis:* a peripheral, inferiorly located *Toxocara* granuloma may be confused with a snowbank. Toxocariasis is usually unilateral, and occurs in a younger age group. Diagnosis can be confirmed by checking *Toxocara* serology.
3. *Fuchs' heterochromic iridocyclitis:* may resemble intermediate uveitis due to mild anterior iridocyclitis without posterior synechia. Fuchs' is always unilateral, demonstrates characteristic KPs and iris heterochromia, and does not develop a peripheral retinal vasculitis.
4. *Senile vitritis:* typically occurs in older patients. The disease presents with vitreous cells without a snowbank or peripheral vascular changes.
5. *Ocular Lyme Borreliosis:* may present with a bilateral vitritis with vitreous snowballs and snowbanking. Patients usually have other features such as granulomatous KPs and posterior synechiae. Diagnosis may be assisted by serologic testing for *Borrelia burgdorferi.*

Treatment

1. Due to the mild anterior segment findings and absence of posterior synechiae there is little if any role for topical steroids and cycloplegics.

2. Treatment is recommended when vision is reduced to the 20/40 level or in patients who complain of severe floaters. The mainstay of treatment involves the use of systemic or periocular steroids. If the disease is unilateral, injections of subtenon methylprednisolone acetate (40 mg) are recommended every 2 to 6 weeks (depending on the clinical response). In patients with bilateral disease or in whom injections have not been effective, prednisone is initially given orally at a daily dosage of 1 mg/kg in divided doses. This dosage is continued for 10 to 14 days, at which time conversion to alternate-day therapy is started, with gradual tapering until the minimum dosage needed to control the inflammation is found. A steroid failure represents a patient who has had at least 4 months of intensive steroid treatment without evidence of clinical improvement.

3. If there is either intolerance or inadequate response to steroid therapy, cryotherapy to the area of pars plana involvement is recommended. One or two rows of cryotherapy are applied under direct visualization utilizing a double freeze-thaw technique. Patients may require retreatment for recurrences. Cryotherapy is also used to treat complicating peripheral retinal neovascularization, especially with an associated vitreous hemorrhage.

4. In cases resistant to steroids and cryoablation, a pars plana vitrectomy to remove inflammatory debris should be considered.

5. As a last resort, treatment with immunosuppressive drugs (e.g., cyclosporin A) should be attempted.

Course and Prognosis   Although the clinical course may be variable, the majority of patients have a chronic smoldering course lasting several years. With appropriate intervention 70% to 80% of patients maintain good visual acuity 10 years after the onset of the disease.

The major vision-threatening complications are chronic cystoid macular edema (CME) and cataract formation. The presence of a snowbank in patients with intermediate uveitis may be associated with more severe vitreous disease and an increased incidence of CME. Other less common complications are secondary glaucoma, band keratopathy, retinal neovascularization, vitreous hemorrhage, retinoschisis, traction retinal detachment, and dragging of the optic nerve vessels and macula (secondary to peripheral vitreous traction bands).

Follow-up   During initial management to control inflammatory activity patients should be seen every 2 weeks. Thereafter, patients should be reexamined at least every 3 to 4 months.

Phacoantigenic Uveitis

Phacoantigenic uveitis is a sterile, autoimmune, zonal granulomatous inflammatory reaction that follows lens trauma or surgery. The pathophysiology is autosensitization to one's own lens protein. Onset generally occurs 1 to 14 days after lens trauma or surgery but has been reported to occur as late as 1 year postoperatively. The inflammation almost always involves only the traumatized eye.

Symptoms   Pain, photophobia, decreased vision.

Ocular Examination

1. *External:* conjunctival chemosis, erythema, and lid swelling.
2. *Anterior segment:* corneal edema, large mutton fat keratic precipitates, moderate to severe flare and cells (rarely a nongranulomatous uveitis), and hypopyon. Residual lens material may be seen in the anterior chamber.
3. *Vitreous:* moderate to severe vitritis.
4. *Fundus:* cystoid macular edema.

Workup

1. History of recent ocular surgery or trauma.
2. Aqueous tap for cytology and culture. Cytology revealing lens material and granulomatous inflammation helps confirm the diagnosis and excludes the possibility of bacterial endophthalmitis.
3. Ultrasound may localize the inflammatory reaction centered around the lens and help evaluate the status of the posterior segment.

Differential Diagnosis

1. Bacterial or fungal endophthalmitis.
2. Sterile endophthalmitis: onset usually 3 to 4 days after surgery and characterized by mild inflammation and hypopyon with little pain or visual loss. Conjunctival chemosis and lid swelling are usually absent.
3. Sympathetic ophthalmia: always bilateral.

Treatment

1. Initial treatment is designed to control the inflammatory response. Topical prednisolone acetate 1% is applied every hour and prednisone (80 mg/d p.o.) is given in divided doses. The dosages are tapered as the condition is brought under control.
2. After the inflammatory response subsides, surgery to remove all residual lenticular material and capsular remnants should be performed.
3. Intraocular pressure elevations can be managed with topical beta-blockers and carbonic anhydrase inhibitors.

Course and Prognosis   The prognosis for vision without treatment is extremely poor as synechia formation, secondary glaucoma, cyclitic membrane formation, hypotony, retinal detachment, and phthisis bulbi may occur. With treatment the prognosis is improved, although many patients still fare poorly.

Presumed Ocular Histoplasmosis Syndrome (POHS)

POHS is believed to be caused by the fungus *Histoplasma capsulatum*. It is most commonly found in the Midwestern United States especially in the Ohio-Mississippi-Missouri Valley region, where the fungus is endemic. Histoplasmosis infection is acquired by inhalation and disseminates via the blood stream to the liver, spleen and choroid. The fungemia is asymptomatic or may cause a mild upper respiratory tract infection. POHS produces no ocular symptoms until many years later if a maculopathy develops. The disease most commonly presents in the second to fourth decades and is more common in whites.

Symptoms   Metamorphopsia or sudden loss of central vision.

Ocular Examination

1. *External:* quiet eye.
2. *Anterior segment:* normal.
3. *Vitreous:* cells are never seen.
4. *Fundus:* the classic triad includes the following:
   a)   Peripapillary and peripheral "histo" spots (chorioretinal scars) secondary to a multifocal choroiditis. These lesions can also appear in the equatorial region as linear streaks running parallel to the ora serrata. Over time, "histo" spots may enlarge, become smaller, or even disappear.
   b)   Peripapillary atrophy.
   c)   Maculopathy: subretinal neovascularization.

Workup   Diagnosis generally based on clinical features.

1. History of travel or residence in areas endemic for histoplasmosis.
2. HLA typing: increased incidence of HLA-B7, especially with associated maculopathy.
3. Fluorescein angiogram: to detect subretinal neovascularization in both eyes.
4. Chest and abdominal x-rays may demonstrate old calcified granulomas involving liver, lungs, and spleen.

5. In atypical cases, consider the histoplasmin skin test to document exposure to *H. capsulatum*. Exacerbation of macular disease has been reported following the histoplasmin skin test.

Differential Diagnosis

1. Myopic degeneration.
2. Angioid streaks: usually associated with a systemic illness such as pseudoxanthoma elasticum, Paget's disease, etc.
3. Sarcoidosis and tuberculosis: usually have associated inflammatory activity in the anterior segment or vitreous or both.

Treatment

1. No treatment is indicated for inactive disease detected on a routine eye examination. However, perimacular histo spots should be followed carefully for the possible development of subretinal neovascularization.
2. For patients with an acute active macular lesion, prednisone (60 mg/d p.o. in divided doses) may be started, although this is not of any proven value.
3. If a subretinal neovascular net is identified on angiography that is located either between 1 and 199 μm from the center of the foveal avascular zone (FAZ) or between 200 and 2500 μm from the center of the FAZ with blood extending within 200 μm of the FAZ center, krypton laser ablation is attempted. If no blood is present within 200 μm of the FAZ and the neovascular net is located 200 to 2500 μm from the center of the FAZ, argon blue-green rather than krypton laser photocoagulation may be performed. Photocoagulation of inactive macular histo spots is not recommended.

Course and Prognosis   Early recognition and ablation of subretinal neovascular membranes threatening the macula significantly improves the chances of maintaining functional vision. Subfoveal and juxtafoveal subretinal neovascular membranes have the poorest prognosis, with 70% of patients having a final visual acuity equal to or less than 20/200. In patients with maculopathy in one eye, there is a 25% chance of involvement of the fellow eye if atrophic histo spots are present in the macular or paramacular region. If histo spots are not present in the macular region of the fellow eye, there is little chance of developing active macular disease in that eye.

Follow-up   To ensure complete ablation of the subretinal neovascular net, patients who have undergone laser treatment should be reexamined 2, 4, and 6 weeks after treatment. Patients should also be seen 3 months and 6 months after treatment, with follow-up every 6 months thereafter. Fluorescein angiograms should be performed as necessary to evaluate any new symptoms or changes in fundus appearance. All treated patients should be instructed in the proper use of an Amsler grid to monitor for signs of metamorphopsia. If inactive histo spots are present in the macular region of the fellow eye, Amsler grid testing should be performed routinely in both eyes.

Sarcoidosis

Etiology A noncaseating granulomatous multisystem disease of unknown etiology most commonly manifested by pulmonary disease, although any organ or tissue may be affected. There is an increased prevalence of sarcoid in the southeastern United States and in Scandinavia. Sarcoid more commonly affects women and blacks (black-white ratio = 10:1). Sarcoid occurs in all age groups but is most common between 20 and 50 years of age. The frequency of ocular involvement in biopsy proven sarcoid ranges from 20% to 25%. A bilateral uveitis is the most common form of ocular sarcoid, with anterior uveitis being the most common manifestation. Posterior segment involvement occurs in approximately 15% to 25% of patients with ocular sarcoid. The uveitis most commonly has an insidious onset and is chronic.

Symptoms Blurred vision, floaters, eye pain, and photophobia. Constitutional symptoms include fever, shortness of breath, cough, chest pain, and weight loss.

Signs
1. *External:* lid margin or conjunctival granulomas, lacrimal gland enlargement (which may be complicated by dry eye), scleritis, or phlyctenular conjunctivitis.
2. *Anterior segment:* band keratopathy, mutton fat granulomatous keratic precipitates, 3 to 4+ cells and flare, Koeppe or Bussaca nodules, posterior synechia, and cataract.
3. *Vitreous:* opacities varying in size from individual cells to aggregates known as snowballs (floating granulomas, Landers sign); snowbanking may occur due to the coalescence of large vitreous opacities that settle on the pars plana.
4. *Fundus:* periphlebitis (sheathing or candle wax drippings) that occasionally is associated with retinal hemorrhages, nodules on the retinal surface, choroidal granulomas, which may lead to pigment epithelial mottling, papilledema (commonly in

association with a facial nerve palsy or other cranial nerve abnormality due to involvement of the central nervous system), papillitis from severe posterior uveitis inducing vascular leakage at the nerve head, or optic nerve granulomas.

Workup No absolute diagnostic criteria exists for sarcoid.

1. Biochemical tests
   a) Elevated serum angiotensin-converting enzyme (ACE)—not specific for sarcoid; may be elevated in diabetes, etc.
   b) Elevated serum lysozyme (nonspecific).
   c) Elevated serum calcium and 24-hour urinary calcium (hypercalcuria is twice as common as hypercalcemia).
2. Immunologic tests
   a) Kveim test (specific for sarcoid with 80% positivity in ocular sarcoid, but reagents usually unavailable and takes 4 to 6 wks to read the result).
   b) Intradermal skin testing with candida, mumps, trichophyton, and PPD. Most patients with active sarcoid are *anergic* due to depression of delayed-type hypersensitivity.
3. Radiologic tests
   a) Chest x-ray: hilar adenopathy or interstitial involvement or both.
   b) Gallium scan of head, neck, and chest (more sensitive than chest x-ray).
   c) CT scan for neurosarcoid: 20% to 35% of patients with posterior segment involvement may have CNS involvement.
4. Fluorescein angiogram if indicated to document retinal vasculitis.
5. Biopsy sites for histologic confirmation
   a) Conjunctiva, especially if a suspicious lesion is present. Blind biopsies have a much lower yield.
   b) Lacrimal gland (especially if the lacrimal glands are enlarged or demonstrate increased gallium uptake).
   c) Other sites include lung, mediastinal lymph nodes, liver, or salivary glands.
6. Schirmer's test: to rule out dry eye.
7. Pulmonologist referral.

Differential Diagnosis

1. Tuberculosis
2. Pars planitis
3. Syphilis
4. Eales' disease
5. Beçhet's disease
6. Juvenile rheumatoid arthritis

Treatment   For anterior uveitis use topical steroids and cycloplegics with dose adjusted for the severity of inflammation. If this does not result in a significant reduction in the level of inflammation, a local anterior subtenon injection (e.g., Depo-Medrol, 40 mg) can be given. Oral steroids are indicated if topical and periocular therapy are ineffective or if posterior segment involvement is present. Doses of 1 to 2 mg/ kg of prednisone every day in divided doses should be given for 7 to 14 days. Once control of the inflammatory reaction has been achieved, an alternate-day regimen should be used by doubling the on-day dose, followed by a slow taper over 2 to 3 months. Since sarcoid is characterized by a chronic course with exacerbations and remissions, it is preferable to treat patients intermittently with high-dose steroids rather than continue them on chronic maintenance doses. The aim of therapy is to prevent vision-threatening complications of the disease. It may not be possible always to eliminate all signs of ocular inflammation.

Prognosis and Complications

1. When bilateral hilar adenopathy is associated with erythema nodosum and anterior uveitis (Lofgren's syndrome) the prognosis is uniformly favorable.

2. In general, prognosis depends on the response to steroid therapy and the proper management of potential complications. Patients with acute iridocyclitis have a better prognosis than those with chronic iridocyclitis.

3. Potential complications of sarcoid involving the anterior segment are secondary glaucoma and cataract formation. Sarcoid in the posterior segment may lead to cystoid macular edema, branch vein occlusion, retinal neovascularization anterior or posterior to the equator, and subretinal neovascularization. In the majority of patients, retinal neovascularization responds to steroid therapy alone, and laser photocoagulation should be reserved for patients with recurrent vitreous hemorrhages unresponsive to medical management. In contrast, subretinal neovascularization should be localized by fluorescein angiogram and, if in a treatable location, ablated with laser.

Sympathetic Ophthalmia

Sympathetic ophthalmia (SO) is a bilateral panuveitis that follows unilateral perforating trauma with inflammation in the injured eye (exciting eye) followed by the development of inflammation in the uninjured eye (sympathizing eye). In 80% of cases, the onset of inflammation in the sympathizing eye occurs within 3 months of injury but has been reported as early as 9 to 10 days and as late as 50 years following the initial injury. The estimated incidence of SO is 0.2% to 1% of nonsurgical penetrating traumatic wounds. The incidence following surgical trauma is felt to be 30 to 50 times less frequent. Sympathetic ophthalmia is more commonly found in men, but this is felt to be secondary to the higher incidence of ocular trauma in men.

Symptoms   Photophobia, blurred vision, and eye pain.

Ocular Examination

1. *External:* the exciting eye shows signs of the original trauma. Ciliary flush is common in the sympathizing eye.
2. *Anterior segment:* moderate to severe anterior uveitis with keratic precipitates (usually granulomatous), flare, cells, posterior synechiae, and iris nodules.
3. *Vitreous:* moderate to severe vitritis.
4. *Fundus:* multiple small drusen-like subretinal lesions (Dalen-Fuchs nodules) present in the peripheral fundus. These lesions may coalesce into large confluent areas, producing an exudative retinal detachment. Papillitis is a prominent feature.

Workup

1. The diagnosis is made on the basis of a history of penetrating ocular trauma associated with the characteristic clinical picture.
2. Histology of the exciting eye if enucleation was performed.
3. Fluorescein angiogram: Dalen-Fuchs nodules may block fluorescence early in the choroidal phase and stain during the late phases or may show hyperfluorescence of the nodules appearing as drusen-like dots. The dye may slowly spread into the subretinal space, demonstrating a serous detachment.

Differential Diagnosis

1. *Vogt-Koyanagi-Harada disease:* more common in Oriental and darkly pigmented patients with no history of trauma. Exudative retinal detachments or extraocular findings are much more common.
2. *Phacoantigenic endophthalmitis:* usually unilateral with inflammation surrounding a ruptured lens *without* involvement of the choroid, retina, or optic nerve. Onset usually 1 to 14 days following lens injury.

Treatment

1. Enucleation. With rare exception, removal of the exciting eye within 10 days of penetrating trauma protects the second eye from developing SO. However, since the overall risk of developing SO is low, enucleation should only be performed in patients for whom the visual prognosis is nil.

2. The role of enucleation *following* the onset of SO is controversial. In some studies, significant improvement in visual prognosis was seen if the exciting eye was enucleated within 2 weeks of the onset of eye symptoms.

3. High-dose corticosteroids are the mainstay of treatment. Oral prednisone at a dose of 100 to 200 mg/day should be used for 1 to 2 weeks, followed by gradual tapering to an alternate-day regimen. This can be supplemented with weekly posterior subtenon injections of 40 mg of methylprednisolone. Patients should be kept on a maintenance steroid dose for 4 to 6 months after the inflammation subsides. Prophylactic steroid use following penetrating ocular trauma does not prevent the development of SO.

4. Topical prednisolone acetate 1% to control anterior segment inflammation and cycloplegia to retard posterior synechia.

5. In cases of steroid-resistant SO or in steroid-induced ocular hypertension, cyclosporin or chlorambucil therapy should be instituted.

Course and Complications   The early stages of SO may result in relatively mild anterior or posterior segment findings. The disease, even if initially brought under control, has a relapsing character necessitating frequent follow-up. Common complications in the sympathizing eye include cataract formation, secondary glaucoma, exudative retinal detachment, and severe chorioretinal scarring. In one long-term study that followed 17 cases of SO, 65% of patients treated with steroids achieved visual acuities of 20/60 or better.

Follow-up   During initial management of the disease, patients should be followed every 1 to 3 days. As the inflammation subsides, patients can be seen every 2 to 3 weeks. Since relapses can occur many years after the initial episode has resolved, continued follow-up is essential.

Syphilis

Etiology   Syphilis is caused by the spirochete *Treponema pallidum*. Congenitally acquired syphilis demonstrates the characteristic fundus appearance of a finely pigmented "salt-and-pepper" retinopathy. A bilateral diffuse interstitial keratitis and anterior uveitis (usually occurring between the ages of 5 and 25 yrs) may occur as a late manifestation of congenital disease. Adult acquired syphylis can be divided into four stages:

1. The primary phase is characterized by a painless ulcer (chancre) usually found on the skin or mucous membranes. Most but not all patients will have a reactive FTA and VDRL.
2. Secondary syphilis occurs 6 to 8 weeks after the primary phase and is characterized by a maculopapular rash involving the palms and soles associated with constitutional symptoms. All serologic markers are reactive in this stage.
3. Latent syphilis follows resolution of secondary syphilis and is characterized by the absence of symptoms, reactive FTA (VDRL may be nonreactive in 30% of patients), and normal cerebrospinal fluid examination.
4. The late or tertiary stage includes neurosyphilis, cardiovascular syphilis, and late benign syphilis (gumma). Many patients in this stage will have a nonreactive VDRL, but all have a positive FTA. Cerebrospinal fluid abnormalities include an elevated protein, pleocytosis, and reactive VDRL.

Ocular complications usually occur during secondary syphilis but may be associated with any of the four stages. Uveitis is the most common ocular disease associated with syphilis, is bilateral in 50% of cases, and occurs in approximately 5% of patients with secondary syphilis. As the ocular manifestations may be protean, an evaluation for syphilis should be included in all initial workups for uveitis.

Symptoms   Blurred vision, eye pain, and photophobia.

Signs   May include several of the following:

1. External: ocular erythema, episcleritis, scleritis.
2. Anterior segment: granulomatous or nongranulomatous iridocyclitis. Engorgement of preexisting iris vascular loops may produce bright red spots on the iris (iris roseata), which may develop into papules (iritis papulosa) or nodules (iritis nodosa). Lens dislocation.
3. Argyll Robertson pupil.
4. Vitritis.
5. Fundus:
   a)   The most common fundus appearance is multifocal or diffuse nonelevated yellow-gray chorioretinal lesions involving the posterior pole and periphery with or without an associated vasculitis.

b) Gass has described a fundus appearance that suggests the diagnosis (acute syphilitic posterior placoid chorioretinitis). Patients had bilateral, large, solitary, flat, yellowish subretinal lesions with faded centers involving the macula and juxtapapillary areas. The fluorescein angiographic pattern was that of early hypofluorescence and late staining.

c) A neuroretinitis can also occur, characterized by a papillitis, retinal edema, and retinal vasculitis, which may be associated with cotton-wool spots, hemorrhages, or paramacular exudates.

d) Retinal artery or vein occlusions, retinal detachments, uveal effusions, primary optic atrophy, choroidal neovascular membranes.

6. Ophthalmoplegia (superior orbital fissure syndrome).

Workup

1. History of recent venereal sore or rash?
2. Check serologic markers:
   a) VDRL or rapid plasma reagin (RPR) and FTA-ABS test (indirect fluorescent assay for antibodies to *T. pallidum*).
   b) Hemagglutination treponemal test for syphilis (HATTS).
   c) Microhemagglutination assay for antibodies to *T. pallidum* (MHA-TP).
3. Lumbar puncture in patients with ocular involvement and serology consistent with late syphilis to rule out neurosyphilis.
4. In HIV-positive patients, syphilis is associated with more extensive ocular disease and is likely to have an accelerated course to nervous system involvement. A lumbar puncture should, therefore, be performed on all HIV-positive patients who may only have serologic or clinical signs of secondary syphilis. HIV-positive patients with secondary syphilis may have a delay in developing a positive response to FTA-ABS and VDRL.
5. Fluorescein angiogram for posterior segment involvement.

Differential Diagnosis

1. Sarcoid
2. Tuberculosis
3. Other causes of necrotizing retinitis (e.g., cytomegalovirus, herpes simplex virus, acute retinal necrosis)

Treatment

1. Consultation with an infectious disease specialist.
2. Ocular syphilis and neurosyphilis should be treated with aqueous crystalline penicillin G 20–24 million units i.v. daily in divided

doses every 4 hours for 10 days followed by 2.4 million units of benzathine penicillin G i.m. weekly for 3 weeks (doses should be decreased in accordance with renal function). Since there is no proven effective alternative in the treatment of neurosyphilis, patients allergic to penicillin should be desensitized before treatment.
3. Laser ablation of treatable choroidal neovascular membranes.

Course and Prognosis Without treatment the disease progresses relentlessly into significant loss of visual function. If treatment is initiated early in the course of the disease the prognosis for visual recovery is improved. The presence of retinal or optic nerve disease worsens the chances of significant visual recovery.

Follow-up Serum VDRL titers should be monitored carefully to determine the adequacy of treatment. In cases of neurosyphilis the cerebrospinal fluid VDRL should be checked every 6 months for 3 years.

Toxocariasis

Ocular toxocariasis is caused by hematogenous invasion of the eye by the larvae of the intestinal roundworm of dogs, *Toxocara canis*. Transmission to humans occurs by ingestion of soil or food contaminated with ova shed in dog feces. Ova hatch in the small intestine; the larvae penetrate the intestinal wall and reach various organs such as the liver, lung, brain, and eyes. Ocular toxocariasis is typically found in children and tends to be unilateral. Three distinct clinical presentations are recognized: endophthalmitis (the most common form), posterior pole retinochoroidal granuloma, and peripheral retinochoroidal granuloma.

Endophthalmitis

Symptoms Painless decrease of vision.

Ocular Examination
1. *External:* minimal injection.
2. Strabismus.
3. *Anterior segment:* anterior uveitis with granulomatous keratic precipitates, flare, cells, and posterior synechiae.
4. *Vitreous:* cells in the anterior vitreous (vitritis) may lead to leukocoria.
5. *Fundus:* a peripheral granuloma or posterior pole granuloma may be seen.

Differential Diagnosis

1. *Retinoblastoma:* usually occurs in younger children and is more commonly bilateral. In contrast to toxocariasis, patients with retinoblastoma have a clear lens, do not form cyclitic membranes, and have calcifications that can be detected by ultrasound.
2. *Pars planitis:* usually bilateral and typically occurs in older children. Although a snowbank may be confused with an inferiorly located *Toxocara* granuloma, a distinct retinochoroidal mass does not develop.
3. *Persistent hyperplastic primary vitreous:* usually diagnosed within the first few weeks of life. The involved eye is usually microphthalmic, a residual hyaloid artery is present, and a vascularized pupillary membrane is often seen.
4. *Coats' disease:* unlike toxocariasis, the vitreous shows little to no inflammatory activity. The typical lesion demonstrates retinal telangiectasia with yellow intraretinal exudation.
5. *Exogenous or endogenous endophthalmitis:* check for history of ocular trauma or immunosuppression.
6. *Retinopathy of prematurity* (ROP): history of low birth weight and supplemental oxygen administration. This condition is almost always bilateral, although frequently asymmetric.

Posterior Pole Granuloma

Symptoms Decreased vision.

Ocular Examination

1. *External:* normal quiet eye, leukocoria.
2. *Anterior segment:* no inflammatory activity.
3. *Vitreous/fundus:* a few vitreous cells may be seen overlying a round elevated yellow-white solitary granuloma (0.5–4 disc diameters) located at the posterior pole, often involving the macula. In chronic granulomas, retinochoroidal anastomosis may be observed within the lesion appearing as large retinal vessels that disappear into the substance of the lesion. A localized serous retinal detachment may overlie the lesion.

Differential Diagnosis

1. *Ocular toxoplasmosis:* healed *Toxoplasma* lesions are flat or depressed, are associated with hyperpigmentation, and commonly are present bilaterally.

2. *POHS:* may be associated with a macular disciform scar resembling a posterior pole granuloma. POHS, however, typically occurs in older patients and also presents with peripapillary atrophy, focal peripheral chorioretinal lesions, and no vitreous cells.

Course and Complications   The extent of visual loss is dependent on the location of the granuloma. Rarely subretinal neovascularization may occur.

Peripheral Retinochoroidal Granuloma

Symptoms   Asymptomatic or decreased visual acuity.

Ocular Examination

1. *External:* quiet eye.
2. *Anterior segment:* no inflammatory activity.
3. *Vitreous/fundus:* a few vitreous cells may be seen overlying a peripherally located yellowish-white granuloma. In the later stages, traction bands may form, extending from the granuloma to the posterior pole, producing retinal folds, macula heterotopia, and occasionally retinal detachment.

Differential Diagnosis

1. Pars planitis: usually bilateral, associated with a more severe vitritis. Whereas the *Toxocara* granuloma may occur in any quadrant, a pars plana snowbank is almost always located in the inferior periphery.
2. Congenital retinal folds: associated with a persistent hyaloid system and no inflammation.
3. Coats' disease.
4. ROP: both *Toxocara* and ROP may produce retinal folds extending from the optic nerve to a white peripheral retinal mass. However, in ROP the retinal dragging usually occurs toward the temporal periphery.

Workup

1. The definitive diagnosis requires the demonstration of *Toxocara* larvae in the eye.
2. Check for history of pica and contact with puppies. History of retinoblastoma in family?
3. Enzyme-linked immunosorbent assay (ELISA) for antibodies to *Toxocara* is the most reliable laboratory test. A titer of 1:8 is

considered positive but lower titers may also be significant. In atypical cases for which the diagnosis is in question due to negative serum titers, aqueous or vitreous samples can also be checked for antibody titers.

4. Cytology: the demonstration of eosinophils in the aqueous or vitreous helps confirm the diagnosis.
5. Ultrasound: to exclude persistent hyperplastic primary vitreous (PHPV) and retinoblastoma.
6. Stool for ova and parasites is *not* useful because the larvae do not mature in the human intestine.

Treatment

1. Patients with minimal to no active inflammation require no treatment.
2. For anterior segment inflammation, topical prednisolone acetate 1% and cycloplegics. If inflammation involves the pars plana region, subtenon injections of 40 mg of methylprednisolone can be given. For severe inflammation, prednisone (60–80 mg/d p.o.) should be administered with gradual tapering.
3. The role of antihelminthic agents such as thiabendazole or diethylcarbamazine is unclear and controversial. They should be used only in conjunction with oral corticosteroids.
4. Pars plana vitrectomy for chronic intraocular inflammation unresponsive to steroids. Scleral buckling or pars plana vitrectomy for tractional or rhegmatogenous retinal detachment or cyclitic membrane formation.
5. Laser photocoagulation may be used in cases in which the intraocular larvae are motile and visible.

Course and Complications   The major complications include cataract, tractional or rhegmatogenous retinal detachment, and cyclitic membrane formation. Rarely subretinal neovascularization may occur.

Toxoplasmosis

Etiology   Toxoplasmosis is caused by the cat parasite *Toxoplasma gondii*. It is almost always congenital (i.e., a previously uninfected female seroconverts during pregnancy and passes the infection transplacentally to the fetus). Maternal infection is caused by exposure to cat feces or by the ingestion of contaminated undercooked meat. The severity of fetal involvement depends on when during pregnancy the infection occurs. Generally if acquired during the third trimester, chorioretinal lesions are totally healed at birth, and unless there is macular involvement, goes undetected. Patients become symptomatic due to recurrences that appear in the form of an active satellite lesion adjacent to an old chorioretinal scar. Toxoplasmosis usually becomes active in only one eye at a time.

Symptoms   Floaters, blurred vision, scotomas.

Signs

1. *External:* quiet eye.
2. *Anterior segment:* cells, flare, and granulomatous or nongranulomatous keratic precipitates may be seen due to spillover from the posterior segment.
3. *Fundus:* the classic lesion is a focal area of exudative retinitis (> 1 disc diameter) adjacent to an old chorioretinal scar with overlying vitritis ("headlight in the fog"). Sheathing of retinal vessels may also be seen in the area of the active lesion. Less commonly, serous retinal elevation may be seen associated with large active lesions. Papillitis may occur due to acute retinitis in the papillary or juxtapapillary area. A deep retinal form with minimal or no vitreal reaction and small multifocal outer retinal lesions usually in the paramacular area has also been described.

Workup

1. Toxoplasmosis titers. Any titer, even in undiluted serum, is significant. In atypical cases where a characteristic fundus lesion is present and serum titers are negative, the aqueous humor can be sampled for the presence of local antitoxoplasmosis antibodies.
2. VDRL-FTA, PPD, chest x-ray, and *Toxocara* titers to exclude other potential causes of exudative retinitis.
3. Fluorescein angiogram for subretinal neovascular lesions.

Differential Diagnosis

1. *Candida endophthalmitis:* usually a multifocal retinitis, not associated with an old chorioretinal scar.
2. *Ocular toxocariasis:* demonstrates an elevated granuloma, not associated with an old chorioretinal scar.
3. *Presumed ocular histoplasmosis syndrome:* never associated with vitreous cells.
4. *CMV retinitis:* lesions are usually associated with retinal hemorrhages at their advancing borders.
5. *Syphilitic chorioretinitis:* usually diffuse or multifocal chorioretinitis which is bilateral in 50% of cases.

6. *Tuberculosis:* usually manifests as a granulomatous anterior uveitis but may also demonstrate focal or multifocal choroiditis with only mild vitreous inflammation.

Treatment Lesions that threaten the macula, involve the optic nerve or papillomacular bundle, or have an associated severe vitritis that may lead to vitreous traction and retinal tear formation *should* be treated. Treatment continues for a total of 6 weeks and includes the following:

1. Pyrimethamine (Daraprim, 75–125 mg loading dose then 25 mg p.o. b.i.d.), or clindamycin (300 mg p.o. q.i.d.). If pyrimethamine is used, pretreatment and weekly complete blood count with platelets should be drawn. Pyrimethamine should be discontinued at the onset of any drop in blood cell or platelet count.
2. Sulfonamides either in the form of sulfadiazine or triple sulfa (if available). Loading dose of 2 to 4 g orally then 1 g orally four times a day.
3. Prednisone (60–80 mg p.o. for 7–10 d) with gradual tapering to 40 mg every other day by 1 month. This dose is maintained until cessation of treatment at 6 weeks. Never use steroids without concomitant antiparasitic therapy.
4. When pyrimethamine is used folinic acid (Leucovorin), 5 mg p.o. three times a week, is taken to prevent bone marrow depression.
5. Topical steroids (e.g., prednisolone acetate 1%) and cycloplegics (e.g., Cyclogyl 2%) to control anterior segment inflammation.

Followup Patients should be followed every week for the first 2 weeks and every 2 weeks thereafter until therapy is completed.

Prognosis and Complications On average patients with ocular toxoplasmosis can anticipate three to four recurrences in their lifetime. With appropriate intervention, the visual prognosis is excellent unless involvement of the macula or papillomacular bundle occurs. Other potential complications affecting the visual prognosis are cystoid macular edema, macular gliosis, subretinal neovascularization, and traction retinal detachment.

Tuberculosis

Etiology Tuberculosis is a chronic granulomatous infection caused by the bacteria *Mycobacterium tuberculosis*. The uvea is involved in about 1.0% of patients with pulmonary disease. Uveal involvement can be seen in the primary, postprimary, and miliary forms of the disease and usually takes the form of an anterior uveitis or disseminated choroiditis.

Symptoms Painless, progressive visual loss.

Signs
1. *External:* rarely conjunctivitis, phlyctenulosis, episcleritis, or scleritis.
2. *Anterior segment:* interstitial keratitis, sclerokeratitis. A chronic iritis or iridocyclitis is usually present, characterized by granulomatous or nongranulomatous keratic precipitates, cells and flare, Koeppe nodules, and posterior synechiae.
3. *Vitreous:* mild vitritis.
4. *Fundus:* focal or multifocal choroiditis, initially small and yellowish lesions with indistinct borders that with time progress to become more distinct, coalesce, and change to a grayish-white color. Occasionally, a large solitary choroidal granuloma may be seen (tuberculoma). Retinal involvement usually occurs secondary to choroidal involvement and presents as a periphlebitis, rarely leading to a vein occlusion.

Workup Usually a presumptive diagnosis due to the lack of histologic confirmation.
1. Elicit history of exposure to tuberculosis.
2. Check PPD using intermediate strength (5 TU) and if negative second strength (250 TU). A response of any size may be significant. A positive PPD may not be significant if a patient has a history of prior BCG injection. In addition, a positive PPD only confirms the clinical impression since it cannot distinguish between previous exposure and active infection.
3. Chest x-ray: a negative x-ray does not rule out tuberculous uveitis.
4. Referral to pulmonary specialist for a positive PPD or chest x-ray. Workup to include sputum collection, gastric washings, and urine culture for acid-fast bacilli.
5. Isoniazid (INH) therapeutic test: may be considered when a uveitis is unresponsive to steroids and tuberculosis uveitis is in the differential diagnosis. INH (300 mg p.o.) is given daily for 3 weeks, with patient examinations performed weekly. If significant clinical improvement is seen, the diagnosis of ocular tuberculosis is likely.

Differential Diagnosis

1. Syphilis: check VDRL, FTA, see Syphilis section, above.
2. Malignant melanoma, metastatic tumor, choroidal hemangioma, granulomatous response to a foreign body: a solitary choroidal tuberculoma may simulate these conditions. Fluorescein angiography and ultrasound can be used to help differentiate these conditions.
3. Sarcoidosis: chest x-ray usually shows hilar adenopathy. Patients are usually anergic. Uncommonly presents as a choroidal granuloma and more often as an anterior uveitis. Check ACE levels, gallium scan.
4. Toxocariasis: typically seen in healthy children. Check ELISA titers.
5. Toxoplasmosis.

Treatment   Consultation with a pulmonary and infectious disease specialist to direct treatment with INH and other antituberculosis drugs such as rifampin and pyrazinamide.

Prognosis   Early diagnosis of tuberculosis uveitis is essential in order to salvage useful vision. Involvement of the macula or optic nerve significantly worsens the prognosis. Since the disease can be successfully treated with specific anti-tuberculosis drugs, it is prudent to err on the side of overdiagnosis. The INH therapeutic test should be performed in any patient with clinical and laboratory findings consistent with tuberculosis uveitis.

Viral Uveitis

Cytomegalovirus Retinitis

CMV retinitis can occur as an acquired disease in immunosuppressed individuals or as a congenital disease in infants.

Congenital CMV is present in 0.5% to 0.2% of all live births and presents with either no symptoms or a nonspecific viral syndrome. Systemic features include fever, pneumonitis, and thrombocytopenia. Central nervous system involvement may cause cerebral periventricular calcifications, deafness, and seizures. Ocular features include optic atrophy, optic nerve hypoplasia, coloboma, microphthalmos or anophthalmos, cataracts, and a multifocal retinochoroiditis (most common feature) resembling toxoplasmosis.

Acquired CMV is most commonly due to AIDS or iatrogenic immunosuppression following organ transplantation or treatment of malignancies.

Symptoms A peripheral lesion may be asymptomatic or cause floaters. A posterior pole lesion leads to blurred vision or scotomas.

Signs

1. *External:* quiet eye.
2. *Anterior segment:* mild to moderate anterior uveitis.
3. *Vitreous:* minimal to mild vitritis.
4. *Fundus:* initially white fluffy retinal infiltrates that are associated with scattered hemorrhages or more granular appearing infiltrates with little associated hemorrhage. Lesions tend to have a perivascular distribution. As the disease progresses, old lesions spread to involve previously normal retina (leading to coalescence), retinal atrophy occurs in older lesions leading to a "brushfire" appearance with retinal pigment epithelial (RPE) stippling centrally, surrounded by the advancing edges of the lesion, which are white and fluffy, and vascular sheathing and hemorrhages become more prominent. When the disease reaches end-stage, the fundus is characterized by a pale optic nerve, atrophic retina, and narrow sheathed retinal vessels.

Workup

1. Elicit risk factors for HIV infection (intravenous drug use, previous blood transfusion, homosexuality, bisexuality, promiscuity).
2. Demonstration of CMV in secretions such as urine, blood, saliva, and buffy coat is important but not diagnostic since it only corroborates active CMV infection. Similarly the presence of serum antibody titers to CMV is not diagnostic because it only indicates previous exposure to CMV. In contrast, the presence in infants of antibodies to CMV after the age of 6 months is more significant.
3. Consider chorioretinal tissue biopsy of a blind eye in bilateral disease of unknown etiology.

Differential Diagnosis

1. *Cotton-wool spots:* the most common ocular finding in AIDS patients. These lesions may spontaneously regress and are rarely associated with hemorrhages.

2. *Ocular toxoplasmosis:* rarely associated with hemorrhages. Usually associated with a more vigorous vitritis (even in immunocompromised patients).
3. *Candida endophthalmitis:* more significant vitritis and no retinal hemorrhages.
4. *Acute retinal necrosis:* generally healthy patients with less hemorrhage.
5. *Herpes simplex retinitis:* usually associated viral encephalitis.

Treatment

1. Decrease the dose of immunosuppressive drugs if possible.
2. Intravenous administration of gancyclovir (5 mg/kg every 12 hrs for 2 wks followed by maintenance I.V. gancyclovir 5 mg/kg in one daily infusion 5 days a week).
3. Neutropenia or other forms of toxicity may preclude intravenous administration but in such circumstances gancyclovir can be given as an intravitreal injection. Induction therapy involves a series of 6 intravitreal injections of 200 micrograms in 0.1 ml per treatment. This is given over an 18-day period followed by weekly intravitreal injections of gancyclovir 200 micrograms in 0.1 ml.
4. In cases of suspected CMV retinitis, weekly ophthalmoscopic examinations with fundus photography should be performed to monitor for progression to a more characteristic fundus appearance.

Course and Prognosis   Untreated CMV retinitis invariably leads to blindness. Once the optic nerve or macula becomes involved, rapid visual deterioration occurs. Visual loss may also occur secondary to a rhegmatogenous retinal detachment. Of patients with CMV retinitis, 80% show clinical improvement or stabilization after gancyclovir treatment. Unfortunately, reactivation of the disease may occur in up to 50% of patients despite aggressive maintenance therapy.

Acute Retinal Necrosis (ARN)

ARN is a necrotizing retinitis that usually affects otherwise healthy patients of all age groups. Bilateral involvement occurs in one-third of cases. Members of the herpes virus family, including herpes simplex, herpes zoster, and CMV, have been implicated as etiologic agents.

Symptoms   Ocular or periorbital pain, floaters, and blurred vision.

Signs

1. *External:* conjunctival and/or diffuse episcleral injection.
2. *Anterior segment:* mild to severe anterior uveitis with either fine or mutton-fat keratic precipitates. In late stages cataract formation, posterior synechiae, rubeosis, and neovascular glaucoma may occur.
3. *Vitreous:* a mild vitritis that becomes increasingly involved, leading to organization and contraction.
4. *Fundus:* multifocal yellow-white patches of retinitis generally located between the midperiphery and ora serrata that usually coalesce within a week. A retinal vasculitis with narrowing and sheathing of vessels, and retinal hemorrhages develop as the disease progresses. Acute optic nerve edema and macular edema may also be seen during the acute stage of the disease.

Workup Diagnosis is based on clinical criteria.

1. Rule out other known causes of retinitis: VDRL, FTA, ANA, toxoplasmosis titers, PPD, chest x-ray, urine for CMV, HIV titers.
2. Ultrasonography to rule out acute optic neuropathy and evaluate the posterior segment with a severe vitritis.
3. Fluorescein angiogram: no retinal perfusion in areas of active retinitis; staining of the optic nerve and macular edema.

Differential Diagnosis

1. Beçhet's disease: associated with genital ulcers, aphthous lesions, arthritis, and other systemic manifestations. The retinal vasculitis generally involves the posterior pole and has a course characterized by exacerbations and remissions.
2. Toxoplasmosis.
3. Syphilis.
4. Bacterial or fungal endophthalmitis: can usually be excluded by clinical history. More significant anterior segment involvement is seen, and in cases of endogenous endophthalmitis, a systemic source of infection is present.
5. Collagen vascular disease (e.g., lupus or periarteritis nodosa).
6. Histiocytic lymphoma: may present with white retinal lesions and a vitritis, but usually has a chronic course and studies including CT scan, lumbar puncture, and vitreous biopsy help establish the diagnosis.
7. CMV retinitis: nearly always in an immunocompromised host. More commonly involves the posterior pole with more retinal hemorrhages and less vitreous reaction.

Treatment

1. Initially, intravenous administration of acyclovir 1500 mg/sq meter every 8 hours for 5 to 10 days followed by oral acyclovir 400–600 mg 5 times a day for 4 to 6 weeks. Patients need baseline complete blood count, blood urea nitrogen, creatinine, and liver function tests.
2. Consider aspirin, 325 mg q day or b.i.d., to help prevent the vascular obstructive complication.
3. Prednisone 60–80 mg/d (p.o. for 1–2 wks with gradual tapering) may be used (only in conjunction with acyclovir) to suppress inflammation. Steroids do not have any beneficial effect on the severity of the retinitis. Topical prednisolone to control anterior segment uveitis.
4. As lesions regress, laser photocoagulation posterior to necrotic retina to create an area of chorioretinal adhesion to help prevent development of a retinal detachment.
5. Optic nerve sheath decompression for acute optic neuropathy.
6. Scleral buckling or pars plana vitrectomy or both should be used for ARN retinal detachments.
7. The role of early vitrectomy, intravitreal acyclovir, and an encircling buckle used prophylactically prior to a retinal detachment is controversial. This option might be considered if vitreous opacification precludes laser treatment.

Course and Prognosis   The acute stage of the disease resolves within 1 to 3 months leaving behind atrophic retina. Due to full-thickness retinal necrosis and vitreous fibrosis, 75% of patients develop rhegmatogenous retinal detachments with varying degrees of proliferative vitreoretino-pathy. The long-term prognosis for vision is adversely affected by the development of ARN optic neuritis, and the development of a retinal detachment.

Follow-up   During hospitalization, patients should be followed daily. Thereafter, patients should be seen every 3 to 4 weeks for approximately 1 year. Both eyes should always be examined since second eye involvement may occur weeks to years after the onset of ARN in the first eye.

Herpes Zoster Uveitis

Herpes zoster uveitis occurs in approximately 40% of patients with cutaneous herpes zoster ophthalmicus (HZO). Onset of the uveitis usually occurs within 2 to 4 weeks following development of the characteristic skin eruption in the ophthalmic division of the trigeminal nerve. Ocular involvement is uncommon unless the nasociliary branch is involved (manifested by vesicles affecting the tip or side of the nose). Herpes zoster ophthalmicus is almost always unilateral, and the accompanying uveitis involves the same side. Ophthalmic zoster generally occurs in either elderly or immunosuppressed patients. The anterior uveitis is felt to occur as a result of ischemia secondary to vascular occlusion.

Symptoms Ophthalmic zoster prodomal symptoms include malaise, headache, nausea, and fever, followed by the development of pain in the area of future skin eruption.

Signs

1. *External:* skin eruption in the distribution of the first division of the trigeminal nerve. Conjunctivitis, episcleritis, scleritis, and ocular motor palsies may also occur.
2. *Anterior segment:* decreased corneal sensation due to neurotrophic keratitis, dendritic, stromal, or disciform keratitis, mild to severe iritis with medium to large keratic precipitates, posterior synechia, "moth-eaten" iris atrophy, hyphema, and hypopyon may occur. Zoster may occur with or without a concomitant uveitis.
3. *Vitreous:* anterior vitreous cells.
4. *Fundus:* usually normal, but choroiditis, occlusive retinal vasculitis, optic neuropathy, and retinal detachment have been reported.

Workup

1. Check for a history of immunosuppression. If occuring in a young healthy patient, consider HIV.
2. Diagnosis made on basis of characteristic appearance of HZO. The uveitis may occur after the skin lesions of HZO resolve.
3. Fluorescein angiogram may show occlusion of iris vessels.

Differential Diagnosis Herpes simplex keratouveitis: no associated skin eruption, iris atrophy with sharply defined borders and scalloped margins, patent iris arteries on angiography, commonly associated with hyphema and secondary glaucoma.

Treatment

1. Oral acyclovir, 600 mg five times a day for 10 days, for active skin lesions (maximum benefit in decreasing the severity of the

uveitis is obtained if started within 72 h after onset of the skin lesions).

2. Cycloplegia to prevent posterior synechiae formation.
3. Topical steroids to control the anterior uveitis. A slow taper is essential to prevent problems of rebound inflammation.
4. Systemic steroids should be considered during the acute phase of HZO to help prevent potential neurologic complications due to cerebral vasculitis and to help prevent postherpetic neuralgia.

Course and Complications   Herpes zoster uveitis usually has a prolonged course lasting several months. Secondary glaucoma and cataract formation may occur.

Vogt-Koyanagi-Harada (VKH) Syndrome

VKH is an idiopathic uveomeningeal syndrome characterized by bilateral anterior and posterior uveitis associated with meningeal and cutaneous findings. VKH syndrome represents the integration of V-K syndrome and Harada's disease (Table 6.5). The disease typically affects darkly pigmented adults (Orientals, blacks, and American Indians) in their third decade.

Symptoms   Pain, photophobia, or painless visual loss.

Signs

1. *External:* ciliary injection, perilimbal vitiligo (Sugiura's sign).
2. *Anterior segment:* granulomatous iridocyclitis with mutton-fat keratic precipitates, iris nodules, peripheral anterior and posterior synechiae.
3. *Vitreous:* vitritis is almost always present.
4. *Fundus:* diffuse multifocal choroiditis frequently resulting in exudative retinal detachments. Following spontaneous reattachment, areas of depigmentation are seen leading to a "sunset glow" appearance to the posterior pole. Optic nerve swelling and hyperemia are common. Peripapillary vasculitis, peripheral periphlebitis, retinal neovascularization, subretinal neovascularization, and retinal arteriovenous anastomoses have been reported.

Systemic Features

1. Cutaneous: poliosis, vitiligo, and alopecia. These signs usually occur weeks to months to years after onset of the ocular disease.

TABLE 6.5

Comparison of V-K syndrome and Harada's disease

	V-K Syndrome	**Harada's Disease**
Age	Early middle age	Early middle age
Race	Oriental, black, heavily pigmented white	Oriental, black, heavily pigmented white
CNS symptoms	Mild or absent	Usually marked
Ocular symptoms	Severe anterior and posterior uveitis (predominantly anterior)	Slight anterior uveitis; marked choroiditis and vitritis; frequent secondary retinal detachment
Prognosis for vision	Poor	Fair to good
Sequelae	Sequelae of other severe uveitis	Spontaneous healing of retinal detachment with albinotic depigmentation of fundus
Auditory disturbances	Common (> 50%)	Common
Alterations of hair	Generally constant (~90%)	Uncommon (< 10%)
Skin changes	Common (> 50%)	Uncommon (< 10%)

From Font RL, Perry HD. Clinical and histopathological observation in severe Vogt-Koyanagi-Harada syndrome. Am J Ophthalmol 1977; 83(2) 244–54.

2. Neurologic: headache, stiff neck (meningeal) which may precede or occur at the onset of the disease. Other neurologic features include coma, delirium, convulsions, ataxia, cranial nerve palsies, tinnitus, deafness.

Workup

1. To establish the diagnosis the following criteria must be present:
   a) No previous history of ocular trauma or surgery.
   b) At least three of the following groups of signs should be present:
      Group 1: cutaneous findings
      Group 2: neurologic findings
      Group 3: anterior uveitis
      Group 4: posterior uveitis
2. Lumbar puncture: Cerebrospinal fluid may show lymphocytosis and elevated protein levels.

3. Neurologic consultation.
4. Fluorescein angiogram: can demonstrate choroiditis, serous retinal detachments, optic nerve leakage, vasculitis, or subretinal neovascularization.
5. HLA testing: increased prevalence of HLA-B22 in Japanese.

Differential Diagnosis

1. Sympathetic ophthalmia: associated with a history of trauma or ocular surgery. No racial predilection.
2. Serous retinal detachments due to toxoplasmosis, posterior scleritis associated with rheumatoid arthritis, and central serous retinopathy.
3. Acute posterior multifocal placoid pigment epitheliopathy: self-limiting and nonrecurrent with spontaneous resolution over several weeks.
4. Serpiginous choroidopathy.
5. Rhegmatogenous retinal detachment: in VKH syndrome, detachments are usually bilateral and are nonrhegmatogenous.

Treatment Anterior uveitis is treated with topical steroids and then gradually tapered. If necessary, periocular and systemic steroid therapy can also be used to control the anterior chamber inflammatory reaction. Posterior uveitis should be treated with prednisone given orally in the range of 100–120 mg/day in divided doses. Maintenance doses may be required for months to years to prevent recurrences. Laser treatment may be necessary for subretinal neovascularization threatening central vision.

Course and Prognosis The course may be severe and chronic. The visual prognosis is poor without appropriate treatment and the early administration of steroids significantly improves the visual outcome. Common causes for visual loss are secondary glaucoma, cataract, macular scarring, and phthisis bulbi.

White Dot Syndromes

Multiple Evanescent White Dot Syndrome (MEWDS)

MEWDS is an acute idiopathic inflammatory disease predominantly found in young women. The disease is usually unilateral and nonrecurrent.

Symptoms   Acute vision loss, stationary black spots, blurred vision, flashing lights.

Signs

1. Afferent pupillary defect may occur.
2. *External:* quiet eye.
3. *Anterior segment:* quiet or mild flare and cells.
4. *Vitreous:* vitreous cells may be seen.
5. *Fundus:* multiple small (100–200 μm) white dots located in the deep retina or RPE, most concentrated in the parafoveal area but may also extend from the posterior pole into the midperiphery. A fine granularity of the macular RPE is also seen. Other findings include mild venous sheathing and disc swelling.

Workup   Diagnosis made on the basis of typical clinical findings.

1. Fluorescein angiogram: demonstrates early hyperfluorescence of the white dots in a wreath-like pattern with late staining. Optic nerve leakage may also be seen.
2. Electroretinogram (ERG): in the acute stage associated with visual loss, the ERG "A" wave and the early receptor potential amplitudes are decreased. These return to normal during the recovery phase of the disease.
3. Visual field: enlargement of the blind spot during the acute stages of the disease with and without associated optic nerve edema, arcuate, central, and cecocentral scotomas and constriction of peripheral isopters.

Differential Diagnosis

1. *Acute posterior multifocal placoid pigment epitheliopathy (APMPPE):* usually bilateral, occuring equally in men and women. The yellow-white lesions involving the RPE are much larger than the white lesions of MEWDS. The angiogram reveals early blocking and late staining of the lesions. When the lesions fade, more prominent RPE changes are seen. Good visual prognosis.
2. *Acute retinal pigment epitheliitis:* presents as an acute visual loss in young and middle-aged patients. The lesions, which cluster around the fovea, appear as dark spots surrounded by a yellow halo of depigmentation. The spots resolve in 6 to 12 weeks. Fluorescein angiogram reveals hypofluorescence surrounded by a rim of hyperfluorescence.

3. *Birdshot retinochoroidopathy:* occurs in an older age group (women 50–70 yrs of age), is bilateral, and does not present with acute visual loss. Posterior segment findings of vitritis and retinal vascular leakage are much more prominent, and patients commonly develop cystoid macular edema. The course is characterized by exacerbations and remissions.
4. *Sarcoid:* usually bilateral with more significant vitreal involvement.
5. *Recurrent multifocal choroiditis:* occurs primarily in young, healthy, myopic women. Acutely, multiple, round, well-circumscribed, grayish lesions appear at the level of the RPE and choriocapillaris in the macula and posterior pole. Optic nerve edema and vitritis may also be present. Resolved lesions resemble old histo spots. Recurrent exacerbations are common, with new lesions developing adjacent to old lesions. Subretinal neovascularization is a common complication of parafoveal lesions. Both inflammatory lesions and subretinal neovascularization are responsive to periocular or systemic steroids or both.
6. *Serpiginous choroidopathy:* typically affects older patients. Course is chronic and recurring, with a poor visual prognosis.

Treatment   None.

Course and Prognosis   The ocular signs usually resolve (leaving only subtle RPE changes) with recovery of vision to normal levels over 2 to 6 weeks. The visual field defects may persist despite return of normal vision and resolution of the fundus findings. Rare recurrences have been reported.

Acute Posterior Multifocal Placoid Pigment Epitheliopathy [APMPPE]

APMPPE typically affects young adults of either sex. A preceding acute viral illness commonly occurs. Most cases are bilateral, with second eye involvement occurring within several days of the first.

Symptoms   Rapid loss of central vision, scotomas.

Signs

1. *External:* usually quiet, episcleritis.
2. *Anterior segment:* mild nongranulomatous iritis may be present.
3. *Vitreous:* mild vitritis is present in 50% of patients.

4. *Fundus:* multiple, noncontiguous, flat yellow-white lesions of varying sizes appear at the level of the RPE. The lesions usually involve the posterior pole or macula area but may extend out to the equatorial region. Other less common fundus manifestations include papilledema, papillitis, venous sheathing, venous tortuosity, and serous retinal detachment.

Workup

1. History of preceding viral illness (e.g., upper respiratory infection, erythema nodosum).
2. Fluorescein angiogram: characteristic pattern of early blocking of choroidal fluorescence with late staining.

Differential Diagnosis   See Multiple Evanescent White Dot Syndrome section, above.

Treatment   None.

Course and Prognosis   Most patients regain excellent vision within 2 to 12 weeks; however, full recovery may not occur, as a result of residual foveal changes. In addition, recurrences may rarely occur, which worsen the visual prognosis.

Follow-up   No follow-up is required once visual recovery occurs.

Birdshot Retinochoroidopathy

Birdshot (vitiliginous) retinochoroidopathy is an idiopathic chronic inflammatory disease that is typically bilateral, affects whites almost exclusively, and affects women more commonly than men. The age of onset ranges from 35 to 70 years. There are no known associated systemic illnesses.

Symptoms   Decreased vision and floaters. Less commonly, nyctalopia, decreased color vision, and photopsias.

Signs

1. *External:* usually quiet eye, rarely erythematous.
2. *Anterior segment:* usually clear, or minimal inflammation.
3. *Vitreous:* vitritis (most pronounced in the posterior vitreous); posterior vitreous separation and keratic precipitates may occasionally be seen on the posterior vitreous surface. No snowballs or snowbanks occur.

4. *Fundus:* multiple cream-colored or depigmented lesions appear at the level of the choroid or RPE. The lesions are seen in the posterior pole and extend to the equatorial region with the highest concentration of lesions noted around the optic disc and nasal to the nerve head. The lesions vary in size and shape but are most frequently oval with a diameter less than one-fourth disc diameter with poorly defined margins. Lesions are not associated with any secondary hyperpigmentation. A retinal vasculitis may lead to cystoid macular edema (CME) and disc edema. Other less common findings include arteriolar narrowing, vascular sheathing, dilation and beading of retinal veins, and small flame-shaped hemorrhages.

Workup   Diagnosis is usually based on clinical findings.

1. HLA typing: HLA-A29 is positive in 80% to 95% of cases.
2. Fluorescein angiogram: to demonstrate CME, disc edema, and leakage from retinal capillaries. The birdshot lesions show mild hyperfluorescence in the late phase of the angiogram.

Differential Diagnosis   See also Multiple Evanescent White Dot Syndrome section, above.

1. *Pars planitis:* depigmented fundus lesions are not seen, and a snowbank is present.
2. *Senile vitritis:* depigmented fundus lesions are not seen.
3. *Harada's disease:* usually presents in darkly pigmented patients, has associated systemic features, and typically demonstrates serous retinal detachments. CME is not generally seen.
4. *Beçhet's disease:* has associated systemic features and more significant anterior segment inflammation.
5. *Histiocytic lymphoma:* lesions are less diffuse and symmetrical compared to birdshot.

Treatment

1. The efficiency of steroids in this disease has not been established. However, patients with evidence of CME and visual acuity less than 20/40 may be treated with either periocular (40 mg of methylprednisolone) or systemic steroids (prednisone, 60–80 mg/d) and tapered slowly.
2. Cyclosporin A for cases unresponsive to steroids.
3. Laser ablation for subretinal neovascularization.

Course and Complications   The course is characterized by recurrent exacerbations and remissions. The most common cause of decreased vision is the development of CME. Less common causes are epiretinal membrane formation, cataract, optic atrophy, vitreous hemorrhage secondary to retinal neovascularization, and subretinal neovascularization.

Prognosis   Due to the poor response to anti-inflammatory therapy, the long-term visual prognosis is guarded.

Serpiginous Choroidopathy

Serpiginous choroidopathy is a chronic recurrent multifocal disease that involves the RPE and choriocapillaris. It typically affects white middle-aged individuals in the fourth to fifth decade of life. The disease is almost always bilateral, but may be markedly asymmetric. There are no associated systemic manifestations.

Symptoms   Blurred vision, metamorphopsia, positive central scotoma, and flashing lights.

Signs

1. *External:* quiet eye.
2. *Anterior segment:* normal or rarely a mild iridocyclitis.
3. *Vitreous:* during active phase, vitreous cells may be present.
4. *Fundus:* lesions usually begin to appear around the optic nerve head and over a period of months to years spread centrifugally in all directions. Less commonly lesions appear in the macula without initial peripapillary lesions or begin in the periphery and spread toward the optic disc. In the active stage of the disease, gray or cream-colored lesions involving the RPE or choriocapillaris or both are found, usually appearing adjacent to old scars. The active stage lasts several weeks and is followed by gradual lightening of the lesions.

Differential Diagnosis   See Multiple Evanescent White Dot Syndrome section, above.

1. Angioid streaks: usually associated with a systemic illness (e.g., Paget's disease, pseudoxanthoma elasticum). Fluorescein angiogram shows early hyperfluorescence of the lesions.
2. POHS: characterized by the absence of vitreous cells, peripapillary atrophy, peripheral punched-out lesions, and subretinal neovascularization involving the macula.

3. Other causes of choroiditis (e.g., sarcoid, tuberculosis, VKH syndrome, and syphilis).

Workup   Diagnosis is made on the basis of clinical appearance. Fluorescein angiogram: the active lesions demonstrate early blockage of fluorescence with late staining. Old atrophic lesions demonstrate early hypofluorescence due to absent choriocapillaris with diffuse staining of the scar in the late phase.

Treatment

1. Although corticosteroids have generally proved ineffective in controlling the disease, a trial of high-dose prednisone (e.g., 60–80 mg/d) for 1 week or posterior subtenon's methylprednisolone (40 mg) or both seems reasonable for active lesions threatening the macula.
2. Laser photocoagulation for subretinal neovascular membranes.
3. Serial fundus photography to follow the course of the disease.

Course and Complications   The disease is characterized by multiple recurrences. Intervals between attacks may vary from weeks to years. Visual loss is related to eventual foveal or parafoveal involvement, and subretinal neovascular membrane formation, which usually occurs at the edge of an old scar.

Selected Readings

Ankylosing Spondylitis

Birkbeck MQ, Buckler WJ, Mason RM, Tegner WS. Iritis as the presenting symptom in ankylosing spondylitis. Lancet 1951;2:802–3.

Beckingsale AB, Davies J, Gibson JM, Rosenthal R. Acute anterior uveitis, ankylosing spondylitis, back pain, and HLA B27. Br J Ophthalmol 1984;68:741–45.

Rosenbaum JT. Characterization of uveitis associated with spondyloarthritis. J Rheumatol 1989;16(6):792–96.

Reiter's Syndrome

Ostler HN, Dawson CR, Schachter J, Engleman EP. Reiter's syndrome. Am J Ophthalmol 1971;71(5):986–91.

Lee DA, Barker SM, Su WPD, Allen GL, Liesegang TJ, Ilstrup DM. The clinical diagnosis of Reiter's syndrome. Ophthalmology 1986;93(3):350–56.

Psoriasis

Lambert JR, Wright V. Eye inflammation in psoriatic arthritis. Ann Rheum Dis 1976;35:354–56.

Knox DL. Psoriasis and intraocular inflammation. Trans Am Ophthalmol Soc 1979;77:210–24.

Juvenile Rheumatoid Arthritis

Kanski JJ. Juvenile arthritis and uveitis. Surv Ophthalmol 1990;34(4):253–67.

Beçhet's Disease

Colvard DM, Robertson DM, O'Duffy JD. The ocular manifestations of Beçhet's disease. Arch Ophthalmol 1977;95:1813–17.

Mishima S, Masuda K, Izawa Y, Mochizuki M. Beçhet's disease in Japan. Trans Am Ophthalmol Soc 1979;77:225–79.

Michelson JB, Chisari FV. Beçhet's disease. Surv Ophthalmol 1982;26(4):190–203.

Benezra D, Cohen E. Treatment and visual prognosis in Beçhet's disease. Br J Ophthalmol 1986;70:589–92.

Binder AI, Graham EM, Sanders MD, Dinning W, James DG, Denman AM. Cyclosporin A in the treatment of severe Beçhet's disease. Br J Rheumatol 1987;26:285–91.

Acute Onset Exogenous Endophthalmitis

Katz LJ, Cantor LB, Spaeth GL. Complications of surgery in glaucoma. Ophthalmology 1985;92(7):959–63.

Driebe WT, Mandelbaum S, Forster RK, Schwartz LK, Culbertson WW. Pseudophakic endophthalmitis. Diagnosis and management. Ophthalmology 1986;93(4):442–48.

Smolin G, Friedlaender MH, eds. Endophthalmitis. Int Ophthalmol Clin 1987;27(2).

Davis JL, Koidou-Tsiligianni A, Pflugfelder SC, Miller D, Flynn HW, Forster RK. Coagulase-negative staphylococcal endophthalmitis. Increase in antimicrobial resistance. Ophthalmology 1988;95(10):1404–10.

Stern GA, Engel HM, Driebe WT. The treatment of postoperative endophthalmitis. Ophthalmology 1989;96(1):62–67.

Delayed Onset Exogenous Endophthalmitis

Roussel TJ, Culbertson WW, Jaffe NS. Chronic postoperative endophthalmitis associated with Propionibacterium acnes. Arch Ophthalmol 1987;105:1199–1201.

Brady SE, Cohen EJ, Fischer DH. Diagnosis and treatment of chronic postoperative bacterial endophthalmitis. Ophthalmol Surg 1988;19:580–83.

Meisler DM, Mandelbaum S. Propionibacterium associated endophthalmitis after extracapsular cataract extraction. Ophthalmology 1989;96(1):54–61.

Theodore FH. Etiology and diagnosis of fungal postoperative
  endophthalmitis. Ophthalmology 1978;85:327–40.
Pettit TH, Olson RJ, Foos RY, Martin WJ. Fungal endophthalmitis following
  intraocular lens implantation. Arch Ophthalmol 1980;98:1025–39.
Pflugfelder SC, Flynn HW, Zwickey TA, et al. Exogenous fungal
  endophthalmitis. Ophthalmology 1988;95(1):19–30.

Nonsurgical Traumatic Endophthalmitis

Parrish CM, O'Day DM. Traumatic endophthalmitis. Int Ophthalmol Clin
  1987;27(2):112–19.
Affeldt JC, Flynn HW, Forster RK, Mandelbaum S, Clarkson JG, Jarus GD.
  Microbial endophthalmitis resulting from ocular trauma. Ophthalmology
  1987;94(4):407–13.
Boldt HC, Pulido JS, Blodi CF, Folk JC, Weingeist TA. Rural endophthalmitis.
  Ophthalmology 1989;96(12):1722–26.

Fungal Endogenous Endophthalmitis

Stern GA, Fetkenhour CL, O'Grady RB. Intravitreal amphotericin B in the
  treatment of *Candida* endophthalmitis. Arch Ophthalmol 1977;95:89–93.
Michelson JB, Friedlaender MH. Endophthalmitis of drug abuse. Int
  Ophthalmol Clin 1987;27(2):120–26.
Brod RD, Flynn HW, Clarkson JG, Pflugfelder SC, Culbertson WW, Miller D.
  Endogenous *Candida* endophthalmitis. Ophthalmology 1990;97(5):666–74.

Bacterial Endogenous Endophthalmitis

Greenwald MJ, Wohl LG, Sell CH. Metastatic bacterial endophthalmitis. A
  contemporary reappraisal. Surv Ophthalmol 1986;31(2):81–101.

Fuchs' Heterochromic Iridocyclitis

Franceschetti A. Heterochromic cyclitis. Am J Ophthalmol 1955;39:50–58.
Kimura SJ. Fuchs' syndrome of heterochromic cyclitis in brown eyed
  patients. Trans Am Ophthalmol Soc 1978;76:76–88.
Liesegang TJ. Clinical features and prognosis in Fuchs' uveitis syndrome.
  Arch Ophthalmol 1982;100:1622–26.
Arffa RC, Schlaegel TF. Chorioretinal scars in Fuchs' heterochromic
  iridocyclitis. Arch Ophthalmol 1984;102:1153–55.
Gee SS, Tabbara KF. Extracapsular cataract extraction in Fuchs'
  heterochromic iridocyclitis. Am J Ophthalmol 1989;108:310–14.

Intermediate Uveitis (Pars Planitis, Chronic Cyclitis)

Smith RE, Godfrey WA, Kimura SJ. Complications of chronic cyclitis. Am
  J Ophthalmol 1976;82(2):277–82.

Aaberg TM, Cesarz TJ, Flickinger RR. Treatment of pars planitis. Surv Ophthalmol 1977;22(2):120–30.

Henderly DE, Genstler AJ, Rao NA, Smith RE. Pars planitis. Trans Ophthalmol Soc UK 1986;105:227–32.

Henderly DE, Haymond RS, Rao NA, Smith RE. The significance of the pars plana exudate in pars planitis. Am J Ophthalmol 1987;103:669–71.

Winward KE, Smith JL, Culbertson WW, Paris-Hamelin A. Ocular Lyme borreliosis. Am J Ophthalmol 1989;108:651–57.

Phacoantigenic Uveitis

Apple DJ, Mamalis N, Steinmetz RL, Loftfoeld K, Crandall AS, Olson RJ. Phacoanaphylactic endophthalmitis associated with extracapsular cataract extraction and posterior chamber intraocular lens. Arch Ophthalmol 1984;102:1528–32.

Wohl LG, Kline OR, Lucier AC, Galman BD. Pseudophakic phacoanaphylactic endophthalmitis. Ophthalmic Surg 1986;17(4):234–37.

Abrahams IW. Phakoanaphylaxis as a cause of granulomatous uveitis following extracapsular cataract surgery. Ann Ophthalmol 1987;19:211–14.

Chan CC. Relationship between sympathetic ophthalmia, phacoanaphylactic endophthalmitis and Vogt-Koyanagi-Harada disease. Ophthalmology 1988;95(5):619–24.

Presumed Ocular Histoplasmosis Syndrome

Braley RE, Meridith TA, Aaberg TM, Koethe SM, Witowski JA. The prevalence of HLA-B7 in presumed ocular histoplasmosis. Am J Ophthalmol 1978;85:859–61.

Olk RJ, Burgess DB, McCormick PA. Subfoveal and juxtafoveal subretinal neovascularization in the presumed ocular histoplasmosis syndrome. Ophthalmology 1984;91(12):1592–1602.

Macular Photocoagulation Study Group. Argon laser photocoagulation for neovascular maculopathy. Arch Ophthalmol 1986;104:694–701.

Macular Photocoagulation Study Group. Krypton laser photocoagulation for neovascular lesions of ocular histoplasmosis. Arch Ophthalmol 1987;105:1499–1507.

Sarcoidosis

Obenauf CD, Shaw HE, Sydnor CF, Klinworth GK. Sarcoidosis and its ophthalmic manifestations. Am J Ophthalmol 1978;86:648–55.

O'Connor GR. Ocular sarcoidosis. Trans New Orleans Acad Ophthalmol 1983;211–22.

Weinreb RN, Tessler H. Laboratory diagnosis of ophthalmic sarcoidosis. Surv Ophthalmol 1984;28(6):653–64.

Callen JP, Eiferman RA. Sarcoidosis: a multisystem disorder with prominent ocular and cutaneous involvement. Int Ophthalmol Clin 1985;25:135–58.

James DG. Ocular sarcoidosis. Ann NY Acad Sci 1986;465:551–63.

Sympathetic Ophthalmia

Makley TA, Azar A. Sympathetic ophthalmia. A long-term follow-up. Arch Ophthalmol 1978;96:257–62.

Marak GE. Recent advances in sympathetic ophthalmia. Surv Ophthalmol 1979;24(3):141–56.

Reynard M, Riffenburgh RS, Maes E. Effect of corticosteroid treatment and enucleation on the visual prognosis of sympathetic ophthalmia. Am J Ophthalmol 1983;96:290–94.

Chan C-C. Relationship between sympathetic ophthalmia, phacoanaphylactic endophthalmitis and Vogt-Koyanagi-Harada disease. Ophthalmology 1988;95(5):619–24.

Jennings T, Tessler HH. Twenty cases of sympathetic ophthalmia. Br J Ophthalmol 1989;73:140–45.

Albert DM, Diaz-Rohena R. A historical review of sympathetic ophthalmia and its epidemiology. Surv Ophthalmol 1989;34(1):1–14.

Syphilis

Spoor TC, Wynn P, Hartel WC, Bryan CS. Ocular syphilis acute and chronic. J Clin Neuro Ophthalmol 1983;3:197–203.

Becerra LI, Ksiazek SM, Savino PJ, et al. Syphilitic uveitis in human immunodeficiency virus infected and noninfected patients. Ophthalmology 1989;96(12):1727–30.

Beauvais DA, Michelson JB, Seybold ME, Friedlaender MH, Boyden DG. Retroviruses and their playpals. Surv Ophthalmol 1989;34(1):59–64.

Tamesis RR, Foster CS. Ocular syphilis. Ophthalmology 1990;97(10):1281–87.

Gass JDM, Braunstein RA, Chenweth RG. Acute syphilitic posterior placoid chorioretinitis. Ophthalmology 1990;97(10):1288–97.

Toxocariasis

Pollard ZF, Jarrett WH, Hagler WS, Allain DS, Schantz PM. ELISA for diagnosis of ocular toxocariasis. Ophthalmology 1979;86:743–52.

Searl SS, Moazed K, Albert DM, Marcus LC. Ocular toxocariasis presenting as leukocoria in a patient with low ELISA titer to *Toxocara canis*. Ophthalmology 1981;88:1302–06.

Hagler WS, Pollard ZF, Jarrett WH, Donnelly EH. Results of surgery for ocular *Toxocara canis*. Ophthalmology 1981;88:1081–86.

Sorr EM. Meandering ocular toxocariasis. Retina 1984;4:90–96.

Shields JA. Ocular toxocariasis. A review. Surv Ophthalmol 1984;28(5):361–79.

Toxoplasmosis

Perkins E.S. Ocular toxoplasmosis. Br J Ophthalmol 1973;57:1–15.

O'Connor GR. Chemotherapy of toxoplasmosis and toxocariasis. In: Srinivasan BD, ed. Ocular Therapeutics. New York: Masson Publishing USA, 1980, chap. 5, pp. 51–58.

Matthews JD, Weiter JJ. Outer retinal toxoplasmosis. Ophthalmology 1988;95:941–46.

Weiss MJ, Velazquez N, Hofeldt AJ. Serologic tests in the diagnosis of presumed toxoplasmic retinochoroiditis. Am J Ophthalmol 1990;109:407–11.

Tuberculosis

Donahue HC. Ophthalmologic experience in a tuberculosis sanatorium. Am J Ophthalmol 1967;64(4):742–48.

Abrams AB, Schlaegel TF. The tuberculin skin test in the diagnosis of tuberculosis uveitis. Am J Ophthalmol 1983;96:295–98.

Fountain JA, Werner RB. Tuberculous retinal vasculitis. Retina 1984;4(1):48–50.

Jabbour NM, Faris B, Trempe CL. A case of pulmonary tuberculosis presenting with a choroidal tuberculoma. Ophthalmology 1985;92(6):834–37.

Grosset JH. Present status of chemotherapy of tuberculosis. Rev Infect Dis 1989;11(suppl 2):5347–51.

Cytomegalovirus Retinitis

Bloom JN, Palestine AG. The diagnosis of cytomegalovirus retinitis. Ann Intern Med 1988;15:963–69.

Gross JG, Sadun AA, Wiley CA, Freeman WR. Severe visual loss related to isolated peripapillary retinal and optic nerve head cytomegalovirus infection. Am J Ophthalmol 1989;108:691–98.

Heinemann MH. Long term intravitreal gancyclovir therapy for cytomegalovirus retinopathy. Arch Ophthalmol 1989;107:1767–72.

Acute Retinal Necrosis

Fisher JP, Lewis ML, Blumenkranz M, et al. The acute retinal necrosis syndrome. Ophthalmology 1982;89(12):1309–16.

Hayreh SS. So-called acute retinal necrosis syndrome—an acute ocular panvasculitis syndrome. Dev Ophthal 1985;10:40–77.

Carney MD, Peyman GA, Goldberg MF, Packo K, Pulido J, Nicholson D. Acute retinal necrosis. Retina 1986;6:85–94.

Blumenkranz MS, Culbertson WW, Clarkson JG, Dix R. Treatment of the acute retinal necrosis syndrome with intravenous acyclovir. Ophthalmology 1986;93(3):296–300.

Duker JS, Blumenkranz MS. Diagnosis and management of the acute retinal necrosis (ARN) syndrome. Surv Ophthalmol 1991;35(5):327–43.

Herpes Zoster Uveitis

Ostler HB, Thygeson P. The ocular manifestations of herpes zoster, varicella, infectious mononucleosis, and cytomegalovirus disease. Surv Ophthal 1976;21(2):148–59.

Womack LW, Liesegang TJ. Complications of herpes zoster ophthalmicus. Arch Ophthalmol 1983;101:42–45.

Cobo LM, Foulks GN, Liesegang T, et al. Oral acyclovir in the therapy of acute herpes zoster ophthalmicus. Ophthalmology 1985;92(11):1574–83.

Vogt-Koyanagi-Harada Syndrome

Perry HD, Font RL. Clinical and histopathological observations in severe Vogt-Koyanagi-Harada syndrome. Am J Ophthalmol 1977;83(2):242–54.

Ohno S, Char DH, Kimura SJ, O'Connor GR. Vogt-Koyanagi-Harada syndrome. Am J Ophthalmol 1977;83(5):735–40.

Snyder DA, Tessler HH. Vogt-Koyanagi-Harada syndrome. Am J Ophthalmol 1980;90(1):69–75.

Friedman AH, Deutsch-Sokol RH. Sugiura's sign. Ophthalmology 1981;88(11):1159–65.

Multiple Evanescent White Dot Syndrome

Jampol LM, Sieving PA, Pugh D, Fishman GA, Gilbert H. Multiple evanescent white dot syndrome. Clinical findings. Arch Ophthalmol 1984;102:671–74.

Sieving PA, Fishman GA, Jampol LM, Pugh D. Multiple evanescent white dot syndrome. Electrophysiology of the photoreceptors during retinal pigment epithelial disease. Arch Ophthalmol 1984;102:675–79.

Aaberg TM, Campo RV, Joffe L. Recurrences and bilaterality in the multiple evanescent white-dot syndrome. Am J Ophthalmol 1985;100(1):29–37.

Mamalis N, Daily MJ. Multiple evanescent white-dot syndrome. Ophthalmology 1987;94(10):1209–12.

Hamed LM, Glaser JS, Gass DM, Schatz NJ. Protracted enlargement of the blind spot in multiple evanescent white-dot syndrome. Arch Ophthalmol 1989;107:194–98.

Acute Posterior Multifocal Placoid Pigment Epitheliopathy

Gass JD. Acute posterior multifocal placoid pigment epitheliopathy. Arch Ophthalmol 1968;80:177–85.

Ryan SJ, Maumenee AE. Acute posterior multifocal placoid pigment epitheliopathy. Am J Ophthalmol 1972;74(6):1066–74.

Kirkham, TH, Ffytche TJ, Sanders MD. Placoid pigment epitheliopathy with retinal vasculitis and papillitis. Br J Ophthalmol 1972;56:875–80.

Lyness AL, Bird AC. Recurrences of acute posterior multifocal placoid pigment epitheliopathy. Am J Ophthalmol 1984;98(2):203–7.

Birdshot Retinochoroidopathy

Ryan SJ, Maumenee AE. Birdshot retinochoroidopathy. Am J Ophthalmol 1980;89:31–45.

Gass JDM. Vitiliginous chorioretinitis. Arch Ophthalmol 1981;99:1778–87.

Fuerst DJ, Tessler HH, Fishman GA, Yokoyama MM, Wyhinny GJ, Vygantaa CM. Birdshot retinochoroidopathy. Arch Ophthalmol 1984;102:214–19.

Brucker AJ, Deglin EA, Bene C, Hoffman ME. Subretinal choroidal neovascularization in birdshot retinochoroidopathy. Am J Ophthalmol 1985;99:40–44.

Priem HA, Kijlstra A, Noens L, Baarsma GS, Laey JJ, Oosterhuis JA. HLA typing in birdshot chorioretinopathy. Am J Ophthalmol 1988;105:182–85.

Hoang PL, Deray BG, Minh HL, et al. Cyclosporin in the treatment of birdshot retinochoroidopathy. Transplant Proc 1988;20(Suppl 4):128–30.

Serpiginous Choroidopathy

Schatz H, Maumenee AE, Patz A. Geographic helicoid peripapillary choroidopathy. Trans Am Acad Ophthalmol Otolaryngol 1974;78:747–61.

Weiss H, Annesley WH, Shields JA, Christopher K. The clinical course of serpiginous choroidopathy. Am J Ophthalmol 1979;87(2):133–42.

Hardy RA, Schatz H. Macular geographic helicoid choroidopathy. Arch Ophthalmol 1987;105:1237–42.

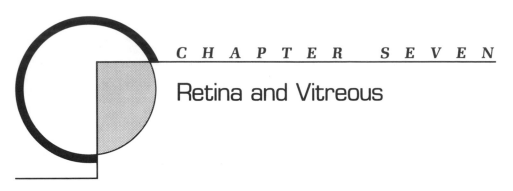

Retina and Vitreous

Vincent S. Reppucci, M.D.

Age-Related Macular Degeneration

Etiology and Symptoms Age-related macular degeneration (ARMD) is the leading cause of visual loss in persons over age 55. A universal definition is lacking, but drusen formation and retinal pigment epithelium (RPE) changes are the sine qua non. Symptoms of ARMD may be subtle but include

1. decreased reading vision,
2. metamorphopsia, and
3. central scotomata.

Signs Can be divided into atrophic and exudative disease.

1. Atrophic (85%)
   a) Drusen
   b) RPE changes
   c) Geographic atrophy

Atrophic disease can be further subdivided into high risk of progression to exudative disease by soft, confluent, or large drusen, and significant RPE clumping.

2. Exudative (15%)
   a) Hemorrhagic or serous RPE detachments
   b) Choroidal neovascularization
   c) Subretinal fibrosis
   d) Disciform scars

Exudative disease accounts for the majority of severe visual loss (20/200).

Workup

1. Amsler grid testing is very sensitive for detecting macular pathology and should be performed to establish a baseline.
2. Fundus examination, for clues of exudative disease such as
   a) hemorrhage,
   b) exudate,
   c) subretinal fluid, and
   d) RPE thickening.
3. Color stereo photos and fluorescein angiography to confirm exudative disease and determine the extent and location of choroidal neovascularization.

Treatment The Macular Photocoagulation Study showed benefit of argon blue-green laser for well-defined, extrafoveal (> 200 μm from the foveal avascular zone) choroidal neovascularization. Unfortunately, most exudative disease presents with ill-defined or subfoveal vessels, for which the benefit of treatment is unknown. Atrophic disease is not treatable, although nutritional supplements such as zinc and antioxidant vitamins have been advocated. Patients should be provided with an Amsler grid.

Patients with bilateral severe visual loss should undergo evaluation for low-vision aids.

Prognosis Over a 5-year period of time, 1% of patients with atrophic and 10% of patients with high-risk atrophic disease progress to exudative disease. The second eye of patients with exudative disease is at a 10% risk of developing exudative changes over 5 years, but the presence of confluent drusen and pigment clumping increase this risk to 50%.

Differential Diagnosis

1. Macular branch vein occlusion
2. Juxtafoveal telangiectasia
3. Chorioretinal scars
4. Central serous chorioretinopathy

Angioid Streaks

Etiology and Symptoms   Spontaneous rupture of a calcified and thickened Bruch's membrane. Usually asymptomatic but may present with central vision loss. May be associated with

1. pseudoxanthoma elasticum (most common),
2. Paget's disease,
3. sickle cell disease,
4. Ehlers-Danlos syndrome,
5. lead poisoning,
6. hyperphosphatemia, and
7. senile elastosis of the skin.

Signs

1. Brownish subretinal lines that emanate in a radial fashion from the disc. They may be mistaken for retinal vessels.
2. Choroidal neovascularization.

Workup

1. Fundus photography for baseline documentation.
2. Fluorescein angiography more fully reveals the degree of angioid streak formation.

Treatment   There is no treatment for the angioid streaks. Choroidal neovascular complexes may be treated by photocoagulation. Patients should be provided with an Amsler grid.

Arterial Occlusions of the Retina

Etiology and Symptoms   Painless, sudden visual loss caused by an obstruction of the central retinal artery (CRAO) or a retinal branch arteriole. Obstruction may be secondary to the following:

1. Emboli: seen in 20% of eyes and may be composed of cholesterol, fibrin, or calcium. Sources of emboli:
   a) Atherosclerotic vascular disease
   b) Cardiac valvular disease
   c) Coagulopathies (including oral contraceptives)
   d) Collagen vascular disease (lupus anticoagulant)
   e) Retrobulbar or periocular intravascular injections (e.g., steroids)
2. Vasospasm (e.g., migraine)
3. Inflammatory (e.g., temporal arteritis)
4. Iatrogenic (e.g., intraocular fluid or gas injection)
5. Extreme elevations in intraocular pressure

Signs

1. Afferent pupillary defect
2. Retinal opacification
3. Macular "cherry red spot"
4. Blood column "box carring"
5. Narrowing of arterioles
6. Disc drusen and prepapillary arteriole loops

Workup

1. Sedimentation rate to rule out temporal arteritis (less than 5% of central retinal artery occlusions).
2. Noninvasive carotid studies and cardiac valvular evaluation via echocardiogram.
3. Medical evaluation for systemic disease as indicated.
4. If diagnosis is in doubt, electroretinogram (ERG) shows loss of B wave with normal A wave.

Treatment

1. For CRAO less than 12 hours old:
   a) Attempt to displace the obstructing embolus distally by rapid decrease of intraocular pressure (IOP) via the following:
      i) Anterior chamber paracentesis
      ii) Ocular massage
      iii) Intravenous hypo-osmotic agents
   b) Retinal vascular dilatation can be accomplished by a rebreathing mask to increase the partial pressure of CO_2 or breathing a mixture of 95% O_2 and 5% CO_2 (carbogen).
2. Branch retinal artery occlusions do not usually respond to treatment.
3. Treat the underlying etiology if identified.

Prognosis   Universally poor for CRAO unless a cilioretinal artery is present serving the macula (about 25% of the population). Rubeosis occurs in 5% of CRAO. Prognosis better for branch retinal arteriole occlusion, for which rubeosis is extremely rare.

Asteroid Hyalosis and Synchysis Scintillans

Both asteroid hyalosis and synchysis scintillans represent intravitreal depositions. Ophthalmoscopically, these depositions may be impressive and may even cause significant obscuring of fundus details. Visual acuity, however, remains quite normal. Asteroid hyalosis is the development of calcium soaps bound to the collagen matrix of the vitreous. It is more common in patients at least 60 years of age and tends to be unilateral. Synchysis scintillans results from cholesterol crystals that form within the vitreous and is most frequently observed following intraocular hemorrhage. It is fairly rare. The crystals tend to settle at the bottom of the vitreous and occur bilaterally.

Treatment   Asteroid hyalosis and synchysis scintillans rarely create significant interference with visual acuity. If the ability to visualize or treat retinal pathology is compromised, the deposits may be removed by vitrectomy.

Best's Disease

Etiology and Symptoms   Best's disease is an autosomal dominantly inherited macular disorder that exhibits characteristic polymorphous foveal lesions which change with time. Although the exact pathophysiology is unknown, the disorder appears to be at the level of the RPE.

Signs (stages that progress with time)

1. Vitelliform "egg yolk": earliest stage appears in childhood; sharply circumscribed subretinal lesion of the fovea. No loss of visual acuity occurs.
2. Pseudohypopyon: onset around puberty; layering of yellow subretinal material.
3. Scrambled egg: diffuse yellow material clumping in the subretinal space. Vision loss occurs to about 20/40 level.
4. Atrophic macular scar: RPE clumping and atrophy, subretinal fibrosis, subretinal neovascularization, vision loss to 20/100 level.

Differential Diagnosis Solitary yellowish subretinal lesions may also occur in the following:

1. Parafoveal retinal telangiectasis
2. Fundus flavimaculatus with central flecks
3. Serous or hemorrhagic RPE detachments
4. Basal laminar drusen
5. Large acute solar maculopathy lesions

Workup

1. Family history of autosomal dominant macular lesions.
2. Fluorescein angiography shows blocking of fluorescence by the vitelliform lesion and minimal to no fluorescence in late views. Angiography is beneficial in determining the presence of choroidal neovascularization.
3. The electro-oculogram (EOG) is abnormal with light-to-dark ratio less than 1.55. Carrier individuals may also exhibit a subnormal EOG. Electroretinogram (ERG) and dark adaptation tests are normal.

Treatment Laser photocoagulation for subretinal neovascularization.

Prognosis Most patients with Best's disease retain good central vision in at least one eye through their lifetime. Significant central visual loss does not occur until the fifth decade. Bilateral cicatricial stage will significantly affect central vision.

Central Serous Retinopathy

Etiology and Symptoms Central serous retinopathy is a disorder of the pigment epithelium that causes accumulation of fluid in the subretinal space. It typically occurs in the macular region in the third to fourth decades. Men are more commonly affected than women. There appears to be a predisposition toward "type A" personality. The exact etiology is unclear but may be related to circulating catecholamines. Patients may complain of the following:

1. Metamorphopsia
2. Visual blurring secondary to an induced hyperopia
3. Partial central scotomata with increased light/dark adaptation time

Signs

1. Detachment of the neurosensory retina
2. Scattered RPE changes (e.g., limited RPE detachments) throughout both fundi
3. Turbid subretinal fluid, occasionally

Workup

1. Fluorescein angiogram:
   a) Classic inverted "smoke stack" sign.
   b) Multiple RPE window defects.
2. Systemic evaluation is not indicated.
3. Stress reduction and cessation of smoking may be of benefit.

Differential Diagnosis

1. Choroidal infarcts (e.g., toxemia of pregnancy); however, these individuals usually have diffuse retinal disease.
2. Exudative age-related macular degeneration in patients over 50 years of age.

Treatment   Central serous retinopathy is a self-limited disorder with spontaneous resorption of the subretinal fluid over a period of several weeks to months. In individuals for whom stereopsis and return of visual function is critical, laser photocoagulation to the regional leak may be considered. There is a risk of developing subsequent subretinal neovascularization with laser treatment.

Prognosis   Usually excellent. Because of the potential for recurring attacks, there may be mild loss of visual function depending on the degree and chronicity of the subretinal fluid. Patients with unilateral disease may describe a permanent color imbalance and loss of contrast sensitivity. Exacerbations may occur during periods of high stress. Of these individuals 5% develop chronic central serous retinopathy with associated RPE changes and moderate central visual loss.

Chloroquine and Hydroxychloroquine Toxicity

Hydroxychloroquine is used in the treatment of rheumatoid arthritis and causes accumulative dose-related pigmentary retinopathy. Chloroquine is commonly used for malaria treatment.

Signs

1. Corneal pigmentation: whorl-like distribution in the epithelium.
2. "Bull's-eye" maculopathy: the macular changes begin as pigmentary mottling.
3. Peripheral retinal involvement with pigmentary changes may result in visual field loss.

Toxic Dose   Toxicity with chloroquine occurs with dosages over 2 mg/lb/day (4.4 mg/kg/day). Toxicity with hydroxychloroquine occurs with dosages over 3.5 mg/lb/day (7.7 mg/kg/day). Toxicity is cumulative.

Workup

1. Baseline photography.
2. Fluorescein angiography shows early pigment changes.
3. ERG and EOG become abnormal in later stages.

Differential Diagnosis

1. Cone rod dystrophies
2. Retinitis pigmentosa
3. Fundus flavimaculatus
4. ARMD

Treatment   Discontinuation of medication if toxicity develops.

Prognosis   The retinal toxicity is irreversible, and careful clinical evaluation is mandatory. Follow-up, at 6-month intervals, should include the following:

1. Visual acuity and Amsler grid
2. Visual fields: Goldmann or automated
3. Color vision
4. Comparison of fundus with baseline photographs

Choroidal Detachment

Etiology and Symptoms   An accumulation of fluid between the choroid and sclera. May be due to a serous or hemorrhagic effusion. This creates an intraocular elevation of the retina and choroid. Serous detachments may occur with:

1. intraocular surgery (including cryopexy or retinal laser) trauma, or hypotony;
2. choroidal tumors (primary or metastatic; and
3. scleritis.

Hemorrhagic detachments may occur with intraocular surgery, especially with a sudden decompression of the globe. Patients who are elderly, hypertensive or highly myopic, and eyes that have undergone previous surgery are at risk.

When the choroidal extends into the visual axis, it may interfere with central vision or even induce a hyperopic shift. Smaller peripheral choroidal detachments may cause some peripheral visual changes. Patients may also complain of pain.

Signs

1. Brown, smooth elevation of the choroid and retina. The choroid is typically anchored to the sclera in the four quadrants by the vortex veins and posteriorly by the disc. This creates a characteristic pattern by ophthalmoscopy and on B-scan ultrasonography.
2. Low IOP: rule out filtering bleb, wound leak, or serous detachment.
3. High IOP: hemorrhagic detachment.

Workup

1. Complete ocular examination.
2. B-scan ultrasound: may distinguish serous from hemorrhagic detachment; large or kissing choroidal detachments may obscure visualization of the posterior pole.
3. Systemic evaluation for collagen vascular disease or neoplasm in the absence of ocular surgery.

Differential Diagnosis

1. Retinal detachment
2. Large choroidal melanomas (especially of the ciliary body) or other choroidal tumors

Treatment   Detachments secondary to postoperative hypotony are best treated by the following:

1. Topical cycloplegics.
2. Topical steroids.
3. Eye shield to minimize unintentional ocular trauma.

4. Repair any wound leakage. This can be done either by pressure patch or by surgical intervention.
5. Systemic prednisone is most beneficial in inflammatory and serous detachments.
6. In the presence of a flat anterior chamber, pupillary block glaucoma, or kissing choroidal detachments unresponsive to medical therapy, surgical drainage should be considered. This is performed by a sclerotomy 7 to 10 mm from the limbus in the quadrant of the choroidal detachment. The maintenance of intraocular pressure via air insufflation or fluid irrigation is adequate to drain the choroidal. In hemorrhagic choroidals, a large fibrous clot may develop, requiring opening of the sclerotomy for removal.

Choroidal Melanoma

Etiology and Symptoms   Choroidal melanoma is the most common primary intraocular malignancy in adults. It arises from uveal melanocytes. Most lesions are diagnosed on routine eye examinations and are asymptomatic. Visual loss develops in macular and peripapillary tumors or secondary to exudative detachments from more peripheral tumors. Ocular pain is uncommon except in advanced or neglected tumors.

Signs
1. Classic finding is a pigmented, elevated, mushroom-shaped mass with an associated exudative retinal detachment. There may be lipofuscin overlying the lesion, and the pigment may be variable or absent.
2. Anterior segment findings include
   a) dilated episcleral blood vessel (sentinel vessel),
   b) secondary glaucoma,
   c) sector cataract, and
   d) iris heterochromia.

Workup   The majority of choroidal melanomas, especially those greater than 5 mm in diameter, are diagnosed most accurately on the basis of ophthalmoscopic appearance, fluorescein angiography, and ultrasonography.

1. Fluorescein angiography demonstrates a double circulation (intrinsic tumor circulation) and extensive late leakage arising from multiple pinpoint regions within the tumor.

2. Ultrasonography, both A and B scan, reveal medium to low internal reflectivity. B scan may show choroidal excavation and retrobulbar shadowing.
3. Radioactive phosphorus (phosphorus-32) testing is fraught with false-positive results but can provide confirmatory information.
4. Rule out extraocular metastases:
   a) Referral to an internist/oncologist
   b) Liver function tests and scanning, including computed tomography (CT)
   c) Bone scan

Differential Diagnosis

1. *Choroidal nevus:* less than 2 mm in height, does not increase in size over time.
2. *Metastatic tumors to the eye:* most common intraocular malignancy (breast and lung most common primary sites) with medium to high internal reflectivity on ultrasonography.
3. *Choroidal hemangioma:* orange mass with overlying hemorrhages, fluorescein angiography demonstrates rapid filling, high internal reflectivity on ultrasonography.
4. *Choroidal hemorrhage:* ocular trauma or surgery, choroidal neovascularization with large subretinal hemorrhage (e.g., ARMD).
5. *Pigmented lesions of the RPE:* congenital hypertrophy or reactive hyperplasia, typically flat and nonprogressive.
6. *Choroidal osteoma:* calcification by ultrasonography, typically in young women.
7. *Melanocytoma of the optic nerve:* jet black optic nerve lesion, more common in blacks.

Treatment   Should be determined by size.

1. Small (less than 3 mm in height): photography, ultrasonography and observation for progression.
2. Medium (3 to 8 mm in height or smaller lesions with documented growth): various treatment modalities have been recommended including photocoagulation, radiotherapy, (either episcleral plaques or external beam radiation), brachytherapy, or local tumor resection. The exact management of these medium-sized tumors including the role of enucleation, which has been suggested to increase the mortality rate, is controversial. The Collaborative Ocular Melanoma Study (COMS), a national randomized controlled study, is comparing radiotherapy to enucleation for such medium-sized tumors.

3. Large (8 mm or higher) tumors in blind eyes: enucleation is the standard approach.

Prognosis Of small to medium-sized melanomas 10% to 30% can be documented to grow during 5-year follow-up. The following are associated with higher metastatic rate and carry a poorer prognosis:

1. Extrascleral extension
2. Large tumor size
3. Epithelioid cell type
4. Ciliary body location

Coats' Disease

Etiology and Symptoms An ideopathic condition in which telangiectatic and aneurysmal retinal vessels are associated with massive subretinal exudation. There is a painless loss of vision, and it affects boys more frequently than girls. It is unilateral in 80% of cases. Two forms of Coats' disease exist based on age at diagnosis:

1. Adolescence
2. Childhood

Signs

1. Localized yellow to greenish subretinal exudative elevation of the retina.
2. Retinal vascular abnormality with telangiectatic, tortuous, aneurysmal dilatations and neovascularization. The degree of exudate, hemorrhage, and vascular changes is extremely variable. The clinical course is variable and generally progressive.

Workup Fluorescein angiography shows telangiectasis and vascular leakage.

Differential Diagnosis

1. Leukocoria
   a) Persistent Hyperplastic Primary Vitreous (PHPV)
   b) Retinoblastoma
   c) Toxocariasis
   d) Congenital cataract
   e) Retinopathy of prematurity
2. Eales' disease

3. Vasculitis
4. Diabetic retinopathy

Treatment   Laser photocoagulation or cryotherapy can be used to control the degree of exudation from abnormal retinal vessels. Abnormal vessels not threatening the macula can be followed.

Prognosis   With photocoagulative treatment, 65% of patients show resorption of exudates and involution of vascular lesions.

Color Vision

Physiology

Color vision, or more accurately color perception, is a complex interplay of visual photo pigments and higher order neuronal processing that allows for the distinguishing of 8 million shades and tints. Within the cones, there are long-wavelength-sensitive (LWS), middle-wavelength-sensitive (MWS), and short-wavelength-sensitive (SWS) photo pigments, which have their peak spectral sensitivities at 566, 543, and 445 nm, respectively. They are also known as "red," "green," and "blue" cones. The interaction of red and green cones is delivered to a "red-green center." The interaction between the blue cones and the red-green center is delivered to a "blue-yellow" center. From here the information undergoes higher neural processing.

Trichromats have normal color vision with all three photo pigments present. Anomalous trichromats have all three photo pigments present but with a deficit in one of three pigments. Dichromats have only two types of photosensitive pigments present, and monochromats have only one photo pigment.

Congenital Color Vision Deficits

The most common color defect is a congenital dichromat. These include the following:

Protanopes: lack LWS or red pigment. See red as black and confuse green and blue/green.
Deuteranopes: lack MWS or green pigment. Cannot distinguish red from green.
Tritanopes: lack SWS or blue pigment. Can see red and green clearly.

Both protanopes and deuteranopes can distinguish blue from yellow and are inherited in a sex-linked recessive pattern. Tritanopes are inherited autosomal dominantly and carry an equal incidence among male and female.

Acquired Color Defects

1. Protan defects: macular retinal disease of degenerative causes (e.g., Stargardt's disease and various cone dystrophies).
2. Deuteron defects: in optic nerve disorders, except glaucoma.
3. Tritan defects: macula disease, on the basis of fluid present (e.g., macular edema, central serous retinopathy, or a shallow retinal detachment). Glaucomatous optic atrophy also tends to manifest as a tritan defect.

Individuals with acquired color defects show greater confusion and variability in naming colors and perform more erratically on color testing. Patients with congenital color deficits name colors more readily and consistently.

Testing

Three major types:

1. Pseudoisochromatic plates primarily for congenital dichromats.
2. The Farnsworth D15 or Farnsworth-Munsell (FM 100) hue testing provides good classification and extreme sensitivity (FM 100).
3. Anomaloscope will accurately classify anomalous trichromats.

Treatment

Congenital color defects are thought to be constant and untreatable. The use of chromatic filters may improve color discrimination. In acquired color defects, treatment of the underlying retinal pathology reverses the defect.

Cotton-Wool Spots

Definition and Symptoms   A microinfarction of the nerve fiber layer produces a cotton-wool spot (soft exudate). Usually asymptomatic but may rarely cause an arcuate scotoma.

Etiology   Of all individuals with cotton-wool spots 95% have a serious underlying systemic disorder. Even a single cotton-wool spot is significant and may be associated most commonly with

1. diabetes,
2. AIDS,
3. hypertension,

4. collagen vascular diseases, and
5. blood dyscrasias.

Workup

1. Systemic medical evaluation required.
2. Blood work to include the following tests:
   a) Complete blood count
   b) Sedimentation rate
   c) Urinalysis
   d) Antinuclear antibody (ANA)
   e) VDRL
   f) Fluorescent treponemal antibody-absorption (FTA-ABS)
   g) Fasting blood sugar

Treatment   Treat the underlying medical condition. Most cotton-wool spots resolve within 8 weeks.

Differential Diagnosis

1. Myelinated nerve fiber
2. Acute retinochoroiditis

Cystoid Macular Edema

Etiology and Symptoms   Diminished central vision due to fluid accumulation within the parafoveal retinal space. Causes of cystoid macular edema (CME):

1. Intraocular surgery: approximately 20% to 40% of individuals undergoing cataract extraction reveal angiographically documented evidence of CME. The majority of these patients do not have visually significant macular edema. Five percent of patients will have noticeable vision loss, usually 2 to 3 weeks after surgery. The onset may be delayed for several months. Anterior chamber intraocular lens implants have a higher incidence of CME when compared with posterior chamber implants, and CME incidence is higher with surgical vitreous loss. Epinephrine may cause transient CME in the aphakic state.
2. Vascular disorders (e.g., diabetes, branch vein occlusion).
3. Trauma.
4. Intraocular inflammation (e.g., uveitis).
5. Retinitis pigmentosa.
6. Idiopathic.

Intraocular surgery and vascular disorders are the most common causes of CME; blurred central vision is the predominant symptom.

Signs Fluid accumulation within Henle's layer results in radially oriented cystic spaces from the fovea.

Workup

1. Postcataract CME: rule out vitreous strands to the wound or any cause of iris irritation (e.g., synechiae or a malpositioned intraocular lens).
2. Fluorescein angiography: early leakage from parafoveal vessels with the accumulation of dye in a petaloid pattern during the late transit phase. Optic disc leakage may be seen.
3. Directed uveitic workup based on suspected etiology; see Chapter 6.

Treatment Often frustrating with no universally accepted regimen. Options:

1. Topical anti-inflammatory agents; steroidal and nonsteroidal.
2. Subtenon injections of steroids.
3. Acetazolamide (Diamox) at low systemic doses, especially in individuals with retinitis pigmentosa.
4. Vitrectomy, both anterior to cut strands and posterior in cases of recalcitrant CME.
5. Vitreolysis of strands by neodymium yttrium-argon-garnet (Nd-YAG) laser.
6. Removal or replacement of anterior chamber intraocular lens.
7. Focal laser photocoagulation for vascular disease.

Prognosis Prognosis for aphakic CME is good, with 80% of patients showing resolution of the macular edema and return of good visual function. Associated disc edema by angiography carries a poorer prognosis. The remaining individuals may develop chronic CME. If CME persists chronic and irreversible retinal changes may occur.

Diabetic Retinopathy

Definition and Symptoms Diabetic retinopathy describes the retinal vascular changes induced by diabetes mellitus and can be divided into three major groups: background, preproliferative, and proliferative. It is the leading cause of new blindness in the United States in persons under the age of 65. The incidence and severity of diabetic retinopathy, while multifactorial, are most directly a function of disease duration. Visual loss may be due to macular edema, ischemia, exudate deposition, proliferative disease, vitreous hemorrhage, and retinal detachments. Unless these changes involve the fovea directly, patients may develop extensive retinopathy without any visual symptoms. This underscores the importance of routine ophthalmoscopic examination in diabetics.

Signs

1. Background retinopathy:
   a) Microaneurysms
   b) Macular edema
   c) Lipid exudates
   d) Intraretinal hemorrhages
2. Preproliferative retinopathy: background changes with evidence of retinal ischemia:
   a) Cotton-wool spot formation
   b) Intraretinal microvascular abnormalities (IRMA)
3. Proliferative diabetic retinopathy (PDR):
   a) New blood vessel formation on the retinal surface.
   b) Background changes are usually evident; however, highly ischemic retinas may be ophthalmoscopically unimpressive.

Workup

1. Routine ophthalmologic examination specifically looking for the development of treatable changes such as macular edema and proliferative retinopathy. The frequency of these visits is dictated by the type of diabetes, the duration of diabetes, and degree of diabetic changes. These are outlined in Table 7.1.
2. Stereo fundus photographs for baseline when background retinopathy is identified.
3. Fluorescein angiography when clinically significant macular edema is suspected or to rule out regions of capillary nonperfusion.
4. The status of the retinopathy should be discussed with the treating primary physician or endocrinologist. Good blood pressure control is of benefit in minimizing exudate formation and the severity of macular edema. Puberty, pregnancy, and sudden initiation of tight metabolic control may accelerate retinopathy, and these patients should be watched more closely.

TABLE 7.1

Timetable for ophthalmologic examination of diabetic patients

Diabetes Type	*Initial Exam*
Type I—pregnant woman	Upon diagnosis
Type I—others	Within 5 yrs of diagnosis
Type II	Upon diagnosis

Fundus Finding	*Follow-up Exam*
Normal or rare microaneurysm	Annually
Moderate background changes	Every 6–9 mo
Preproliferative lesions or severe background changes	At least every 4 mo

Examination to include detailed direct and indirect ophthalmoscopy through a widely dilated pupil; fluorescein angiography where warranted; and a search for other ocular conditions for which diabetic persons are at increased risk (especially cataract and glaucoma). Minimally acceptable interval shown. More frequent examinations may be preferred.

Differential Diagnosis Changes such as microaneurysm formation and capillary closure can be seen in the following:

1. Radiation retinopathy
2. Collagen vascular diseases
3. Localized vascular abnormalities such as vein occlusions and arteriole venous malformations

Proliferative changes can be seen in the following:

1. Hemoglobinopathies
2. Uveitis
3. Vasculitis
4. Carotid artery disease

Treatment

Laser photocoagulation

1. Macular photocoagulation is used to treat clinically significant macular edema (CSME). The Early Treatment Diabetic Retinopathy Study (ETDRS) has shown that treatment is beneficial in decreasing visual loss by 50%. CSME is defined as follows:

a) Retinal thickening or hard exudate deposition within 500 μm (one-third disc diameter) of the fovea.

b) Retinal thickening of one disc area or greater in size within one disc diameter of the fovea.

Treatment can be directed either at localized areas of leakage or in a grid fashion to more diffuse areas of leakage as defined by fluorescein angiography.

2. Scatter (panretinal) photocoagulation is used to treat proliferative diabetic retinopathy with the presence of three of the four high-risk criteria for severe vision loss as determined by the DRS:

a) Any new vessel formation

b) Neovascularization at or within one disc diameter of the disc (NVD)

c) NVD greater than 30% of disc area or neovascularization elsewhere (NVE) greater than one-half disc area

d) Vitreous or preretinal hemorrhage

A Venn diagram can be constructed to differentiate between risk factors and high-risk factors (Fig. 7.1).

3. Side effects of scatter photocoagulation:

a) Decreased peripheral vision

b) Diminished night vision

c) Transient worsening of macular edema

d) Partial loss of accommodation

e) Choroidal effusion with angle closure glaucoma immediately after treatment

Pars Plana Vitrectomy

1. Nonclearing vitreous hemorrhage of more than 6-weeks' duration
2. Traction retinal detachment involving or threatening the macula

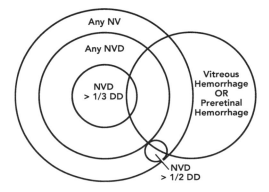

FIGURE 7.1. Venn diagram illustrating various risk factors of diabetic retinopathy. Any risk factor or combination of risk factors that lies within three circles is considered at high risk for severe vision loss due to diabetic retinopathy. For example, NVD $>\frac{1}{3}$ DD lies within three circles, but any NV [e.g., NVE] with vitreous hemorrhage is only two risk factors and hence not at high risk for severe vision loss.

3. Retinal traction causing macular distortion
4. Type I diabetic patients with severe PDR and extensive neovascular membranes with formed and firmly attached vitreous

---

Eales' Disease

Etiology and Symptoms   Eales' disease is an idiopathic disorder characterized by bilateral peripheral retinal neovascularization. It occurs primarily in the third to fourth decade with a male predominance. Eales' disease is widespread in the Indian subcontinent, with a suggested association to tuberculosis. The macula usually remains free of disease until late in the course. Often the initial manifestation is vitreous hemorrhage secondary to peripheral neovascularization. Intraocular inflammation frequently manifests as vascular sheathing.

Signs

1. Peripheral retinal neovascularization, sparing the macula until late in the course.
2. Vitreous hemorrhage: may be the presenting sign.
3. Vascular sheathing.
4. Uveitis.
5. Optic disc swelling.

Workup

1. Systemic evaluation to rule out other forms of proliferative vaso-occlusive neovascularization.
2. Fluorescein angiography reveals the regions of peripheral nonperfusion.

Differential Diagnosis

1. Sarcoidosis and other vasculitides
2. Hemoglobinopathies
3. Diabetic retinopathy

Treatment   Panretinal photocoagulation typically results in a good response with regression of peripheral neovascularization. Repeated vitreous hemorrhages with the development of retinal detachment may require vitrectomy.

Prognosis   Prognosis for Eales' disease is fairly good if photocoagulative treatment can be instituted in time. Typically, the peripheral occlusive disorder spares the macular region, allowing for retention of moderate central acuity.

Electrophysiology

Electroretinogram

The Electroretinogram (ERG) measures the change in resting potential across the retina occurring with light stimulation. It is a measured mass response of the retina and consists of A, B, C, and D waves.

1. A wave is produced by the photoreceptors and is a function of outer retinal viability.
2. B Wave is produced by Müller cells and corresponds to inner nuclear layer function.
3. C and D waves are not seen during usual clinical conditions.

The photopic (cone-mediated) and scotopic (rod-mediated) responses make distinct contributions to the ERG, with the photopic response occurring first. Primary cone-versus-rod disorders can be isolated via a dark-adapted ERG and a flicker or scotopic ERG.

The ERG is best used as a diagnostic aid. For example:

1. Flat ERG:
   a) Retinitis pigmentosa
   b) Diffuse chorioretinitis
   c) Choroideremia
   d) Amaurosis congenita of Leber
2. Decreased B wave, increased A wave: central retinal artery occlusion, affecting primarily the inner retinal layer.
3. Diffuse decrease of ERG:
   a) Toxic retinal states such as administration of chloroquine or quinine drugs
   b) Intraocular toxic substances such as chalcosis or siderosis
   c) Vitamin A deficiency or other systemic diseases such as mucopolysaccharidosis, hypothyroidism, and anemia
4. Elevated ERG:
   a) Early siderosis
   b) Corneal opacity or cataract formation
5. Normal ERG:
   a) Cortical blindness
   b) Dyslexia

    c) Hysteria
    d) Optic nerve disease

Recent electronic advances and computer-aided testing allow for focal ERGs to aid in the diagnosis of various macular disorders.

Electro-oculogram

The Electro-oculogram (EOG) measures the cornea/fundus potential as the eye moves between two electrodes. The changes in the potential from light to dark represent a combined picture of photoreceptor and RPE activity. The light-to-dark ratio of normal persons is 1.7 or greater. It is abnormal at 1.6 or less and considered flat below 1.2.

    The EOG is a useful adjunct to the ERG. An abnormal EOG is the rule with an abnormal ERG. However, the hallmark of Best's disease is an abnormal EOG with normal ERG. This has also been seen in early chloroquine toxicity and metalosis bulbi and in cases of fundus flavimaculatus, dominant drusen, and pattern dystrophies of the RPE.

Visual Evoked Response

The visual evoked response (VER) is the electrical response of the visual cortex to visual stimulation. The VER is measured with scalp surface electrodes rather than ocular electrodes and is dominated by the central 20° of retina. Although highly variable among individuals, it varies less than 10% from the fellow eye. The VER is therefore most sensitive if one optic pathway is normal, as in unilateral amblyopia or optic nerve disease. VER abnormalities may result from retinal, optic nerve, optic tract, optic radiation, or visual cortex pathology. The VER response consists of two positive and two negative waves. The peak of the second positive wave is referred to as the implicit time. Abnormal VERs show decrease of amplitude and increase of implicit time.

Pattern VER

The Pattern VER (PVER) is evoked by a checkerboard grid, which alternates at a frequency of 2 to 10 Hertz. The principal feature is a positive wave with a peak delay or implicit time of about 100 ms (P100). This response is dependent on the resolution of the pattern. A delay in the appearance of P100 is a classic but not specific finding of optic neuritis and may persist after resolution of the acute process. Interpretation of results is most accurate when a response asymmetry suggests unilateral visual system pathology. The PVER may provide a gross test of visual acuity for infants or uncooperative patients.

Fluorescein Angiography

Fluorescein Characteristics

Sodium fluorescein absorbs blue light at 465 to 490 nm and emits green-yellow light at 520 to 530 nm. This allows sodium fluorescein injected intravenously to be photographed through a blue filter allowing green-yellow fluorescent light to pass but block the blue flash. The sodium fluorescein molecule will not diffuse through the blood retina barrier, although it will diffuse into the choroid through the fenestrated choriocapillaries.

Indications for Fluorescein Angiography

Fluorescein angiography allows for the visualization of normal and abnormal retinal microcirculation. It is invaluable for determining regions of blood retina barrier breakdown as in intraretinal vascular leakage or defects of the RPE complex. The following are specific indications.

1. Any suspected vascular disorder of the retina:
   a) Diabetic retinopathy
   b) Hypertensive retinopathy
   c) Branch vein occlusion or arteriole occlusions
   d) Branch arteriole occlusion
   e) Retinal edema
2. Blocking or window defects of the RPE:
   a) Pattern dystrophies
   b) Angioid streaks
   c) Fundus flavimaculatus
3. Neovascularization, both preretinal and subretinal, shows early and sustained fluorescence due to plasma leakage.
4. Macular laser photocoagulation.
5. Cystoid macular edema.

Fluorescein Patterns

A detailed description of the interpretation of fluorescein angiograms is beyond the scope of this text. The normal times for the various phases of a retinal angiogram are as follows:

Time After Injection	Phase
Approx. 8 s	Pre-arterial choroidal flush
Approx. 9–11 s	Arterial
11–14 s	Arteriovenous
11–25 s	Venous
> 25 s	Recirculation

Abnormal patterns include the following:

1. Hypofluorescence:
   a) Blockage by pigment, blood, exudate, or scar.
   b) Vascular filling defect: arteriole occlusion.
2. Hyperfluorescence:
   a) Transmission of fluorescein ("window" defect):
      i) Drusen: *early,* bright; *late,* dims slowly; *border,* sharp.
      ii) Choroidal new vessels: *early,* bright; *late,* bright; *border,* fuzzy.
      iii) RPE detachment: *early,* dim; *late,* bright; *border,* sharp.
   b) Preinjection fluorescence.
   c) Retinal edema: late fluorescence.

Complications

Intravenous fluorescein is usually well tolerated, with nausea being the most frequent side effect, occurring in 5% of patients. The nausea occurs approximately 30 seconds after injection, lasts for several minutes, then disappears. An occasional patient may vomit. The most frequent allergic reactions are hives and itching, occurring about 5 to 10 minutes after injection. Bronchospasm and anaphylaxis have been reported but are extremely rare.

Fundus Flavimaculatus (Stargardt's Disease)

Etiology and Symptoms Fundus flavimaculatus is an autosomally recessive inherited disorder characterized by lipofuscin accumulation within the RPE. During childhood or early adulthood, patients will develop bilateral visual loss. These flecks vary in size, shape, and distribution and have been described as disciform in nature. With time their color changes from yellow to gray, and they may increase in size.

Signs There are two forms of the disorder. One is characterized by atrophic macular changes with minimal or no fleck formation. The other reveals extensive midperipheral fleck formations.

The macular RPE may have a beaten bronze appearance in either an oval or bull's-eye fashion. There is an increased incidence of choroidal neovascularization.

Workup
1. Careful ophthalmoscopic examination of the macula especially in the absence of flecks.
2. Fluorescein angiography reveals a dark choroid (due to blockage by lipofuscin). The flecks are hypofluorescent.
3. ERG: subnormal in some.
4. EOG: subnormal in some.

Differential Diagnosis   Other conditions showing flecked retina:

1. Drusen.
2. Fundus albipunctatus—small white dots in midperiphery, macula remains normal, nyctalopia.
3. Retinitis punctata albescens.
4. Multiple vitelliform lesions.
5. Pseudoxanthoma elastica.
6. Chloroquine retinopathy.
7. Functional vision loss—normal examination and fluorescein angiography.
8. Cone dystrophy—distinctive ERG pattern, color vision loss.

Treatment   None, other than low-vision aids, genetic counseling.

Prognosis   These patients typically exhibit central vision in the 20/200 to 20/400 range. Less severe vision loss in patients with normal electrophysiology.

Hypertensive Retinopathy

Etiology and Symptoms   Hypertension may be a result of unknown causes (essential, 90% of cases) or secondary to other conditions:

1. Pheochromocytoma
2. Kidney disease
3. Pre-eclampsia
4. Coarctation of the aorta

The hallmark of hypertensive changes within the retina is the constriction of arterioles, either focal or generalized.

Signs

1. Prolonged duration of particularly elevated blood pressure may cause breakdown of the blood retina barrier with formation of the following:
   a) Retinal hemorrhages, usually flame-shaped
   b) Cotton-wool spots
   c) Intraretinal lipid deposition
   d) Development of a macular scar
   e) Capillary closure
2. Acute and severe elevations of blood pressure may also cause:
   a) Fibrinoid necrosis of choroidal arterioles (Elschnig spots)
   b) Optic disc edema
3. Arteriolar narrowing is the earliest sign, from thickening of the arteriolar wall or arteriolosclerotic changes. This creates a reduction of the arteriole-to-venule ratio, which is normally 2:3.
4. A-V nicking: thickening of the arteriolar wall leads to compression of the vein especially at arteriole-venous (A-V) crossings, where a common adventitia is shared. Severe compression may cause branch retinal vein occlusion.
5. Retinal microaneurysm.
6. Retinal macroaneurysm.
7. Central retinal vein occlusion.

Two major classifications of hypertensive and arteriolosclerotic changes exist:

1. Keith-Wagener-Barker classification:

   Group 1: constriction of retinal arterioles.
   Group 2: focal arteriolar narrowing and A-V nicking.
   Group 3: changes of group 1 and 2 along with hemorrhage, exudate, and cotton-wool spot formations.
   Group 4: papilledema and Elschnig spots.

2. The Scheie system classifies hypertension and arteriolosclerosis separately:
   a) Hypertensive changes:

      Stage 0:   no retinal vascular changes.
      Stage I: diffuse arteriolar narrowing.
      Stage II: focal regions of arteriolar constriction.
      Stage III: focal and diffuse arteriolar narrowing with retinal hemorrhages.
      Stage IV: retinal edema, hard exudates, and papilledema.

b) Arteriolosclerotic changes:

Stage 0: normal.
Stage 1: broadened arteriolar light reflex.
Stage 2: A-V nicking.
Stage 3: copper wire arteriolar appearance.
Stage 4: silver wire arterioles.

Workup

1. Medical evaluation of hypertension looking for an underlying cause.
2. Emergency referral for diastolic blood pressure of > 120 mmHg (malignant hypertension).

Treatment Blood pressure control under the direction of the patient's primary physician.

Differential Diagnosis

1. Diabetic retinopathy: arteriolar narrowing less common. Many diabetics may have hypertension as well.
2. Radiation retinopathy.
3. Collagen vascular disease.

Prognosis Patients with advanced hypertensive retinopathy have a significantly diminished life span owing to concurrent severe cardiac and renal disease. Severe visual loss does not usually occur on the basis of hypertensive retinopathy except for ischemic papilledema associated with accelerated malignant hypertension.

Macular Hole

Etiology and Symptoms Defect of the retina within the foveal region. The etiology of idiopathic macular holes is unclear. However, evidence suggests local vitreoretinal tractional forces are involved. Idiopathic macular holes are most frequently seen in individuals in their sixth to seventh decade of life. Seventy percent are women. It usually presents as a decrease in reading vision with a small central scotoma.

Signs

1. Full-thickness, round, sharply defined defect of the fovea
2. Surrounding cuff of subretinal fluid
3. Overlying operculum

Workup

1. Slit lamp biomicroscopy to determine the status of the posterior vitreous especially in the fellow eye.
2. Peripheral retinal examination to rule out retinal tear formation.
3. Baseline photography.

Differential Diagnosis

1. Pseudomacular hole or a lamellar hole: in these incidences, there is usually obvious epiretinal membrane formation and the visual acuity is in the 20/50 range.
2. Chronic cystoid macular edema with cystic changes in the fovea.

Treatment   There is increasing evidence that surgical removal of pre-retinal fibrosis may be protective against the formation of macular holes. A study is under way to determine the appropriate indications and effectiveness of surgical intervention. Patients should be provided with an Amsler grid to monitor vision in the fellow eye. Macular holes may rarely progress to rhegmatogenous retinal detachments, and in these cases pars plana vitrectomy with air-fluid exchange is indicated. Patients usually do well with low-vision aids.

Prognosis   Most patients with idiopathic macular hole formation retain vision in the 20/80 to 20/200 range. Surrounding subretinal fluid may limit the vision further. The risk of developing a macular hole in the second eye is less than 10%. The presence of a posterior vitreous separation in the fellow eye appears to be protective.

Macular Pucker

Etiology and Symptoms   Synonyms include cellophane retinopathy and preretinal fibrosis. A wrinkling of the retinal surface secondary to contracture of a preretinal membrane or of the posterior vitreous hyaloid. Peripheral retinal tears, previous intraocular inflammation, or recent retinal detachment surgery are known causative factors. In 50% of individuals, the cause is idiopathic. Symptoms include progressive painless loss of central vision with metamorphopsia. Macropsia is pathognomonic for this condition.

Signs

1. Distorted and tortuous retinal vessels
2. Irregular foveal light reflex
3. Macular edema by fluorescein angiography

Workup

1. Careful peripheral retinal examination looking for retinal tears.
2. Photographs for documentation.
3. Fluorescein angiogram.
4. If suspicion of previous intraocular inflammation, consider uveitis workup.

Treatment   When the visual acuity is significantly hampered, pars plana vitrectomy with removal of the preretinal membrane successfully improves vision in approximately 80% of cases. Approximately 5% of puckers recur following surgical removal.

Optic Pit

Etiology and Symptoms   Optic pits are felt to be due to incomplete closures of the embryonic fissure. They occur in approximately 1 of 10,000 eyes. Theories of pathogenesis include:

1. leakage of cerebrospinal fluid into the subretinal space,
2. leakage of liquified vitreous into the subretinal space, and
3. schisis of the inner plexiform layer.

May result in distorted or blurred central vision.

Signs

1. Defect within the temporal aspect of the disc.
2. Serous retinal detachment in 40% to 50% of patients; most frequent in early adulthood, low in height, confined to the vascular arcades.

Workup   Fluorescein angiography: extension of the serous elevation to the disc with the appearance of an optic pit is fairly conclusive.

Differential Diagnosis

1. Central serous retinopathy
2. Peripapillary subretinal neovascularization
3. Choroidal infarcts

Treatment   Various medical and surgical interventions have been suggested. Photocoagulation may allow for retinal reattachment, although the final visual acuity may not improve. Recent use of vitrectomy with gas-fluid exchange may result in a better long-term prognosis.

Peripheral Retinal Neovascularization

Etiology and Symptoms Peripheral retinopathies can be broken down into three groups:

1. Vascular diseases
   a) Diabetes
   b) Hemoglobinopathies
   c) Branch retinal vein occlusions
   d) Eales' disease
   e) Dysproteinemias
   f) Hyperviscosity syndromes
   g) Multiple retinal embolization (e.g., cardiac myxoma)
   h) Aortic arch syndrome
   i) Carotid cavernous fistulas
2. Inflammatory diseases
   a) Sarcoidosis
   b) Vasculitis
   c) Pars planitis
   d) Collagen vascular disease
3. Various miscellaneous causes
   a) Multiple sclerosis
   b) Chronic retinal detachments
   c) Familial exudative vitreoretinopathy
   d) Incontinentia pigmenti

Signs

1. Vitreous hemorrhage
2. Retinal detachment

Workup

1. Complete physical examination with special attention to carotid and cardiac valvular disease
2. Hemoglobin and serum protein electrophoresis
3. Complete blood count
4. Chest x-ray
5. Fasting blood sugar
6. Antinuclear antibody test
7. Lupus anticoagulant antibody

Treatment Scatter photocoagulation remains the mainstay of treatment for ischemic neovascularization. Correction of any underlying systemic disease may also be of benefit.

Phakomatoses

These conditions have multiple ocular (including retinal) as well as systemic findings.

Neurofibromatosis (von Recklinghausen's Disease)

1. Incidence: the most common phakomatosis. Incidence varies between 1 in 1500 and 1 in 3000 live births.
2. Inheritance: autosomal dominant with equal male and female incidence.
3. Systemic findings:
   a) Café-au-lait spots: pigmented macular spots usually on the trunk.
   b) Subcutaneous tumors: fibroma molluscum.
   c) Elephantiasis neurofibromatosis.
   d) Axillary freckling: pathognomic. Other systemic findings include neurofibromas, bilateral optic nerve gliomas, meningiomas.
   e) Bone hypertrophy.
4. Eye findings:
   a) Plexiform neurofibromas of the lid.
   b) Pulsating exophthalmos.
   c) Myelinated corneal nerves.
   d) Congenital glaucoma: affected side only.
   e) Lisch nodules: iris nevi.
   f) Uveal melanoma.
   g) Retina: angiomas, retinal detachment, neovascularization.
   h) Optic nerve gliomas.

Workup   Should include careful family history, CT scan, and electroencephalogram (EEG).

Treatment
1. Genetic counseling.
2. Specific eye findings require treatment.

Encephalotrigeminal Angiomatosis (Sturge-Weber Syndrome)

1. Heredity sporadic but occasionally autosomal dominant.
2. Systemic findings:
   a) Skin: nevus flameus (port-wine stain) with unilateral involvement of the first two divisions of the fifth cranial nerve.

    b) Skull: facial hemihypertrophy.

    c) Central nervous system: intracranial hemangioma; intracranial calcifications result in seizures.

3. Eye findings:

    a) Episcleral hemangiomas.

    b) Amblyopia secondary to ptosis or a tropia.

    c) Glaucoma.

    d) Ectopic lentis.

    e) Choroidal hemangioma: "tomato ketchup fundus."

    f) Exudative retinal detachment.

Workup Should include magnetic resonance imaging (MRI) scan of the brain and a general medical and neurologic evaluation.

Treatment

1. Glaucoma surgery is fraught with complication because of the risk of expulsive hemorrhage.

2. Other ophthalmic problems are treated as indicated.

Tuberous Sclerosis (Bourneville's Disease)

1. Incidence is approximately 1 in 200,000.

2. Inheritance: autosomal dominant.

3. Typical triad of findings:

    a) Mental retardation

    b) Epilepsy

    c) Adenoma sebaceum

4. Systemic findings:

    a) Skin: ash leaf white spot that is pathognomic, adenoma sebaceum.

    b) Central nervous system: seizures, mental retardation, intracranial calcification ("brain stones").

    c) Others include thyroid tumors and multiple endocrine adenomas.

5. Ocular findings:

    a) Optic nerve drusen.

    b) Astrocytic hamartomas of the retina—elevated and nodular. Hamartomas can be mistaken for retinoblastoma.

    c) Exudative retinal detachment.

Workup Family history, MRI scan, general physical examination, and neurologic evaluation.

Cerebroretinal Angiomatosis (von Hippel-Lindau Disease)

1. Lindau designation denotes central nervous system involvement.
2. Inheritance: roughly 20% autosomal dominant.
3. Systemic findings:
   a) Central nervous system.
      i) Cerebellar hemangiomas
      ii) Spinal chord hemangiomas
   b) Other hemangiomas of pancreas, liver, and kidneys are possible.
4. Eye findings: retinal hemangioma, von Hippel lesion; 50% are bilateral. The earliest lesions appear as microaneurysms and leak with fluorescein angiography. Later more hemorrhaging occurs and a retinal detachment or secondary glaucoma can occur.

Workup

1. Careful family history and complete ocular examination with special attention to rule out bilateral hemangiomas. Hemangiomas will develop and enlarge in size with time and new ones may develop.
2. Medical workup including MRI of brain and abdominal MRI scan.
3. Fluorescein angiography.

Treatment   Laser photocoagulation or cryotherapy of retinal hemangiomas if vision is affected.

Racemose Hemangiomatosis (Wyburn-Mason Syndrome)

1. Systemic findings:
   a) Arteriovenous malformations of the midbrain, which are congenital and nonprogressive.
   b) Mental retardation.
2. Ocular findings:
   a) Seventh nerve palsy.
   b) Strabismus.
   c) Pulsating exophthalmos.
   d) Gaze palsies.
   e) Vascular malformations can extend from the midbrain to the optic nerve.
3. Inheritance: sporadic.

Workup

1. General medical evaluation
2. MRI of the brain.

Treatment   These retinal lesions do not progress and therefore do not require treatment.

Ataxia Telangiectasia (Louis-Bar Syndrome)

1. Inheritance: autosomal recessive.
2. Systemic findings: skin—arteriole telangiectasias of the nose and ears.
3. Central nervous system findings:
   a) Cerebellar and cortical degeneration
   b) Meningeal telangiectasias
   c) Cerebellar ataxia
4. Hematologic findings:
   a) Leukemia
   b) Decreased gammaglobulins
5. Eye findings:
   a) Telangiectasias of bulbar and peripheral conjunctiva
   b) Nystagmus
   c) Strabismus—ocular motor apraxia with ophthalmoplegias
   d) Dilated conjunctival vessels

Workup   Family history, complete medical evaluation, and MRI of the brain.

Retinal Detachment

Etiology   Separation of the neurosensory retina from the retinal pigment epithelium. There are three mechanisms.

> *Rhegmatogenous or tear-induced:* separation of the vitreous gel may create a break, tear, or hole, in the sensory retina. This then allows fluid to seep into the subretinal space, creating a detachment.
>
> *Tractional:* vitreous contracture pulls or tents the retina off the retinal pigment epithelium. They are always concave in nature. It is a slowly progressive disorder without acute symptoms.
>
> *Exudative:* result from choroidal tumors, inflammatory or exudative choroidal lesions. They are quite rare and behave

much like rhegmatogenous detachments except that no retinal break can be found and a choroidal mass can often be seen.

The incidence of retinal detachment is approximately 1 in 15,000 per year. The following are predisposing factors to retinal detachment:

1. Prior retinal detachment: 5% rate of redetachment.
2. Prior cataract surgery: 5% rate with intracapsular surgery and 1% rate with extracapsular surgery.
3. Moderate myopia greater than 8 diopters: 0.1%.
4. Lattice degeneration: less than 1%.
5. Family history of detachment.
6. Previous ocular trauma.

Symptoms

1. New or an increased number of floaters: typically small in size.
2. Light flashes: brief and resemble lightning bolts or arcs of light.
3. Loss of peripheral vision, which increases as the detachment progresses. Patients may describe a curtain blocking their peripheral vision.

Signs

1. Elevation of the retina with loss of choroidal vascular pattern.
2. Shifting subretinal fluid in exudative or long-standing rhegmatogenous detachments.
3. Relative decrease in intraocular pressure compared with the fellow eye.
4. Pigmented vitreal cells (Shafer's sign).

Workup   Rhegmatogenous detachments: careful and thorough ophthalmoscopy is required to identify all retinal breaks. If a retinal break cannot be identified and an exudative retinal detachment is suspected, then ultrasonography may aid in identifying a choroidal mass.

Differential Diagnosis

1. Retinoschisis: a splitting within the neurosensory retina. It is a smooth, bilateral, glistening elevation typically located inferotemporally. Inner or outer layer breaks may be seen.
2. Choroidal detachment: a brown elevation with preservation of choroidal markings, see Choroidal Detachment section, above.

Treatment   Ninety-five percent of detachments are treatable. With rhegmatogenous detachments, retinal breaks must be closed (apposing the choroid to the retina). This stops fluid seepage through the break and retards futher detachment. Retinal breaks may be closed via external or internal tamponade.

1. The external method or scleral buckling is the "gold standard." A silicone element is sutured to and indents the sclera to appose the break. The area surrounding the break is treated with cryotherapy to induce a long-term retinal adhesion.
2. Pneumatic retinopexy provides for internal tamponade via an intravitreal gas bubble. Retinal breaks are pretreated with cryotherapy or laser and an expanding gas is injected intravitreally. The patient's head is positioned so the bubble apposes and "seals" the break.
3. Vitrectomy is reserved for complicated detachments involving proliferative vitreoretinopathy, giant retinal tears, opaque media, or vitreoretinal traction.

Prognosis Progression of a retinal detachment is variable but may be swift. Visual prognosis depends on the preoperative state of macula. "Macula on" detachments have the best prognosis. "Macula off" detachments left untreated for longer than a week have a poorer prognosis.

Retinitis Pigmentosa

Etiology and Symptoms Retinitis pigmentosa (RP) describes a spectrum of generalized chorioretinal disorders with variable onset, progression, severity, and inheritance patterns. It can be classified in several ways:

1. Typical and atypical.
2. Hereditary pattern (autosomal dominant, autosomal recessive, or X-linked recessive).
3. Psychophysical characteristics (rod-cone vs. cone-rod). Typical RP manifests with
   a) nyctalopia,
   b) progressive contraction of peripheral visual field, and
   c) loss of central or color vision.

Signs Progressive photoreceptor and RPE atrophy is the common characteristic. Other findings:

1. Posterior subcapsular cataract
2. Optic disc pallor

3. Pigment clumping "bone spiculization" of the RPE, along with areas of depigmentation
4. Edematous appearance to the fundus (early finding)
5. Narrowed retinal arterioles
6. Cystoid macular edema
7. Vitreous opacification "veil"

Atypical RP includes closely related or incomplete forms of RP, some with associated systemic and metabolic diseases:

1. RP sine pigmentosa: typical RP without apparent RPE changes.
2. Cone-rod dystrophy: central and color vision loss and nyctalopia in early life. Photopic ERG is primarily affected.
3. Leber's congenital amaurosis: presents at birth and is essentially a congenital form of RP.
4. Goldmann-Favre disease: autosomal recessive with retinoschisis, vitreous veil, and retinal detachment.
5. Kearns-Sayre syndrome: autosomal recessive, restriction of extraocular movements, ptosis, heart block (cardiology consultation for management).
6. Treatable forms of RP:
   a) Bassen-Kornzweig syndrome (hereditary abetalipoproteinemia): poor absorption of the fat-soluble vitamins (A, K, and E) leads to ataxia, diarrhea, limited extraocular muscle movement, acanthocytosis, and abetalipoproteinemia. Treatment: vitamin A, K, and E supplementation with restriction of dietary fat.
   b) Refsum's disease (autosomal recessive): deficiency in phytanic acid oxidation results in cerebellar ataxia, polyneuropathy, deafness, extraocular muscle movement restriction, and skin disease. Treatment: low phytanic acid diet (restrict green leafy vegetables and milk products).

Workup

1. Careful history including family pedigree with examination of family members for findings consistent with a carrier state.
2. Goldmann visual fields.
3. ERG: scotopic is absent or greatly attenuated.
4. Dark adaptation.
5. Fluorescein angiography for suspected CME.
6. Blood work:
   a) FTA-ABS
   b) Serum phytanic acid level
   c) Lipid profile
   d) Peripheral blood smear (for acanthocytes)
7. Electrocardiogram.

Differential Diagnosis

1. Choroideremia: X-linked recessive, distinctive retinochoroidal degenerative pattern which spares the macula. Late in the disease can resemble RP.
2. Gyrate atrophy: autosomal recessive, nyctalopia, fundus shows scalloped areas of complete retinal atrophy, high myopia, with elevated serum ornithine levels.
3. Syphilis: bone spiculization of the retina with positive serology, often other ocular findings, see Syphilis section in Chapter 6.
4. Congenital rubella: deafness, microphthalmos, cataract, heart defects with a pigmentary retinopathy.
5. Congenital stationary night blindness: no RPE changes, ERG shows normal A wave.
6. Cone dystrophy: normal scotopic ERG.
7. Drug toxicity (e.g., phenothiazine).

Treatment   No treatment is available other than to treat the underlying systemic problem (see above). Consider the following:

1. Genetic counseling.
2. Low-vision aids.
3. Cataract extraction.
4. Acetazolamide (Diamox) may help CME.

Prognosis   Varies with the underlying etiology. Control of diet in Refsum's disease may prevent the progression of vision loss.

Sickle Cell Retinopathy

Etiology and Symptoms   Sickle cell retinopathy is seen in individuals who have SS, S-thal, and SC hemoglobinopathy. Sickle carriers may rarely manifest disease. Sickling characteristics of the erythrocytes lead to microinfarctions creating an ischemic form of retinopathy resulting in proliferative disease. Most patients are black or of Mediterranean ancestry. Usually asymptomatic, but patients may notice

1. vision loss and
2. vitreous floaters.

Signs   Nonproliferative manifestations of sickle cell retinopathy:

1. Salmon-colored retinal hemorrhages, which may be subretinal, intraretinal, or preretinal. As these hemorrhages resorb, they leave black sunbursts, iridescent spots, and schisis cavities

corresponding to subretinal, intraretinal, and preretinal hemorrhages, respectively.
2. Retinal arteriole occlusion, especially during sickling crisis.
3. Choroidal infarctions.
4. Elevated intraocular pressure.
5. Central retinal artery occlusion due to increased IOP.
6. Angioid streaks: in individuals with SS and sickle trait.

Proliferative sickle retinopathy can be classified as follows:

Stage 1: peripheral arteriole occlusion
Stage 2: arteriole-venous anastomoses
Stage 3: neovascularization that extends into the vitreous base and has a "sea-fan" appearance
Stage 4: traction or rhegmatogenous retinal detachment

Proliferative retinopathy is most common in SC compared to S-thal, with SS having the least severe changes. This is because of the increased blood viscosity of SC disease compared with SS disease.

Workup

1. Sickle cell preparation and hemoglobin electrophoresis (sickle cell trait may have a negative sickle cell preparation).
2. Fluorescein angiography.

Differential Diagnosis Peripheral proliferative retinopathies may also be seen in the following:

1. Other hemoglobinopathies
2. Eales' disease
3. Diabetes
4. Branch retinal vein occlusion
5. Hyperviscosity syndromes (e.g., collagen vascular disease)
6. Dysproteinemias
7. Aortic arch syndrome
8. Retinal embolization (e.g., talc)
9. Carotid cavernous fistulas

Treatment

1. Peripheral scatter photocoagulation for peripheral neovascularization.
2. Vitrectomy and scleral buckling is indicated for patients with nonclearing vitreous hemorrhages and traction or rhegmatogenous retinal detachments. There is a high incidence

of anterior segment ischemia in patients who undergo standard scleral buckling procedures; exchange blood transfusions are indicated preoperatively to minimize this complication.

Prognosis   Although SC disease is a more benign systemic disease it carries the worst ocular prognosis.

Venous Occlusions of the Retina

Etiology and Symptoms   Venous occlusions generally develop as a result of one of the following mechanisms:

1. Generalized arteriosclerosis secondary to hypertensive disease causes a mechanical compression of the vein from the juxtaposed arterial wall.
2. Elevated intraocular pressure may have a similar compressive effect.
3. Inflammatory disease (e.g., vasculitis) or diabetes.

Patients typically notice a sudden, painless loss of vision. If the branch occlusion does not involve the macular region, it may be asymptomatic.

Signs   Vein occlusions can be divided into two categories, central retinal vein occlusion (CRVO) and branch retinal vein occlusion (BRVO). Both manifest as an occlusive disease of the venous network, causing intraretinal hemorrhage and edema formation along the distribution of the involved vein. Other findings:

1. Cotton-wool spots
2. Neovascularization of the retina or anterior segment (CRVO)
3. Optociliary shunt vessels of the optic nerve

Workup

1. Search for systemic etiology:
   a) Hypertension—check blood pressure.
   b) Diabetes—fasting blood sugar.
   c) Vasculitis—complete blood count, FTA-ABS, erythrocyte sedimentation rate, prothrombin and partial thromboplastin times, antinuclear antibodies, serum protein electrophoresis.
2. Complete ophthalmic examination:
   a) Especially IOP and gonioscopy.
   b) Rule out rubeosis.

   c) Rule out relative afferent pupillary defect. Presence correlates strongly with severe ischemic disease and the development of neovascularization.

3. Fluorescein angiography: rule out macular edema and the degree of nonperfusion (capillary drop out) within the retinal vasculature.

Differential Diagnosis

1. *Diabetic retinopathy:* may mimic a small macular branch vein occlusion, changes confined more to the posterior pole, bilateral.
2. *Carotid stenosis (ocular ischemia):* rubeosis and dilated veins, midperipheral hemorrhages, low IOP.
3. *Increased intracranial pressure:* disc edema with less hemorrhage.

Treatment

1. CRVO:
   a) Treat underlying systemic condition.
   b) Lower IOP.
   c) Panretinal photocoagulation, for ischemic CRVO based on fluorescein angiography or rubeosis.
   d) Low-dose aspirin.
2. BRVO: individuals with branch retinal vein occlusions and macular edema will benefit from grid photocoagulative treatment if the following criteria are met:
   a) Vision of 20/50 or worse.
   b) Foveal capillary net intact.
   c) No hemorrhage in fovea.
   d) Documentation of macular edema involving 180° or less of the fovea.
   e) The deposition of foveal exudate is also amenable to photocoagulation.

Prognosis   Those patients at high risk of developing neovascularization should be followed closely at monthly intervals looking for neovascularization.

Vitreous Hemorrhage

Symptoms

1. Floaters
2. Cobwebs
3. Light flashes
4. Partial or total visual loss

Signs

1. Blood in the vitreous usually obscures the red reflex.
2. Old dehemoglobinized hemorrhage is ochre-colored.

Workup

1. Careful vitreo-retinal examination for posterior vitreous detachment, retinal tears, neovascularization, and vascular anomalies.
2. Ultrasound will detect retinal detachment if ophthalmoscopy is obscured.

Etiology

1. Retinal neovascularization:
   a) Diabetes
   b) Sickle cell disease
   c) Eales' disease
2. Retinal tear or detachment
3. Posterior vitreous detachment
4. Trauma
5. Vascular anomalies (angiomas etc.)
6. Retinal macroaneurysms
7. Choroidal neovascularization
8. Subarachnoid hemorrhage (Terson's syndrome)

Treatment   Most hemorrhages will clear with expectant management. Bed rest, head elevation, elimination of medically unnecessary anticoagulants, and bilateral patching may be dramatically effective. Hemorrhages obscuring fundus details should be followed by ultrasonography. Erythroblastic glaucoma may occur, requiring treatment. Pars plana vitrectomy is indicated for the following:

1. Nonclearing hemorrhage (after 6 months)
2. Retinal detachment
3. Retinal traction threatening fovea

Selected Readings

Age-Related Macular Degeneration

Macular degeneration. Preferred practice patterns. American Academy of Ophthalmology, 1990.
Macular photocoagulation study group. Argon laser photocoagulation for neovascularization maculopathy. Arch Ophthalmol 1986;104:694–701.

Angioid Streaks

Jaeger EA. Miscellaneous diseases of the fundus. In: Duane TD, ed. Clinical ophthalmology. Philadelphia: Harper and Row, 1983, vol. 3, chap. 36, pp. 4–10.

Arterial Occlusions of the Retina

Brown GC. Retinal arterial obstructive disease. In: Ryan SJ, ed. Retina. St. Louis: CV Mosby, 1989, vol. II, chap. 73.

Brown GC, Margagal LE, Sergott R. Acute obstruction of the retinal and choroidal circulations. Ophthalmology 1986;93:1373–82.

Asteroid Hyalosis and Synchysis Scintillans

Roy FH. Ocular differential diagnosis, 3rd ed. Philadelphia: Lea and Febiger, 1984, p. 295.

Best's Disease

Hereditary macular dystrophies. In: Tasman W, ed. Duane's clinical ophthalmology. Philadelphia: JB Lippincott, 1990, vol. 3, chap. 9.

Curry HF, Moorman LT. Fluorescein photography of vitelliform macular dystrophy. Arch Ophthalmol 1968;79:705.

Central Serous Retinopathy

Watzke RC. Acquired macular disease. In: Duane TD, Jaeger EA, eds. Clinical ophthalmology. Philadelphia: Harper and Row, 1988, vol. 3, chap. 23, pp. 4–9.

Chloroquine and Hydroxychloroquine Toxicity

Fraunfelder FT. Drug-induced ocular side effects and drug interactions, 3rd ed. Philadelphia: Lea and Febiger, 1989, p. 60.

Choroidal Detachment

Bellows AR, Chylack LT Jr, Hutchinson BT. Choroidal detachment. Clinical manifestation, therapy, and mechanism of formation. Ophthalmology 1981;88:1107–15.

Ruiz RS, Salmonsen PC. Expulsive choroidal effusion. A complication of intraocular surgery. Arch Ophthalmol 1976;94:69–70.

Choroidal Melanoma

Shields JA. Diagnosis and management of intraocular tumors. St. Louis: CV Mosby, 1983.

COMS Manual of Procedures. Springfield, Virginia: National Technical Information Service; 1989. NTIS Accession No. PB90-115536.

Coats' Disease

Coats G. Forms of retinal disease with massive exudation. R Lond Ophthal Hosp Rep 1907–1908;18:440–525.

Harris GS. Coats' disease: evaluation of management. Ophthalmology 1970; 5:311–20.

Color Vision

Benson WE. Introduction to color vision. In: Duane TD, Jaeger EA, eds. Clinical ophthalmology. Philadelphia: Harper and Row, 1988, vol. 3, chap. 6.

Pokorney J, Smith VC, Verriest G, Pinckers AJLG, eds. Congenital and acquired color vision defects. New York: Grune and Stratton, 1979.

Cotton-Wool Spots

Ashton N. Pathophysiology of retinal cotton wool spots. Br Med Bull 1970;26:143–50.

Brown GC, Brown MM, Hiller T, Fischer D, Benson WE, Margagal LE. Cotton-wool spots. Retina 1985;5:206–14.

Cystoid Macular Edema

Gass JDM, Norton EWD. Cystoid macular edema and papilledema following cataract extraction: a fluorescein fundoscopic and angiographic study. Arch Ophthalmol 1966;76:646–61.

Fung WE. Aphakic cystoid macular edema. In: Ryan SJ, ed. Retina. St. Louis: CV Mosby, 1989, vol. 2, chap. 111.

Diabetic Retinopathy

Early Treatment Diabetic Retinopathy Study Research Group. Photocoagulation for diabetic macular edema, ETDRS report No. 1. Arch Ophthalmol 1985;103:1796–1806.

Diabetic Retinopathy Study Research Group. Photocoagulation treatment of proliferative diabetic retinopathy: the second report of DRS finding. Ophthalmology 978;85:82–106.

American Academy of Ophthalmology. Diabetic retinopathy, preferred practice patterns. San Francisco: American Academy of Ophthalmology, 1989.

Eales' Disease

Spitznas M. Eales' disease: clinical picture and treatment with photocoagulaton. In: L'Esperance FA Jr, ed. Current Diagnosis and Management of Chorioretinal Diseases. St. Louis: CV Mosby, 1977, pp. 513–21.

Gieser SC, Murphy RP. Eales' disease. In: Tasman W, ed. Clinical Ophthalmology. Philadelphia: JB Lippincott, 1990, vol. 31, pp. 1–5.

Fluorescein Angiography

Berkow JW, Kelley JS, Orth DH. Fluorescein angiography: a guide to the interpretation of fluorescein angiograms. San Francisco: Manuals Program, American Academy of Ophthalmology, 1984.

Fundus Flavimaculatus (Stargardt's Disease)

Noble KG, Carr RE. Stargardt's disease and fundus flavimaculatus. Arch Ophthalmol 1979;97:1281–85.

Hadden OB, Gass JDM. Fundus flavimaculatus and Stargardt's disease. Am J Ophthalmol 1976;82:527–39.

Ernest JT, Krill AE. Fluorescein studies in fundus flavimaculatus and drusen. Am J Ophthalmol 1966;62:1–6.

Hypertensive Retinopathy

Scheie HG. Evaluation of ophthalmoscopic changes of hypertension and arteriolar sclerosis. Arch Ophthalmol 1953;49:117–38.

Ashton N. The eye in malignant hypertension. Trans Am Acad Ophthalmol Otolaryngol 1972;76:17–40.

Irinoda K. Colour atlas and criteria of fundus changes in hypertension. Philadelphia: JB Lippincott, 1970.

Macular Hole

Gass JDM. Stereoscopic atlas of macular diseases diagnosis and treatment, St. Louis: CV Mosby, 1987, pp. 690–705.

Johnson RN, Gass, JDM. Idiopathic macular holes: observations, stages of formation, and implications for surgical intervention. Ophthalmology 1988;95:917–24.

Macular Pucker

Michels RG. Vitrectomy for macular pucker. Ophthalmology 1984;91:1384–88.

Wise GN. Clinical features of idiopathic preretinal macular fibrosis. Am J Ophthalmol 1975;79:349–57.

Optic Pit

Watzke RC. Acquired macular disease. In: Duane TD, Jaeger EA, eds. Clinical ophthalmology. Philadelphia: Harper and Row, 1988, vol. 3, chap. 23, pp. 10–13.

Peripheral Retinal Neovascularization

Jampol LM, Goldberg M. Peripheral proliferative retinopathies. Surv Ophthalmol 1980;25:1–14.

Retinal Detachment

Glaser BM, Michels RG. Surgical retina. In: Ryan SJ, ed. Retina. St. Louis: CV Mosby, 1989, vol. 3.
Lincoff H, Kriessig I. Retinal detachment. In: Fraunfelder FT, Roy, FH. Current ocular therapy 2. Philadelphia: WB Saunders, 1985, pp. 474–76.

Retinitis Pigmentosa

Weleber RG. Retinitis pigmentosa and allied disorders. In: Ryan SJ, ed. Retina. St. Louis: CV Mosby, 1989, vol. 1, chap. 20.
Heckenlively JR, ed. Retinitis pigmentosa. Philadelphia: JB Lippincott, 1988.

Sickle Cell Retinopathy

Goldberg MF. Sickle cell retinopathy. In: Duane TD, Jaeger AE, eds. Clinical ophthalmology. Philadelphia: Harper and Row, 1979, vol. 3, chap. 17.
Goldberg MF. Classification and pathogenesis of proliferative sickle retinopathy. Am J Ophthalmol 1971;71:649–65.

Venous Occlusions of the Retina

Branch Vein Occlusion Study Group. Argon laser photocoagulation for macular edema in branch vein occlusion. Am J Ophthalmol 1984;98:271–82.
Hayreh SS, Rojas P, Podhajsky P, Montague P, Woolson RF. Ocular neovascularization with retinal vascular occlusion: III. Incidence of ocular neovascularization with retinal vein occlusion. Ophthalmology 1983;90:488–506.

Vitreous Hemorrhage

Winslow RL, Taylor BC. Spontaneous vitreous hemorrhage: etiology and management. South Med J 1980;73:1450–52.
Jaffe NS. Complications of acute posterior vitreous detachment. Arch Ophthalmol 1968;79:568–71.

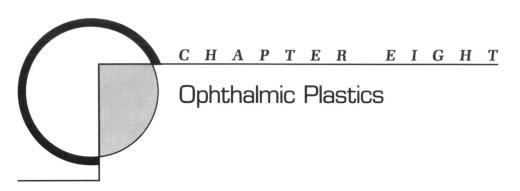

C H A P T E R   E I G H T

Ophthalmic Plastics

Keith D. Carter, M.D.
Gene R. Howard, M.D.

Anatomy

Eyelid Anatomy

Upper Eyelid

The anatomy of the upper eyelid is shown in Figure 8.1. The relevant clinical points are as follows:

1. The anterior lamellae consist of the skin and orbicularis muscle, and the posterior lamellae consist of the tarsus and conjunctiva.
2. In the upper lid, the tarsal plate is 12 mm high centrally.
3. The orbital septum meets the levator aponeurosis 2 to 3 mm above the tarsus and separates the orbit from the anterior eyelid.
4. The levator aponeurosis separates the lacrimal gland into the palpebral and orbital lobe and inserts on the anterior portion of the tarsal plate.
5. The preaponeurotic fat pad lies anterior to the levator aponeurosis and is a key landmark in eyelid surgery.
6. The eyelid crease forms as a result of anterior extensions of the levator aponeurosis.

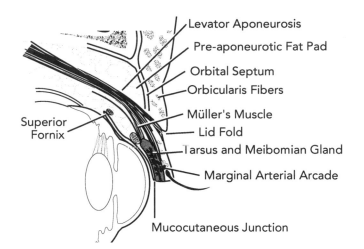

FIGURE 8.1. Upper Eyelid Anatomy

7. The orbicularis muscle (protractor) is innervated by cranial nerve (CN) VII and closes the eyelid.
8. Müller's muscle is sympathetically innervated and inserts into the superior edge of the tarsus. It accounts for approximately 2 mm of lid elevation, and its malfunction, as in Horner's syndrome, results in a ptosis.

Lower Eyelid

The anatomy of the lower eyelid is shown in Figure 8.2. The relevant clinical points are as follows:

1. The capsulopalpebral fascia is analogous to the levator aponeurosis of the upper lid.

FIGURE 8.2. Lower Eyelid Anatomy

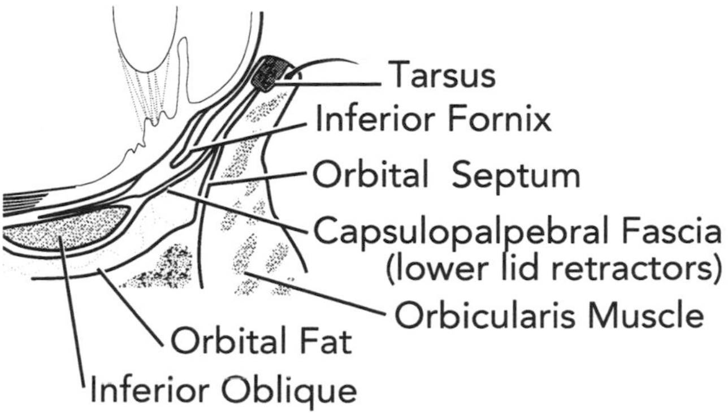

2. The tarsal plate is approximately 5 mm in height centrally.
3. The inferior tarsal muscle (analogous to Müller's muscle) retracts the lower eyelid. In Horner's syndrome the lower eyelid may be higher (upside-down ptosis).

Lacrimal Anatomy

The lacrimal system is shown in Figure 8.3.

1. Lacrimal gland
   a) Two lobes (orbital and palpebral) of the gland are separated by the levator aponeurosis.
   b) Ductal system: ducts from orbital lobe go through the palpebral lobe before emptying into the superior cul-de-sac. Surgical resection of the palpebral lobe can damage the orbital lobe's secretory ducts.
2. Tear film—the following glands contribute to the three-layer tear film:
   a) Meibomian glands—anterior oil layer
   b) Accessory glands (Krause and Wolfring)—aqueous layer
   c) Lacrimal gland—aqueous layer
   d) Glands of Moll and Zeis—posterior mucin layer

FIGURE 8.3. Lacrimal System

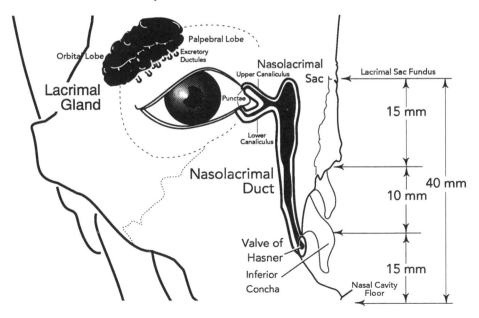

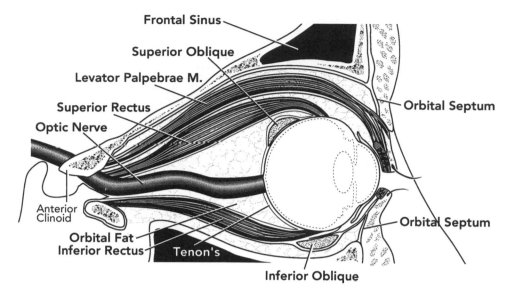

FIGURE 8.4. Orbital Anatomy, Axial View

    3. Lacrimal excretory system
      a) Important dimensions
        i) Puncta—approximately 0.3 mm in diameter
        ii) Canaliculi, upper and lower—8 to 10 mm in length
        iii) Lacrimal sac—15 mm (fundus 3–5 mm, body 10 mm)
        iv) Nasolacrimal duct (empties beneath the inferior turbinate)—15 mm in length
      b) Valves
        i) Rosenmüller—at the common canaliculus
        ii) Hasner—at the distal end of the nasolacrimal duct

Orbital Anatomy

The orbital anatomy is shown in Figures 8.4 and 8.5.

    1. Embryology: parts of the orbit derived from neural crest include the maxillary process, lateral nasal process, mesenchyme, and the base of the skull.
    2. Bones of the orbit (Figs. 8.6–8.9).
      a) Orbital margin
        i) Superior orbital margin—frontal.
        ii) Medial orbital margin—maxillary process of frontal, lacrimal, frontal process of maxilla.

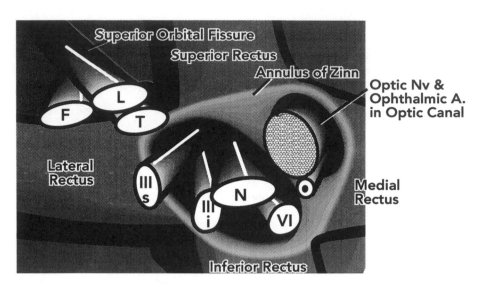

FIGURE 8.5. Orbital Anatomy, Coronal View

    iii) Inferior orbital margin—maxilla and zygoma.
    iv) Lateral orbital margin—zygomatic process of the frontal
         and the frontal process of the zygoma (the lateral orbital
         tubercle, or Whitnall's tubercle, is located 10 mm below
         the zygomaticofrontal suture).
  b) Superior orbital wall—frontal and sphenoid.

FIGURE 8.6. Medial Orbital Wall

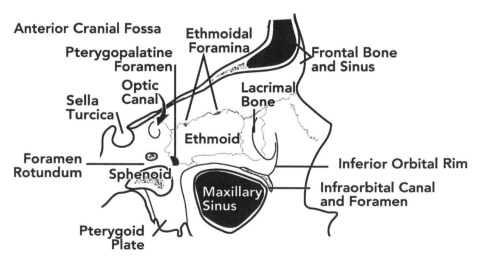

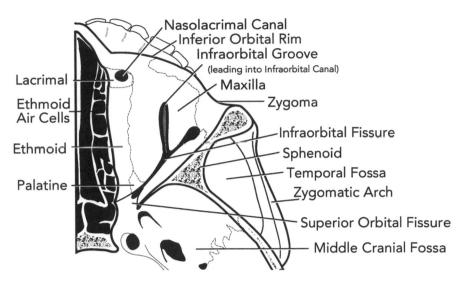

FIGURE 8.7. Orbital Floor

FIGURE 8.8. Lateral Orbital Wall

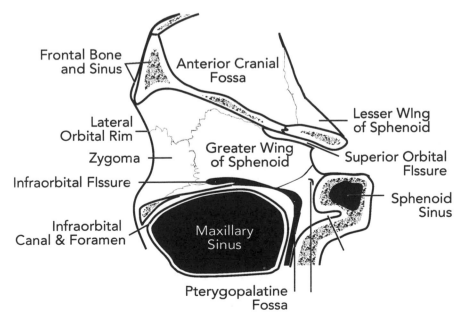

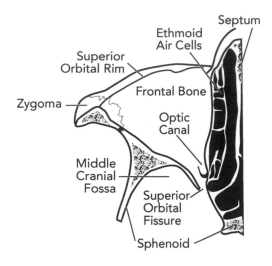

FIGURE 8.9. Orbital Roof

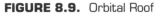

    c) Medial orbital wall—frontal process of the maxilla lacrimal, sphenoid, lamina papyracea of the ethmoid
    d) Inferior orbital wall (orbital floor)—maxilla, zygoma, palatine
    e) Lateral orbital wall—zygoma, greater wing of the sphenoid
3. Orbital dimensions

Volume: 30 cc
Entrance height: 35 mm
Entrance width: 40 mm
Medial wall length: 45 mm
Posterior globe to optic foramen: 18 mm
Length of orbital segment of optic nerve: 25 mm

Anesthesia

Preoperative Medications

The primary forms of preoperative medications involve the tranquilizer and narcotic analgesic groups. Several combinations are possible for preoperative reduction of anxiety and pain control.

    1. Tranquilizers
        a) Benzodiazepines: diazepam (Valium), midazolam (Versed)
        b) Hydroxyzine pamoate (Vistaril)
        c) Promethazine hydrochloride (Phenergan)
    2. Narcotic analgesics: meperidine hydrochloride (Demerol), morphine sulfate

3. Common approaches may include
   a) Valium p.o. (5–15 mg p.o. 45 min preoperatively),
   b) Demerol, 1 mg/kg (50–100 mg) and Vistaril (25–50 mg i.m.),
   c) morphine (0.1 mg/kg i.m.) and Versed (2–6 mg i.m.), and
   d) Versed i.v. (use slowly, infuse over 2 min).

Local Anesthetic

1. Topical agents
   a) Tetracaine hydrochloride
   b) Proparacaine hydrochloride
   c) Cocaine 4% solution for nasal packing in adults
   d) Oxymetazoline (Afrin) or Neo-Synephrine (0.25%) for nasal packing in infants and young children
2. Infiltrative anesthesia options include
   a) lidocaine 2% with epinephrine 1:100,000 units mixed 50:50 with 0.5%–0.75% bupivacaine for local cases; and
   b) lidocaine 1% with epinephrine 1:100,000 units for cases under general anesthesia when hemostasis is important.

   Toxic adult doses are 15 cc of 2% lidocaine without epinephrine (300 mg) and 25 cc of 2% lidocaine with epinephrine (500 mg).

General Anesthesia

Most eyelid, nasolacrimal, and some anterior orbital biopsies can be done under local anesthesia in a cooperative adult. General anesthesia is used primarily for pediatric and orbital cases or in cases of anxious adults who might otherwise refuse surgery.

Eyelid Malposition

Entropion

Definition Inversion of the eyelid margin such that the margin, the lashes, and sometimes the external skin surface are turned inward. Remember the normal position of the meibomian gland orifices is upright.

Classification

1. Congenital
2. Involutional
3. Spastic
4. Cicatricial

Etiology

1. Laxity of canthal tendons.
2. Disinsertion or attenuation of lid retractors—the inferior tarsus loses stability as a result of weakened retractors.
3. Spasm of preseptal orbicularis, which overrides the pretarsal orbicularis.
4. Shortening of posterior lamellae due to chemical burn, Stevens-Johnson syndrome, cicatricial pemphigoid, or trachoma (upper lid).

It is important to accurately identify the etiology of the entropion so the proper corrective procedure is selected.

Presentation

1. Epiphora
2. Foreign body sensation
3. Corneal trauma and ulceration

Evaluation

1. Routine eye examination with special attention to the cornea, looking for trauma, fornix shortening, and symblepharon.
2. Pinch test (if one can pull the eyelid 6 mm or more from globe, this indicates an abnormal excess of laxity).
3. Squeeze test (repeated eyelid squeezing may induce spastic entropion).

Differential Diagnosis

1. Trichiasis
2. Distichiasis
3. Epiblepharon (excessive lower lid skin and orbicularis muscle, which may cause inversion of lashes toward the cornea)

Treatment

1. Immediate management includes antibiotic ointments and bland lubricants.
2. Congenital entropion is rare and is generally caused by a tarsal kink. This is managed with a Wies procedure or rotational sutures.
3. Involutional entropion displays little or no movement of the lower lid on downgaze, which should have approximately 3 to 4 mm of excursion. Reinsertion of the lower eyelid retractors and lateral canthal tendon strengthening procedures is curative.

Remember the lower lid retractors are located under the preaponeurotic fat, just as the levator aponeurosis is in the upper lid.

4. Spastic entropion is often an early stage of involutional entropion and is accompanied by ocular inflammation and lid swelling. Treatment with Quickert sutures or lateral tarsal strip usually resolves the problem.

5. Cicatricial entropion may be managed with multiple procedures including full-thickness incision and repositioning of lower eyelid or lengthening of posterior lamella with a mucous membrane graft.

Follow-up

1. Aggressive lubrication and observation for corneal trauma with treatment of any corneal infection.

2. Quickert sutures should be followed closely because of high rate of recurrence.

Ectropion

Definition   The eversion of the eyelid margin, usually with a separation of the eyelid from the globe. When in doubt about the eyelid margin, look at the position of the meibomian gland orifices, which are normally upright.

Classification and Etiology

1. Involutional ectropion: horizontal tarsal laxity, or medial canthal tendon laxity (can determine this entity by the ability of pulling the punctum laterally past the limbus).

2. Paralytic: denervation of the lid protractors or paralysis of orbicularis muscle (CN VII palsy).

3. Cicatricial: shortening of the eyelid skin or both the eyelid skin and muscle (anterior lamella).

4. Congenital: associated with the congenital eyelid syndrome.

5. Mechanical: loss of tissue from trauma, surgery, or thermal and chemical burns.

Presentation

1. Epiphora

2. Corneal desiccation, keratopathy, and ulceration

3. Keratinization of palpebral conjunctiva

Evaluation

1. Routine eye history (noting any previous eyelid trauma, surgery, nerve palsy, or contact dermatitis) and examination.
2. Snap back test: normally when the lid is pulled from the globe it should snap back into its normal position with one blink. Abnormal laxity is present when it takes two or more blinks to reestablish the lid's normal position.

Treatment

1. Corneal lubrication.
2. Temporary taping of lateral eyelid.
3. Cicatricial: release the cicatrix or a full-thickness skin graft.
4. Congenital: a mild condition may not require treatment, otherwise treat as a cicatricial process.
5. Involutional:
   a) Punctal ectropion: medial spindle—use a 5-0 double armed chromic suture.
   b) Total lid ectropion: lateral tarsal strip with a medial canthal tendon plication.
6. Paralytic:
   a) Temporary paralysis: lubricants, moist chamber glasses, taping the lid closed.
   b) Permanent paralysis: tarsorrhaphy, lateral tarsal strip.
7. Mechanical: excision of mass and horizontal tightening. With traumatic or postsurgical ectropion, skin grafting and horizontal tightening are required.

Trichiasis and Distichiasis

Definition   Trichiasis is the misdirection of eyelashes from the anterior lamella, which rub on the cornea and conjunctiva. Distichiasis is the growth of a second row of lashes from the meibomian gland orifices in the posterior lamella.

Etiology

1. Congenital
2. Eyelid trauma
3. Chronic inflammation
4. Tumor distortion of eyelid

Presentation

1. Epiphora
2. Foreign body sensation
3. Corneal trauma (superficial punctate keratitis)

Differential Diagnosis

1. Epiblepharon: an extra fold of skin near the margin of the lower eyelid, which may result in lashes rubbing against the eye
2. Entropion

Treatment

1. Mechanical epilation: single lash or isolated lashes.
2. Electrolysis (hyfrecation): single lash or isolated lashes. Requires local anesthesia with a setting of 25 to 30, which may be increased as needed. The argon laser has also been used.
3. Cryotherapy: useful with a large segment of lashes. The double freeze-thaw technique is the most effective. A thermocouple is useful and a temperature of $-20°C$ is required. Warn patient that the eyelid will swell.
4. Lid splitting and excision (distichiasis).
5. Full-thickness wedge resection.

Follow-up As needed for further lash removal.

Essential Blepharospasm and Hemifacial Spasm

Definition Essential blepharospasm is a bilateral episodic involuntary spasm of the orbicularis muscle, causing eyelid closure and progression to complete eyelid closure over months to years. Hemifacial spasm is involuntary unilateral eyelid and facial spasm.

Etiology For essential blepharospasm, a lesion rostral to the facial nucleus has been suggested but not clearly identified. Most cases of hemifacial spasm are due to a vascular loop or mass pressing on the facial nerve as it exits the brainstem.

Presentation Essential blepharospasm manifests as an increased rate of blinking, which may begin unilaterally but progresses to bilateral disease. Meige's disease describes an orofacial extension of the spasm. Hemifacial spasm manifests as unilateral tonoclonic spasms of eyelid and face.

Evaluation

1. Inquire about a history of neurologic disease, drugs (dopaminergic stimulating drugs, nasal decongestants, antihistamines, phenothiazines), or habit spasm.
2. Computed tomography (CT) or magnetic resonance imaging (MRI) scan (hemifacial spasm).
3. Neurology referral (hemifacial spasm).

Differential Diagnosis

1. Parkinson's disease
2. Corneal irritation
3. Spastic entropion
4. Blepharitis
5. Keratoconjunctivitis sicca
6. Aberrant regeneration of CN VII
7. Myokymia

Treatment

1. Medical: botulinum toxin injections is the treatment of choice; Baclofen (Lioresal) and orphenadrine citrate (Norflex) have been used with some success.
2. Surgical:
   a) Hemifacial spasm: decompression of mass or vascular loop.
   b) Blepharospasm—neurectomy, orbicularis myectomy.

Facial Palsy

Definition   Decreased function of CN VII.

Etiology

1. Congenital
2. Idiopathic (Bell's palsy)
3. Neoplasm—acoustic neuroma
4. Herpes zoster (Ramsay Hunt syndrome)
5. Trauma
6. Infection of the parotid gland
7. Cerebrovascular accident

Presentation

1. Mask faces
2. Brow droop
3. Ectropion
4. Epiphora
5. Drooling

Physical Examination

1. Complete eye examination with attention to corneal surface
2. Schirmer's test
3. Assessment of orbicularis function

4. Test for Bell's phenomena (upward movement of the eyes with lid closure)
5. Cranial nerve examination

Evaluation

1. MRI scan of the head
2. Electroneuronography of the facial nerve as part of a full neurology evaluation
3. Pontogram (blink reflex)
4. Audiologic tests

Treatment

1. Initial management should be directed toward optimizing corneal lubrication and reducing epiphora by taping of the lateral canthal region or a temporary surgical tarsorrhaphy. A definite surgical repair of the eyelid should be delayed until no further improvement in function has occurred for 6 months.
2. Definitive management options include a lateral tarsal strip for ectropion, palpebral spring or gold weight placement, a temporalis muscle sling, or browplasty.

Blepharoptosis

Definition Drooping of upper eyelid, which may be unilateral or bilateral.

Etiology

1. Congenital
2. Acquired
   a) Aponeurotic
   b) Neurogenic
   c) Myogenic
   d) Mechanical
   e) Traumatic

Presentation

1. Congenital: accounts for about 50% of all cases of ptosis. May show the following associated features:
   a) Normal or weak superior rectus (limitation of upgaze).

b) Blepharophimosis syndrome—narrowing of the palpebral fissure with epicanthus inversus, ectropion, and telecanthus (autosomal dominant).

c) Congenital fibrosis syndrome—a condition in which the ocular muscles including the levator muscle become fibrosed. The most commonly involved muscle is the inferior rectus. The patient usually has a chin-up position. Treatment is usually directed toward the inferior rectus muscle followed by appropriate ptosis surgery.

d) CN III palsy

e) Aberrant CN III function

f) Horner's syndrome

g) Jaw-winking (Gunn's syndrome)—lid movement with chewing

2. Acquired:

a) Aponeurotic: elevated lid crease due to attenuation or dehiscence of the levator aponeurosis.

b) Myogenic

i) Chronic progressive external ophthalmoplegia

ii) Myasthenia gravis

iii) Oculopharyngeal dystrophy

iv) Myotonic dystrophy

c) Neurogenic

i) CN III palsy

ii) Horner's syndrome

iii) Synkinetic

iv) Neurotoxins

History and Examination

1. History. Important questions to ask:

a) When was it first noted?

b) Has it progressed?

c) Does it worsen during the day?

d) Are there any systemic health problems?

e) Has there been any trauma or surgery to the eyelid?

f) Is there a history of malignant hyperthermia?

2. Routine examination with special attention to the following:

a) Head position

b) Brow use in maintaining lid elevation

c) Interpalpebral fissure height

d) Levator function

e) Lagophthalmos

f) Upper lid crease height

g) Lid lag on downgaze

   h) Extraocular muscle motility: in congenital ptosis the levator
       muscle is unable to relax
   i) Corneal surface
   j) Visual field test, with and without lid taped, to document
       loss of vision making the ptosis more than just a cosmetic
       problem
3. Other tests may be included if a specific etiology is suspected:
   a) Cranial nerve examination
   b) Pupillary testing for Horner's syndrome
   c) Tensilon test for myasthenia gravis
   d) Forced duction test for entrapment versus paresis
   e) Jaw movement for synkinetic lid movement
4. Quantitation of ptosis:
   a) 2 mm—mild
   b) 3 mm—moderate
   c) 4 mm or more—severe
5. Quantitation of levator function:
   a) 8 mm or more—good
   b) 5 to 7 mm—fair
   c) 4 mm or less—poor

Differential Diagnosis   Pseudoptosis:

1. Contralateral lid retraction
2. Enophthalmos
3. Anophthalmia
4. Microphthalmia
5. Phthisis
6. Dermatochalasis

Treatment   Management depends on the etiology and amount of
ptosis as well as the levator function. Multiple surgical procedures have
been developed; however, the basic mechanical principles are similar.
Table 8.1 is a basic guideline for selection of corrective procedures. One
should be especially conservative with myogenic ptosis. Other options
include a ptosis crutch built into glasses and taping the eyelid.

Complications of Ptosis Surgery

1. Undercorrection (most common)
2. Overcorrection
3. Suture granuloma
4. Erosion of suture onto cornea
5. Entropion or ectropion
6. Conjunctival prolapse

TABLE 8.1

Correction of ptosis

Surgical Technique	Indications
Fasanella-Servat Conjunctiva—Müller's resection	Minimal ptosis (1–2 mm) Good levator function (8–15 mm)
Aponeurosis advancement	Ptosis worse than 3 mm Levator function better than 5 mm
Levator resection	Ptosis worse than 4 mm Levator function (3–8 mm)
Frontalis suspension	Ptosis worse than 4 mm Levator function worse than 3 mm

Eyelid Tumors

History

1. Onset of lesion and patient awareness of it
2. Malignancy elsewhere
3. Previous radiation exposure
4. Growth rate
5. Bleeding from the lesion
6. Ulceration
7. Change in color

Examination

1. Visual examination: the lesion's size, color, shape, location, and its effect on lashes or other structures should be documented. Features of malignancy:
   a) Induration
   b) Irregular borders
   c) Ulceration
   d) Pearly borders
   e) Telangiectasia
   f) Variation in color
2. Palpation: to determine if the lesion is mobile or fixed, also check for regional lymph nodes.

3. Systemic evaluation in certain cases:
   a) Sebaceous cell cancer—regional nodes
   b) Melanoma—liver, lung, bone, and skin

Differential Diagnosis Some of the more common benign as well as malignant tumors are listed below with some of their key features.

Benign tumors

Hordeolum: inflammation and infection of either the glands of Zeis (external) or meibomian glands.

Chalazion: chronic lipogranulomatous reaction of the meibomian glands. In cases of recurrent chalazion one must think of the possibility of sebaceous cell carcinoma.

Epidermal inclusion cyst: elevated, well-defined lesion of the eyelid.

Nevus: pigmentation of the lids, which may involve both the upper and lower lid simultaneously, does not change in size.

Xanthelasma: flat yellow lesions of the eyelids that may be associated with abnormal serum lipoprotein levels.

Molluscum contagiosum: viral infection results in multiple waxy nodules which are umbilicated. A chronic follicular conjunctivitis is often seen.

Capillary hemangioma: presents as an enlarging red nodule early in life and is composed of solid groups of benign endothelial cells (see "Selected Orbital Tumors" in Orbital Disease section, below).

Keratoacanthoma: extremely rapid growth with a central crater filled with keratin.

Actinic keratosis: long exposures to the sun results in dysplasia of the epidermis. Malignant transformation is possible.

Seborrheic keratosis: epidermal growth disturbance in the elderly with an oily, "stuck on" appearance.

Malignant tumors

Basal cell carcinoma: the most common malignant tumor of the eyelid. Typically has a pearly elevated nodular border with telangiectatic vessels on the surface. Rarely metastasizes.

Squamous cell carcinoma: typically occurs in sun-exposed areas, often in a site of previous actinic keratosis. These tumors can metastasize.

Sebaceous cell carcinoma: highly malignant tumor arising from either the meibomian glands or Zeis glands. Often mimics chronic blepharitis (especially if unilateral) or a chalazion.

Malignant melanoma: very uncommon tumor of the eyelid, as
    nevi rarely undergo malignant transformation.

Workup   Many of the lesions listed above have a classical clinical presentation. Frequently, however, it is difficult to distinguish between benign and malignant or premalignant forms. When in doubt, it is necessary to perform a biopsy.

Treatment

Benign lesions

Hordeolum: hot compresses three times a day, topical antibiotics
    (erythromycin, bacitracin), systemic antibiotics (tetracycline).
Chalazion: steriod injections, 0.1 cc of triamcinolone diacetate (5
    mg/ml) (may repeat in 1 wk if lesion has not decreased),
    surgical incision, and curettage.
Epidermal inclusion cyst: simple excision.
Nevus: observation.
Xanthelasma: observation, serum lipid screen, excision may
    require full-thickness skin graft.
Molluscum contagiosum: excision and curettage.
Capillary hemangioma: observation is initially indicated, as most
    will begin to involute after 1 year of age (see "Selected
    Orbital Tumors" in Orbital Disease section, below).
Keratoacanthoma: may undergo spontaneous resolution or can be
    simply excised.
Actinic keratosis: observation or simple excision.
Seborrheic keratosis: simple excision.

Malignant lesions   We recommend that all suspected basal cell
and squamous cell carcinomas be evaluated and treated by Mohs' microsurgical technique. Other techniques include resection with frozen
section control and cryosurgery. Suspected sebaceous cell carcinoma
should be initially managed by a wedge or map biopsy and submitted
as fresh tissue for oil red O stain. Alert the pathologist to your clinical
suspicion. The treatment for malignant melanoma of the skin is surgical excision with wide margins based on the depth, location, and size
of the lesion.

Follow-up   Every 6 months to 1 year after excision.

Prognosis   Mohs' microsurgical excision results in a 1% to 4% recurrence rate of primary basal cell or squamous cell carcinoma.

Lacrimal Gland Disorders

Diagnostic Techniques for Lacrimal System Disease

Measurement of tear production can be determined by the following:

1. Schirmer 1 (reflex and basic secretion)
2. Schirmer 2 (stimulate the turbinate)
3. Basic secretion test (topical anesthesia applied prior to Schirmer test)

Tear outflow can be measured by the following:

1. Functional tests:
   a) Fluorescein dye disappearance test: 2% fluorescein dye is placed in the conjunctival fornices and its presence or absence is noted 5 minutes later.
   b) Jones 1 test: fluorescein is placed in the conjunctival cul-de-sac. The test is positive if dye is found in the inferior meatus of the nose 5 minutes later by placing a cotton-tipped applicator into the nose.
   c) Jones 2 test: residual fluorescein is irrigated out of the conjunctiva. The lacrimal system is irrigated with a cannula. If fluorescein is recovered, an incomplete block is present; if unstained fluid is recovered, an inadequate lacrimal pump is present; if no fluid appears, a complete obstruction is identified.
   d) Dacryocystography.
   e) Dacryoscintigraphy.
   f) CT and MRI scan.
2. Structural tests:
   a) Irrigation
   b) Probing of upper lacrimal system (only the canaliculi and sac)

Congenital Lacrimal System Drainage Disorders

Definition   Obstruction of tear drainage outflow system. This may occur in up to 6% of newborns.

Etiology

1. Obstruction of the nasolacrimal duct
2. Atresia of the lacrimal puncta
3. Absence or atresia of canaliculi
4. Congenital lacrimal amniotocele
5. Facial anomalies

Presentation

1. Epiphora
2. Discharge on eyelids
3. Conjunctivitis
4. Dacryocystitis

Physical Examination   Special attention to the following:

1. Gentle compression of lacrimal sac to express contents
2. Examination of eyelids for presence of upper and lower puncta

Evaluation

1. Dye disappearance test
2. Culture discharge from sac

Differential Diagnosis

1. Allergy
2. Congenital glaucoma
3. Conjunctivitis
4. Corneal disease or trauma
5. Eyelid malposition
6. Trichiasis or distichiasis

Treatment   The primary goal is opening and maintaining a patent tear drainage system.

1. Obstruction of nasolacrimal duct (membrane). The majority will resolve by 6 weeks of age. Initial management consists of massage of the nasolacrimal sac two to four times per day followed by instillation of topical antibiotic drops. Persistent symptoms over several weeks or parental anxiety may warrant early probing. The success of primary probing decreases significantly after 13 months of age. Extreme care is required to avoid creating a false passage. Approximately 5% to 10% of probings fail and require repeat probing. Silicone stents are used in repeat probings. Inferior turbinate infracture may be necessary. Important distances to recall when probing:
   a) Punctum to end of nasolacrimal duct:
      Infant—20 mm
      Adult—35 mm
   b) Entrance of nose to opening of the nasolacrimal duct:
      Children—20 to 25 mm
      Adult—35 mm

2. Atresia of lacrimal punctae requires cutdown over punctae with or without intubation.

3. Absence or atresia of canaliculi requires cutdown, probing, and intubation. Frequently no system can be found, and the child may need a dacryocystorhinostomy (DCR) with Jones tube placement.

4. Congenital lacrimal amniotocele typically presents at birth, and early probing can be curative.

5. Facial anomalies may require probing, intubation, and DCR after craniofacial reconstructive surgery in the midface region.

Follow-up Stents remain in place for 6 to 12 months. Recurrence of symptoms after repeated probings may necessitate treatment with a DCR.

Prognosis The majority of obstructions can be resolved with probing and intubation or DCR.

Acquired Lacrimal System Drainage Disorders: Obstruction of Tear Outflow System

Symptoms and Signs

1. Epiphora
2. Discharge on eyelids
3. Conjunctivitis
4. Dacryocystitis
5. Telecanthus (history of trauma)
6. Mass above or below the medial canthal tendon

Etiology

1. Trauma: obliteration of anatomic structures from injury or radiation necrosis and fibrosis
2. Pharmacologic: punctal phimosis and obstruction can occur with chronic exposure to antiviral (idoxuridine) or antiglaucoma (phospholine iodide) agents
3. Inflammation (i.e., sarcoidosis, Wegener's granulomatosis, or pseudotumor)
4. Infection: either bacterial or fungal canaliculitis, dacryocystitis, or sinusitis
5. Systemic disease (i.e., Paget's disease)
6. Primary acquired nasolacrimal duct obstruction
7. Lacrimal sac tumors: either primary (papilloma, squamous cell carcinoma, hemangiopericytoma, etc.) or secondary (lymphoma, basal cell carcinoma, maxillary sinus tumors, etc.)

Workup

1. Gentle compression on the lacrimal sac looking for discharge from the puncta, which should be sent for gram stain and culture.
2. Dye disappearance test.
3. Jones 1 test.
4. Jones 2 test.
5. Dacryocystography and dacryoscintigraphy (optional).
6. CT scan or MRI scan (rule out lacrimal sac mass).

Differential Diagnosis

1. Allergy.
2. Conjunctivitis.
3. Keratoconjunctivitis sicca.
4. Trichiasis or distichiasis.
5. Eyelid malposition.
6. Canaliculitis: the puncta is usually swollen and inflamed.

Treatment

1. Management options vary when there is concurrent infection, whether the obstruction is partial or total, if a canalicular system is actually present or in the presence of a lacrimal sac neoplasm.

2. Canaliculitis is managed by irrigation with a penicillin solution (60,000–160,000 units/ml) and curettage for *Actinomycetes* (most common organism). Rifampin and erythromycin are alternatives.

3. Dacryocystitis: obstructions with concurrent bacterial infections are treated with warm compresses and topical antibiotic drops and ointments. Oral antibiotics (dicloxacillin, 500 mg q.i.d.) are also recommended for mild infections and intravenous antibiotics (penicillin G, 4.8×10^6 units/d, or nafcillin, 1 g q. 4h) are recommended for moderate to severe infections. The nasolacrimal duct (NLD) system should not be irrigated due to the risk of rupturing an inflamed sac resulting in widespread cellulitis. Incision and drainage of any abscess should be performed. After the acute infection is controlled a DCR is indicated.

4. Partial obstruction may be managed with probing and silicone intubation. Total obstruction is treated with a DCR and intubation.

5. Absence of a canalicular system may require treatment with a DCR and Jones tube. Lacrimal sac neoplasms may require a dacryocystectomy.

Follow-up   Patients treated with DCR and lacrimal intubation who have an uncomplicated course may be seen during the first postoperative week and in 4 to 6 months for follow-up. Some surgeons may remove the silicone tubes at 6 weeks in non-trauma-related cases. Others prefer to wait 6 to 12 months before tube removal.

Complications

1. Treatment failure of the infectious process
2. Recurrent extubation
3. Corneal trauma from silicone tubes
4. Punctal erosion from silicone tubes
5. Scarring and closure of canalicular system after removal of silicone tubes
6. Spontaneous closure of nasal ostium after DCR
7. Failure to achieve clear surgical margins from tumor in a dacryocystectomy

Prognosis   A DCR with silicone intubation generally results in long-term patency and elimination of symptoms in 90% of cases.

Lacrimal Gland Masses

Etiology (More Common)

1. Infectious agents (acute dacryoadenitis)
   a) Bacterial: staphylococcal, streptococcal, neisseria
   b) Viral: mumps, mononucleosis, herpes zoster
   c) Fungal: tuberculosis, syphilis, leprosy
2. Inflammatory (chronic dacryoadenitis): Sjögren's disease, sarcoidosis, Graves' disease, pseudotumor
3. Lymphomatous: benign reactive lymphoid hyperplasia, atypical lymphoid hyperplasia, lymphoma
4. Epithelial tumor: benign mixed tumor (pleomorphic adenoma), malignant mixed tumor, adenoid cystic carcinoma
5. Dermoid cyst
6. Cystic masses
7. Childhood tumors: granulocytic sarcoma, leukemia, neuroblastoma, rhabdomyosarcoma

Presentation   See Table 8.2.

Evaluation   A thorough history must be taken for any systemic disease. Consider ordering the following laboratory tests:

TABLE 8.2

Presentation of lacrimal gland masses

Etiology	Duration	Signs/Symptoms
Inflammatory	Acute	Swelling, pain, redness; usually unilateral
Infectious	Acute	Swelling, pain, redness; preauricular node; usually unilateral; malaise, fever; leukocytosis
Lymphomatous	Variable	Variable
Benign mixed	More than 12 mo	Painless swelling; lid droop
Malignant mixed	Less than 12 mo	Painful swelling
Adenoid cystic	Rapid onset	Painful

1. Complete blood count with differential, antinuclear antibody (ANA), serum lysozyme
2. Purified protein derivative (PPD) skin test
3. Thyroid function tests
4. Chest x-ray
5. CT or MRI scan of the orbits

Treatment

1. Acute dacryoadenitis with unilateral red, painful swelling is usually of bacterial or viral origin. Treatment includes hot compresses, antipyretics, and oral or intravenous antibiotics.

2. Chronic dacryoadenitis of systemic origin warrants evaluation and treatment for systemic disease. Initial treatment may involve an oral antibiotic or a short course of oral steroids.

3. Lacrimal gland duct cysts can be excised or marsupialized.

4. Lymphoid lesions require incisional biopsy. Pathologic evaluation should include immunohistochemical studies. These studies require fresh tissue so the specimen should be divided for permanent sections and for immunohistochemical studies. All patients should have a systemic workup to rule out systemic lymphoma.

5. Benign reactive lymphoid hyperplasia and atypical lymphoid hyperplasia require radiation therapy. Malignant lymphoma requires evaluation for systemic disease. If systemic lymphoma is detected, the appropriate chemotherapy is recommended. If the orbital lesion does not respond to chemotherapy, then local radiation is warranted. A hematologist or oncologist should be involved.

6. Benign mixed tumors are the most common epithelial tumor of the lacrimal gland. It is slow growing. If one suspects this tumor, an excisional (en bloc) biopsy via a lateral orbitotomy is done to avoid risk of malignant transformation of remaining cells and recurrence.

7. Malignant mixed tumors require an incisional biopsy followed by en bloc resection.

8. Adenoid cystic carcinoma is the most common malignant tumor of the lacrimal gland. The pain associated with this tumor is due to perineural invasion. The classic "Swiss cheese" pattern is seen histopathologically. The treatment of this tumor is orbital exenteration.

Follow-up

1. Acute dacryoadenitis is frequently self-limited.
2. Chronic dacryoadenitis requires referral to internal medicine department.
3. Lymphomatous tumors are referred to hematology or oncology specialists.
4. Epithelioid tumors should be followed yearly with examination and radiologic studies.

Complications Incisional biopsy of a benign mixed tumor can result in malignant transformation. Tumor recurrence can result in death.

Prognosis

1. Acute and chronic dacryoadenitis cases usually resolve with treatment.
2. Benign mixed tumors have a good prognosis.
3. Malignant mixed tumors and adenoid cystic tumors have a poorer prognosis.

Orbital Disease

Diagnostic Techniques

When evaluating orbital disease a complete eye examination is necessary with special attention to the following:

1. Globe position
2. Proptosis
3. Globe ptosis
4. Lid appearance

5. Palpation of orbit for masses
6. Auscultation of orbit for bruits

Diagnostic equipment and techniques of particular use in examination of orbital problems include the following:

1. Visual fields and Amsler grid
2. Color vision
3. Cranial nerve examination
4. Exophthalmometry
5. Echography—excellent for frequent follow-up examinations
6. CT or MRI scan
7. Selected laboratory work based on the suspected etiology

Selected Orbital Inflammatory Conditions

Signs and Symptoms

1. Preseptal cellulitis: eyelid edema, erythema, and tenderness; ocular examination is normal.
2. Orbital cellulitis: eyelid edema, erythema, and tenderness. Decreased ocular motility with pain on motion, proptosis, fever, malaise.
3. Orbital abscess: usually a late sequela of orbital cellulitis, see above.
4. Subperiosteal abscess: presentation may be similar to orbital cellulitis.
5. Cavernous sinus thrombosis: marked limitation of ocular motility, visual loss, dilated pupil with sluggish response to light, palsy of CN III, IV, V (first division), and VI, bilateral extension of symptoms and signs.
6. Idiopathic inflammatory pseudotumor: acute severe pain with loss of vision or double vision, usually unilateral with restriction of extraocular muscles. The inflammation can involve any component of the orbit (sclera, fat, lacrimal gland, etc.). Patients are typically afebrile.

Etiology

1. Contiguous infection from the paranasal sinuses, a dental abscess, intracranial infection, or the skin. Think of mucormycosis in diabetic patients.
2. Trauma.
3. Postsurgical.
4. Systemic infection.
5. Idiopathic.

Evaluation See "Diagnostic Techniques," above. In addition, one should obtain the following in all of the above-mentioned conditions except in an adult with preseptal cellulitis.

1. A complete blood count with differential white cell count
2. Cultures of the conjunctiva, any infectious site, and the nasopharynx
3. CT scan of orbits and central nervous system

Differential Diagnosis

1. Trauma
2. Mucocele of paranasal sinus
3. Orbital neoplasm (rhabdomyosarcoma, leukemia, etc.)
4. Dacryoadenitis
5. Dacryocystitis
6. Systemic vasculitis (Wegener's granulomatosis, etc.)

Treatment

1. Preseptal cellulitis
   a) Children: hot compresses, admit to the hospital for intravenous antibiotics (nafcillin, chloramphenicol), oral antibiotics (Cefaclor, cefuroxamine, or amoxicillin/clavulanate [Augmentin] 40 mg/kg in three divided doses).
      Antibiotics should cover *Streptococcus* (especially S. *pyogenes*), *Diplococcus pneumoniae*, and *Haemophilus influenzae* (especially in children 6 mo to 3 yrs of age).
   b) Adults: can be managed as outpatients with hot compresses and oral antibiotics (Cefaclor, dicloxacillin, or amoxicillin/ clavulanate [Augmentin]).
2. Orbital cellulitis: all patients should be admitted to the hospital for intravenous antibiotics (Ceftriaxone, cefazolin, or nafcillin). Frequent examination of vision, pupils, and motility (q. 2–4 h) is necessary.
3. Orbital and subperiosteal abscesses: admit for intravenous antibiotics with surgical drainage.
4. Cavernous sinus thrombosis: admit for intravenous antibiotics with careful observation for neurologic deterioration.
5. Pseudotumor: oral prednisone with radiation treatment in those cases unresponsive to steroids after histologic confirmation.

Follow-up Antibiotic coverage for adults with preseptal cellulitis may only require 7 to 10 days of oral antibiotics. The patients initially should be seen every few days until improvement occurs, then weekly until signs and symptoms resolve. Children with preseptal cellulitis and all other forms of orbital inflammatory disease may require up to 2 weeks of intravenous antibiotics and 1 week of oral antibiotics after discharge.

Prognosis   Orbital cellulitis can rapidly progress to an orbital abscess or cavernous sinus thrombosis. The latter may result in blindness, permanent neurologic damage, or death.

Selected Orbital Tumors

The diagnosis and management of each tumor in this section are discussed separately.

Cystic Tumors

Dermoid Cyst   Represents dermal structures that are trapped along suture lines during development. The cysts are lined with keratinized epidermis and can have any of the dermal appendages. The cysts are mobile, soft, painless masses. The location is usually the lateral orbit at the zygomaticofrontal suture or nasally at the nasofrontal suture.

A medially located cyst could represent an encephalocele so a CT scan is warranted prior to surgical excision.

Treatment involves complete excision with care not to rupture the cyst because of the potential inflammatory reaction to the cyst contents.

Lipodermoid   A benign mass that is usually located subconjunctivally on the lateral aspect of the globe. This tumor can extend into the orbit making complete excision difficult.

These are generally observed; if the tumor becomes cosmetically unacceptable, then the visible portion of the tumor is excised.

Meningocele   Not a true tumor but a protrusion of the meninges through defects in the orbital bones. If brain tissue is included, then it is called a meningoencephalocele. The mass is smooth, soft, and occasionally pulsates. It is usually located nasally and can be confused with an orbital dermoid.

Echography, CT, or MRI are useful diagnostic tools. Surgical repair with a neurosurgeon is indicated.

Mucocele   Develops from a chronic sinus infection with obstruction of the draining ostium and in children with cystic fibrosis. These cystic masses enlarge owing to accumulation of mucus and extend into the orbit by eroding the orbital bones. The frontal and ethmoid sinuses are most often affected.

Sinus series x-rays or CT scans are diagnostic. Treatment involves surgical excision with total removal of the sinus mucosa to prevent recurrences with obliteration of the sinus and the creation of a drainage passage into the nose.

Vascular Tumors

Capillary Hemangioma   A benign vascular tumor. It presents in the first few weeks of life, then slowly involutes over the next 4 to 6 years. The most common location is the periocular area, particularly the eyelids. It occasionally is located in the anterior orbit. The appearance is a reddish-blue mass that blanches with pressure. An eyelid lesion can cause astigmatism leading to amblyopia.

Observation is indicated if the lesion is asymptomatic and there is no evidence of astigmatism or amblyopia. Corticosteroid therapy is indicated if astigmatism, strabismus, amblyopia, or severe cosmetic deformity is present. Treatment is given by local injection directly into the lesion. Care is taken to aspirate before injecting the steroids. Triamcinolone, 40 mg (Kenalog), and betamethasone, 6 mg (Celestone), mixed in a 3 cc syringe with a 23 to 25 gauge needle are typically used. Some resolution should be seen within 1 to 3 weeks. Complications of steroid injections include skin atrophy and intravascular injection.

Cavernous Hemangioma   This is the most common orbital vascular tumor in adults. The clinical presentation is slow progressive proptosis. Composed of dilated cavernous spaces containing blood, the tumor is encapsulated. CT findings show a round, well-defined mass, usually located in the intraconal space. The lesion can be surgically excised if symptomatic.

Lymphangioma   The exact origin of this tumor remains unknown. It is composed of fluid-filled cystic spaces lined with endothelial cells. Its onset is within the first decade of life, usually as an acute orbital mass that is filled with blood ("chocolate cyst"). These lesions involve the conjunctiva, eyelids, oropharynx, and orbit.

The clinical presentation is gradual proptosis. The lesion may increase during upper respiratory infections. Lymphangiomas are infiltrative in nature, which makes surgical removal impossible. Observe lesions that are asymptomatic; surgical debulking is warranted if treatment is necessary. The use of the carbon dioxide laser has improved surgical treatment of these lesions.

Neural Tumors

Neurofibroma   Tumor of peripheral nerves composed of Schwann cells, endoneural fibroblasts, and axons. One of the findings in neurofibromatosis (autosomal dominant, café-au-lait spots, axillary freckling, fibroma molluscum, plexiform neurofibroma can give the classic S-shaped lid, pulsating exophthalmos from sphenoid bone dysplasia, optic nerve glioma). Observe if asymptomatic. Debulking of the tumor is indicated if vision is threatened or the mass is disfiguring.

Optic Nerve Glioma (Juvenile Pilocystic Astrocytoma)   See "Compressive Optic Neuropathy," in Optic Neuropathies section, Chapter 9. This is a benign tumor of children with a slow, progressive proptosis with vision loss. Twenty-five to fifty percent of cases are associated with neurofibromatosis.

Intradural tumor growth causes expansion of the optic nerve, unlike a meningioma that compresses the nerve.

Workup includes CT scan (classic fusiform appearance of the nerve), MRI (excellent for following the extent of the tumor), and echography and biopsy if the diagnosis is in question. One can observe these patients when the vision is good and the glioma is intraorbital. Patients are followed every 6 months, with CT or MRI scan yearly.

Surgical excision is indicated if the tumor is extending into the orbital apex (intracanalicular section) or there is evidence of intracranial extension. Radiation therapy is useful with extensive intracranial involvement, and resection is not a viable option.

Meningioma   See "Compressive Optic Neuropathy" in Optic Neuropathies section, Chapter 9. Tumor origin is the arachnoid layer; can be primary from the optic nerve sheath or secondary from surrounding structures (e.g., the sphenoid wing). Orbital extension is possible and contributes to the clinical signs based on the tumor's location.

Clinical findings include slow, progressive proptosis, loss of vision, and optociliary shunt vessels. This tumor is more common in adults but is more aggressive in children. CT scan shows calcification ("railroad track sign") of the optic nerve. Observation is indicated if the tumor is confined to the orbit and vision is good.

Surgical removal may be required if the vision is poor and the tumor is not confined to the orbit.

Myogenic Tumors

Rhabdomyosarcoma   This is a tumor of striated muscle in different stages of development. Types include

1. *pleomorphic,* rarely in orbit;
2. *embryonal,* most common in orbit;
3. *alveolar,* metastasis common; and
4. *botryoid.*

Acute onset of progressive proptosis due to rapid growth of the tumor typically in children. Biopsy of the tumor for diagnosis is followed by systemic evaluation. Immunohistochemical tests are useful diagnostic aids. Treatment should be coordinated with a pediatric oncologist and includes chemotherapy and radiation.

Metastatic Tumors

Any systemic carcinoma can metastasize to the orbit. Proptosis, pain, and orbital bone destruction are common findings. The clinical suspicion must be present if the appropriate history is to be obtained.

Neuroblastoma   Acute onset of proptosis with periorbital ecchymosis. Often, a history of neuroblastoma elsewhere can be elicited but the initial presentation can be orbital. Urine vanillylmandelic acid (VMA) is often elevated. Treatment is coordinated with a pediatric oncologist and includes chemotherapy and radiation.

Leukemia   Acute myelogenous leukemia presents in the orbit as granulocytic sarcoma (chloroma), which is often diagnosed prior to the systemic leukemia. A biopsy is necessary if there is no history of leukemia. Treatment includes consultation with a pediatric oncologist for systemic disease.

Bronchogenic Carcinoma   The most common metastatic carcinoma in males; a smoking history is often positive. Treatment involves systemic chemotherapy and orbital radiation.

Breast Carcinoma   The most common metastatic carcinoma in women. Usually there is a positive history of breast carcinoma. Proptosis, pain, and ptosis are common. Some cases have enophthalmos from scirrhous breast carcinoma. Treatment includes systemic hormonal therapy, chemotherapy, and orbital radiation.

Prostate Carcinoma   Signs include progressive proptosis, with the CT scans revealing osteoblastic changes. Workup should include examination of the prostate, chest x-ray, and serum acid phosphatase level. Treatment involves orbital radiation. The prognosis with orbital involvement is poor.

Graves' Orbitopathy

Definition   An ophthalmic condition resulting in exophthalmos, which may be associated with a hyperthyroid, euthyroid, or hypothyroid state.

Classification   See Table 8.3.

TABLE 8.3

Thyroid ophthalmopathy findings: Werner classification system

Class	Findings
0	No signs or symptoms
1	Only signs (periorbital edema, chemosis, injection, upper eyelid lag on downgaze—von Graeffe's sign, upper eyelid retraction—Dalrymple's sign)
2	Signs and symptoms
3	Proptosis
4	Extraocular muscle involvement (strabismus)
5	Corneal involvement (exposure keratitis)
6	Sight loss

Etiology   Currently thought to be an autoimmune disease resulting in lymphocytic infiltration and edema of extraocular muscles and orbital tissue with eventual fibrosis and contraction.

Presentation   The female-to-male ratio is 4:1, with the average age of onset 50 years. It may initially be unilateral but generally becomes bilateral.

Evaluation

1. Routine eye examination.
2. Visual field examination.
3. Color plate test.
4. Hertel exophthalmometry.
5. Thyroid function tests: 80% of patients with Graves' disease are hyperthyroid, 10% hypothyroid, and 10% euthyroid.
6. CT scan.
7. Echography.

Differential Diagnosis

1. Orbital idiopathic inflammatory pseudotumor
2. Orbital neoplasm
3. Orbital cellulitis
4. Systemic disease: lymphoma, sarcoidosis, amyloidosis, vasculitis
5. Orbital vascular malformation

Treatment

1. Medical evaluation by an internist to manage the thyroid dysfunction.

2. Corneal protection and lubrication: artificial tears during the day with a lubricating ointment at night.
3. Corticosteroids: usually in very symptomatic patients with acute orbital findings or in those with acute compressive optic neuropathy. The dosage of prednisone varies between 40 and 80 mg daily. Avoid long-term management with steroids.
4. Orbital radiation: used in acute cases when steroids are contraindicated or for compressive optic neuropathy if the patient is a poor candidate for surgical decompression or refuses surgery.
5. Surgical
   a) Tarsorrhaphy: for corneal exposure.
   b) Lid retraction surgery: should wait until disease activity has been quiet for at least 6 months.
      i) Upper eyelid operations include levator muscle recession, Müller's muscle extirpation, or use of spacer material (cartilage, sclera, fascia, hard palate).
      ii) Lower eyelid operations include retractor muscle extirpation or use of spacer material as indicated above.
   c) Strabismus surgery: based on the ocular deviation. The goal would be to obtain fusion in the primary position and in downgaze if possible. Again, the disease process should be stable for 6 months prior to surgery.
   d) Orbital decompression: the orbital walls are removed to increase the orbital volume and relieve the pressure on the optic nerve. All four walls can be removed, but the walls most commonly removed are the orbital floor and medial wall. Some surgeons advocate doing orbital decompression for cosmetic purposes before any lid or strabismus surgery.

Follow-up   Should include baseline optic nerve function tests such as color vision, visual fields, and pupillary examination. Follow-up should be every 3 to 6 months, based on severity of the disease. Once stable, yearly examinations are adequate.

Selected Readings

Anatomy

Doxanas MT, Anderson RL, eds. Clinical orbital anatomy. Baltimore: Williams and Wilkins, 1984.

Zide BM, Jelks GW. Surgical anatomy of the orbit. New York: Raven Press, 1985.

Lemke BN. Anatomy of the ocular adnexa and orbit. In: Della Rocca RC, ed. Ophthalmic plastic and reconstructive surgery. St. Louis: CV Mosby, 1987, pp. 3–74.

Anesthesia

Donlon JV. Local anesthesia for ophthalmic surgery: patient preparation and management. Ann Ophthalmol 1980;12:1183–91.

White PF, Vasconex LO, Mathes SA, et al. Comparison of midazolam and diazepam for sedations during plastic surgery. Plast Reconstr Surg 1988;81:703–10.

Wackym PA, Dubrow TJ, et al. Malignant hyperthermia in plastic surgery. Plast Reconstr Surg 1988;82:878–82.

Entropion

Wies FA. Spastic entropion. Trans Am Acad Ophthalmol Otolaryngol 1955;59:503–6.

Quickert MH, Wilkes DI, Dryden, RM. Nonincisional correction of epiblepharon and congenital entropion. Arch Ophthalmol 1983;101:778–81.

Benger RS, Frueh BR. Involutional entropion: a review of the management. Ophthalmic Surg 1987;18:140–42.

Baylis HI, Silkiss RZ. A structurally oriented approach to the repair of cicatricial entropion. Ophth Plast Reconstr Surg 1987;3:17–20.

Nerad JA. Eyelid malpositions. In: Linberg JV, ed. Lacrimal surgery. New York: Churchill Livingstone, 1988.

Ectropion

Tenzel RR, Buffam FV, Miller GR. The use of the lateral canthal sling in ectropion repair. Can J Ophthalmol 1977;12:199–202.

Frueh BR, Schoengarth LD. Evaluation and treatment of the patient with ectropion. Ophthalmology 1982;89:1049–54.

Tse D. Surgical correction of punctal malposition. Ophthalmol 1985; 100:339–41.

Nerad JA. Eyelid malpositions. In: Linberg JV, ed. Lacrimal surgery. New York: Churchill Livingstone, 1988, pp. 61–89.

Trichiasis and Distichiasis

Sullivan JH, Beard C, Bullock JD. Cryosurgery for treatment of trichiasis. Am J Ophthalmol 1976;82:117–21.

Wood JR, Anderson RL. Complications of cryosurgery. Arch Ophthalmol 1981;99:460–63.

Essential Blepharospasm and Hemifacial Spasm

Gillum WN, Anderson RL. Blepharospasm surgery: an anatomical approach. Arch Ophthalmol 1981;99:1056–62.

Dutton JJ, Buckley EG. Botulinum toxin in the management of blepharospasm. Arch Neurol 1986;43:380–82.

Garland PE, Patrinely JR, Anderson RL. Hemifacial spasm. Results of unilateral myectomy. Ophthalmology 1987;94:288–94.

Kalra HK, Magoon EH. Side effects of the use of botulinum toxin for treatment of benign essential blepharospasm and hemifacial spasm. Ophthalmic Surg 1990;21:335–38.

Facial Palsy

Mausolf FA. Techniques for the repair of orbicularis oculi palsy. Ophthalmic Surg 1978;9(3):67–70.
May M. Surgical rehabilitation of facial palsy: total approach. In: May M, ed. The facial nerve. New York: Thieme, 1986, pp. 695–777. Gold weights, lid springs.
Seiff SR, Sullivan JH, Freeman LN, Ahn J. Pretarsal fixation of gold weights in facial nerve palsy. Ophth Plast Reconstr Surg 1989;5:104–109.
Stamler JF, Tse DT. A simple and reliable technique for permanent lateral tarsorrhaphy. Arch Ophthalmol 1990;108:125–27.

Blepharoptosis

Crawford JS. Repair of ptosis using frontalis muscle—conjunctiva resection ptosis procedure. Ophthalmic Surg 1977;8:31–40.
Wiggs EO. The Fasanella-Servat operation. Ophthalmic Surg 1978;9:48–57.
Frueh BR. The mechanistic classification of ptosis. Ophthalmology 1980;87:1019–21.
Older JJ, Dunne PB. Silicone slings for the correction of ptosis associated with progressive external ophthalmoplegia. Ophthalmic Surg 1984;15:379–85.
Beard C. Ptosis surgery past, present, future. Ophth Plast Reconstr Surg 1985;1:69–72.
Leone CR, Shore JW. The management of the ptosis patient. Ophthalmic Surg 1985; 16:666–70. Part 2. 1985;16:720–27.
Mauriello JA, Wagner RS, Caputo AR, Natale B, Lister M. Treatment of congenital ptosis by maximal levator resection. Ophthalmology 1986;93:466–69.
Berlin AJ, Vestal KP. Levator aponeurosis surgery. Ophthalmology 1989;96:1033–36.
Shore JW, Bergin DJ, Garrett SN. Results of blepharoptosis surgery with early postoperative adjustment. Ophthalmology 1990;97(11):1502–11.

Eyelid Tumors

Baylis HI, Cies WA. Complications of Mohs' chemosurgical excision of eyelid and canthal tumors. Am J Ophthalmol 1975;80:116–22.
Beard C. Malignancy of the eyelids. Am J Ophthalmol 1981;92:1–6.
Doxanas MT, Green WR, Iliff CE. Factors in successful surgical management of basal cell carcinoma of the eyelids. Am J Ophthalmol 1981;91:726–36.
Fraunfelder FT, Zacarian SA, Wingfield DL, Limmer BL. Results of cryotherapy for eyelid malignancies. Am J Ophthalmol 1984;97:184–88.
Yeats RP, Waller RR. Sebaceous carcinoma of the eyelid: pitfalls in diagnosis. Ophth Plast Reconstr Surg 1985;1:35–42.

King RA, Ellis PP. Treatment of chalazia with corticosteroid injections. Ophthalmic Surg 1986;17:351–53.

Doxanas MT, Iliff WJ, Iliff NT, Green WR. Squamous cell carcinoma of the eyelids. Ophthalmology 1987;94:538–41.

Sloan GM, Reinisch MD, Nichter LS, Saber WL, Lew K, Morwood DT. Intralesional corticosteroid therapy for infantile hemangiomas. Plast Reconstr Surg 1989;83:459–66.

Diagnostic Techniques for Lacrimal System Disease

Hornblass A, Ingis TM. Lacrimal function tests. Arch Ophthalmol 1979;97:1654–55.

Taylor HR, Louis WJ. Significance of tear function test abnormalities. Ann Ophthalmol 1980;12:531–35.

Clinch TE, Benedetto DA, Felberg NT, Laibson PR. Schirmer's test. A closer look. Arch Ophthalmol 1983;101:1383–86.

Congenital Lacrimal System Drainage Disorders

Kushner BJ. Congenital nasolacrimal system obstruction. Arch Ophthalmol 1982;100:597–600.

Welham RAN, Hughes S. Lacrimal surgery in children. Am J Ophthalmol 1985;99:27–34.

Katowitz, JA, Welsh MG. Timing of initial probing and irrigation in congenital nasolacrimal duct obstruction. Ophthalmology 1987;94:698–705.

Acquired Lacrimal System Drainage Disorders

Putterman AM, Epstein G. Combined Jones tube—canicular intubation and conjunctival dacryocystorhinostomy. Am J Ophthalmol 1981;91:513–21.

Angrist RC, Dortzbach RK. Silicone intubation for partial and total nasolacrimal duct obstruction in adults. Ophth Plast Reconstr Surg 1985;1:51–54.

Linberg J, McCormick SA. Primary acquired nasolacrimal duct obstruction. A clinicopathologic report and biopsy technique. Ophthalmology 1986;93:1055–62.

Hawes MJ, Dortzbach RK. Trauma of the lacrimal drainage system. In: Linberg JV, ed. Lacrimal surgery. New York: Churchill Livingstone, 1988.

Rosen N, Sharir M, Moverman DC, Rosner M. Dacryocystorhinostomy with silicone tubes: evaluation of 253 cases. Ophthalmic Surg 1989;20:115–19.

Jordan DR, Nerad JA, Tse DT. The pigtail probe, revisited. Ophthalmology 1990;97:512–19

Lacrimal Gland Masses

Hurwitz JJ. A practical approach to the management of lacrimal gland lesions. Ophthalmic Surg 1982;13:829–36.

Jakobiec FA, Hallerveo J, Trokel S, et al. Combined clinical and computed tomographic diagnosis of primary lacrimal fossa lesions. Am J Ophthalmol 1982;94:785–807.

Shields CL, Shields JA, Eagle RC, Rathmell JP. Clinicopathologic review of 142 cases of lacrimal lesions. Ophthalmology 1989;96:431–35.

Selected Orbital Inflammatory Conditions

Macy JI, Mandelbaum SH, Minckler DS. Orbital cellulitis. Ophthalmology 1980;87:1309–13.

Weiss A, Friendly D, Eglin K, Chang M, Gold B. Bacterial periorbital and orbital cellulitis in childhood. Ophthalmology 1983;90:195–200.

Harris GJ. Subperiosteal abscess of the orbit. Arch Ophthalmol 1983; 101:751–57.

Selected Orbital Tumors

Sherman RP, Rootman J, LaPointe JS. Orbital dermoids: clinical presentation and management. Br J Ophthalmol 1984;68:642–52.

Kushner BJ. Intralesional corticosteroid injection for infantile adnexal hemangioma. Am J Ophthalmol 1982;83:496–506.

Ruchman MC, Flanagan JC. Cavernous hemangioma of the orbit. Ophthalmology 1983;90:1328–36.

Wright JE, Steward WB, Krohel GB. Clinical presentation and management of lacrimal gland tumors. Br J Ophthalmol 1979;63:600–6.

Boldt HC, Nerad JA. Orbital metastases from prostate carcinoma. Arch Ophthalmol 1988;106(10):1403–8.

Shields JA. Diagnosis and Management of orbital tumors. Philadelphia: WB Saunders, 1989.

Graves' Orbitopathy

Cooper WC, Harris GJ. Orbital surgery (orbital decompression). In: Jones IS, Jakobiec, FA, eds. Disease of the orbit. New York: Harper and Row, 1979, pp. 600–3.

Grove AS. Upper eyelid retraction and Graves' disease. Ophthalmology 1981;88:499–506.

Brennan MW, Leone CR, Janaki L. Radiation therapy for Graves' disease. Am J Ophthalmol 1983; 96:195–99.

Char DR. Thyroid Eye Disease. Baltimore: Williams and Wilkins, 1985.

Neigel JM, Rootman J, Belkin RI, et al. Dysthyroid optic neuropathy. Ophthalmology 1988;95:1515–21.

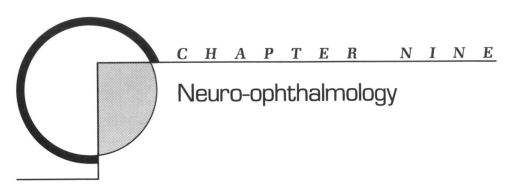

Neuro-ophthalmology

Richard E. Appen, M.D.
Michael P. Vrabec, M.D.

Amaurosis Fugax

Definition and Symptoms   Transient unilateral impairment of vision lasting several minutes, which indicates a disturbance of the arterial perfusion of the eye. Clarify if the patient tested each separately.

Etiology

1. Occlusive carotid artery disease (emboli or hypoperfusion)
2. Emboli from cardiac disease (myxoma, mural thrombi, valve disease, talc—intravenous drug abuse)
3. Temporal arteritis
4. Migraine—retinal
5. Idiopathic (especially young, healthy patient) without sequelae
6. Impending vein occlusion
7. Hyperviscosity states

Workup

1. Retinal examination: emboli, signs of ocular ischemic syndrome (neovascularization of retina, retinal hemorrhage), ophthalmodynamometry of central retinal artery.
2. Carotid evaluation: listen for bruits, Doppler ultrasound if symptoms are atypical or digital subtraction angiogram if patient is an acceptable risk for endarterectomy.
3. Blood work: Sedimentation rate, and if elevated, temporal artery biopsy complete blood cell count; blood sugar; blood lipids.
4. Cardiac evaluation: electrocardiography, echography.

Treatment

1. Carotid disease: endarterectomy—risks may outweigh possible benefits in some patients and pertinent clinical trial is under way; aspirin; smoking cessation; control hypertension; lower cholesterol.
2. Temporal arteritis: prompt oral prednisone.
3. Migraine: avoid beta-blockers, consider amitriptyline at bedtime.

Diplopia

Definition and Symptoms Monocular diplopia, present when one eye is occluded and caused by irregularity of the ocular media (cataract, keratoconus), does not indicate a neurologic disorder. Binocular diplopia, occurring only with both eyes open, indicates a misalignment of the visual areas. Clarify whether images are separated vertically or horizontally and in what direction of gaze they are farthest apart. Associated symptoms including limb weakness, paresthesias, ptosis, anisocoria (suggesting a neurologic cause), diurnal variation (myasthenia), heat or cold intolerance (dysthyroid disease), subjective bruit (carotid-cavernous fistula), or malaise and headache (temporal arteritis) should be elicited.

Examination

1. Careful orbital and lid examination including palpebral fissure measurement, orbital resiliency, exophthalmometry, and corneal sensation.
2. Careful measurement of the deviation with prism and cover test in all fields of gaze and head tilt.
3. Forced duction testing.

Differential Diagnosis and Workup

1. Cranial nerve (CN) palsies: see section on this topic, below.
2. Orbit disorder or dysthyroid disease. Laboratory tests: free thyroxin index (FTI), triiodothyronine radioimmunoassay (T3RIA), thyroid stimulating hormone (TSH), antithyroglobulin, antithyroid microsomal antibodies, orbital computed tomography (CT) or magnetic resonance imaging (MRI) scan.
3. Myasthenia gravis: edrophonium intravenously (Tensilon test); Prostigmin intramuscularly; CT of chest to rule out thymoma.
4. Temporal arteritis: erythrocyte sedimentation rate (ESR), temporal artery biopsy; mechanism of diplopia is thought to be muscle ischemia.
5. Central nervous system (CNS) causes of diplopia:
   a) Internuclear ophthalmoplegia (INO) is caused by a lesion involving the medial longitudinal fasciculus (MLF) in the pons as it passes from the pontine horizontal gaze center adjacent to the CN VI nucleus to the CN III subnucleus innervating the medial rectus (Fig. 9.1). Clinical findings:
      i) Weakness of the medial rectus (MR) on attempted horizontal gaze to the opposite side while convergence remains intact (posterior INO). With a mild INO, a rapid horizontal saccade may be necessary to demonstrate weakness of the affected medial rectus.
      ii) Nystagmus of the abducting eye on gaze direction that demonstrates the INO.
      iii) Convergence may be affected (anterior INO, 20% of cases).

   If the MLF and horizontal gaze center are involved, a "one and a half" syndrome occurs with gaze paralysis to the ipsilateral side and an INO on gaze to the opposite side. A unilateral INO is typically secondary to vascular disease,

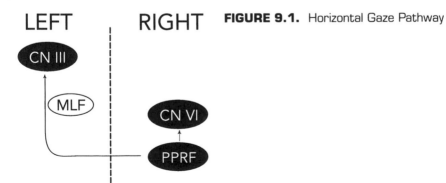

LEFT   RIGHT   **FIGURE 9.1.** Horizontal Gaze Pathway

CN III

MLF

CN VI

PPRF

while a bilateral INO is caused by the demyelination of multiple sclerosis (MS); rarer causes include neoplasm, infection, drug toxicity, and trauma. MRI scan is the study of choice.

b) Skew deviation: a vertical imbalance of the eyes that is not caused by an actual muscle weakness. The imbalance may measure the same in all directions of gaze. Nystagmus may occur. MRI scanning is the study of choice to examine the cerebellum and brainstem.

c) Parinaud's syndrome (Sylvian aqueduct or dorsal midbrain syndrome). Clinical findings:
   i) Paralysis of convergence and of voluntary upward gaze, with intact Bell's phenomenon.
   ii) Dilated pupils that constrict to a near stimulus but not to light.
   iii) A small exotropia despite normal horizontal eye movements.
   iv) Globe retraction within the orbit on attempted upward gaze.

MRI scanning is the study of choice. Lesion involves the midbrain near the quadrigeminal plate and is typically caused by a pinealoma in young persons and by vascular or metastatic disease in older persons.

Treatment

1. Monocular occlusion: part-time to encourage reestablishment of binocular fusion if the condition is thought to be temporary.
2. Prism.

Headache

Definition and Symptoms   Headache is a complaint very commonly heard by ophthalmologists, and the patient's history is extremely important. Questions to ask patients regarding their headaches:

1. Quality of headaches: dull ache versus knife-like pain.
2. Quantity of pain: is it the worst headache of the patient's life?
3. Location: frontal? periorbital (sinus)? Note that if a headache occurs consistently in the same location, it may indicate serious pathology.
4. Timing and setting: a pain that occurs consistently at the same time or awakens a patient from sleep is potentially serious.
5. Associated features of serious concern include nausea, vomiting, mental status changes, or other neurologic signs or symptoms (paresis, etc).

Etiology and Signs   The list of potential causes of headache is extremely long; discussed are several conditions important because of their common occurrence or potential for serious consequences.

1. Uncorrected refractive error: typically causes a dull headache with reading and can be easily treated with the proper glasses.
2. Angle closure glaucoma: eye pain with halos, nausea, and vomiting.
3. Ocular or orbital inflammation: herpes zoster may cause severe facial pain before the rash. Ramsay Hunt syndrome is due to the virus attacking CN VII with external ear pain and vesicles. Postherpetic neuralgia is easier to diagnose with pain and dysesthesia along a trigeminal nerve dermatome.
4. Sinus disease: periorbital pain located over the sinuses.
5. Tic douloureux (trigeminal neuralgia): brief knife-like pain in the area of CN V, often triggered by an external stimulus (wind, touch, etc.).
6. Increased intracranial pressure: severe generalized pain with optic disc swelling (see Papilledema section, below).
7. Central nervous system pathology: will usually have associated neurologic signs or alteration of mental status.
   a)   Subarachnoid or subdural hemorrhage: typically severe pain.
   b)   Tumor: constant location of pain is characteristic.
8. Malignant hypertension: retinal hemorrhages with disc swelling.
9. Temporal arteritis: weight loss, malaise (see section on this topic, below).
10. Migraine: very common condition that typically has a positive family history. Patients may also remember having "sick headaches" as a child. It is unusual for patients to develop migraine headaches in mid to late life. Migraines may be aggravated in some by pregnancy, birth control pills, and certain foods (alcohol, cheese, chocolates, and nuts). Different categories of migraine:
    a)   *Common migraine*—throbbing headache without an aura. The most common form of migraine is unilateral and should affect both sides on different occasions; if not, consider other causes.
    b)   *Classic migraine*—the headache is preceded by a loss of vision (aura), typically a scintillating scotoma that lasts from 15 to 30 minutes before the headache. Auras occurring after or during the headache are not typical of migraine.
    c)   *Complicated migraine*—the headache is associated with other, possibly permanent, neurologic symptoms (paresis of extraocular muscles, hearing loss).

    d) *Acephalgic migraine*—the aura occurs without the headache especially in older patients with a past history of classic migraine.

    e) *Retinal migraine*—a monocular, transient gray-out of vision, usually with no sequela.

11. Cluster headache: a unilateral throbbing pain with associated tearing, sweating, and rhinorrhea that typically occurs in cycles with daily occurrences (often awakening a patient from sleep) for several weeks and can repeat or resolve. A Horner's syndrome may also be seen.

Workup

1. Complete eye examination including refraction for near vision, slit lamp examination for narrow angles, optic nerve evaluation for swelling, and spontaneous venous pulsations (SVP)—note that 25% of normal subjects lack SVP.
2. Palpate temporal arteries for tenderness and signs of arteritis.
3. Visual fields if the vision is considered abnormal, or if a neurologic lesion is suspected.
4. Vital signs, especially blood pressure and brief neurologic examination (especially cranial nerves).
5. Neurologic referral if history and physical examination point to a possibly serious etiology.
6. MRI scan is indicated when history or physical examination suggests potential serious cause.

Treatment Should be directed toward the underlying etiology with avoidance of chronic analgesics, which have the potential for addiction and may mask the evaluation of a serious problem.

1. Migraine treatment falls under two categories (generally managed by a neurologist):
    a) Prophylactic medications include propranolol, nifedipine, tricycle antidepressants, and aspirin.
    b) Therapeutic medications include analgesics and ergotamine (a vasoconstrictor that should be used with caution in patients with classic migraine).
2. Cluster headaches are treated similarly to migraine with ergotamine; corticosteroids, methysergide, or lithium may also be effective.
3. Postherpetic neuralgia may sometimes be relieved with prednisone, tricyclic antidepressants, or cimetidine.

Visual Fields

Anatomy of the Visual Pathway

See Figure 9.2.

Visual Field Assessment

1. Confrontation: finger counting in various quadrants, gross assessment.
2. Goldmann perimetry: assesses the peripheral field kinetically, moving a visual stimulus from the nonseeing periphery toward central fixation until it is perceived. In addition, a supra-threshold spot of light is used to explore statically for areas of nonseeing within the peripheral boundary of the field of vision. Preferred when there is marked vision impairment or for patients who are less able to maintain good concentration.
3. Automated perimetry: assesses visual field statically, measuring how progressively bright a stationary light must be for it to be seen (its threshold) within the periphery of the field of vision. Automated perimetry is more sensitive to and accurate for subtle deficits within the central 25° of the visual field, but requires better patient alertness and cooperation.

FIGURE 9.2. Visual Pathways

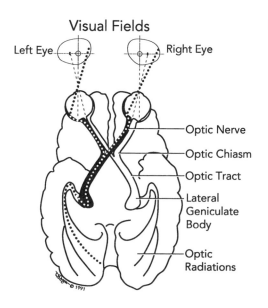

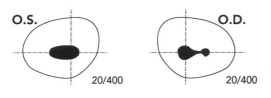

FIGURE 9.3. Monocular Field Defects OS, central scotoma; OD, cecocentral scotoma.

Visual Field Anomalies

Monocular Deficit

See Figure 9.3. A monocular defect indicates a disturbance of the retina or optic nerve anterior to the chiasm. In general, retinal lesions do not respect the vertical or horizontal meridians; optic nerve lesions can respect the horizontal but not the vertical meridians, and cause visual field defects connecting with the blind spot. Central scotomas are associated with reduced visual acuity; etiologies typically include macular disease, optic neuritis, and toxic optic neuropathies (Fig. 9.3, OS). If a central scotoma extends temporally to include the blind spot, it is termed cecocentral and occurs commonly with tobacco-alcohol or nutritional amblyopia (Fig. 9.3, OD).

Nerve Fiber Bundle Defect [Arcuate, Bjerrum]

See Figure 9.4. Focal damage to the optic nerve results in a field defect that communicates with the blind spot and generally has an arcuate shape above or below central fixation corresponding with the path of nerve fibers passing from the optic disc to the retina (Fig. 9.4, OS). More extensive damage to the nerve, especially mediated by vascular insufficiency, can result in an altitudinal field defect with no vision above (or below) the horizontal midline (Fig. 9.4, OD). Etiologies:

1. Glaucoma
2. Ischemic optic neuropathy
3. Optic nerve drusen

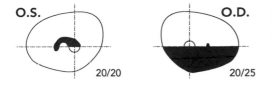

FIGURE 9.4. Nerve Fiber Bundle Defects OS, arcuate scotoma; OD, altitudinal defect.

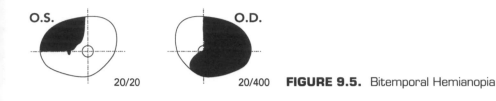

FIGURE 9.5. Bitemporal Hemianopia

Optic Chiasm Lesions

See Figure 9.5. Crossing fibers from the nasal retina (55% of all fibers, and note that macular fibers cross posteriorly in the chiasm) are predominantly involved, resulting in defects in the temporal half of the field of each eye, a bitemporal hemianopia. The deficits are commonly asymmetric. Etiologies:

1. Pituitary adenoma
2. Meningioma
3. Craniopharyngioma
4. Aneurysm

Note that persons with tilted optic discs or high myopia with bilateral ectasia of the nasal fundus may seem to have a bitemporal hemianopsia, which does not respect the vertical midline, as an artifact of perimetry.

Postchiasmal Lesions

See Figure 9.6. Lesions of the optic tract (which are rare) and optic radiations affect the same side of the visual field in each eye, resulting in a homonymous hemianopia. The more posterior the lesion, the more identical or congruous the homonymous hemianopic defect becomes. Note that a complete defect is nonlocalizing.

Parietal lobe lesions result in damage to the superior optic radiations and a subsequent homonymous defect denser inferiorly with hemiplegia. Temporal lobe lesions damage inferior fibers causing homonymous deficits more dense superiorly ("pie in the sky"), often with memory loss and formed hallucinations.

Occipital lobe lesions commonly are caused by occlusive posterior cerebral artery disease and typically produce a congruous homony-

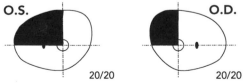

FIGURE 9.6. Homonymous Hemianopia

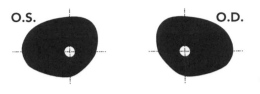

FIGURE 9.7. Generalized Constriction of the Visual Fields

mous defect without other cerebral impairment. Cortical blindness may result if bilateral occipital insults occur, resulting in total bilateral homonymous hemianopias. Such patients may deny that they are blind (Anton's syndrome) or perceive motion but not form (Riddock's phenomenon). Partial bilateral homonymous hemianopic defects are more common, with which visual acuity may remain normal.

General Constriction of the Fields

See Figure 9.7. One must differentiate between organic lesions (such as retinitis pigmentosa, glaucoma, bilateral occipital strokes, and chronic papilledema) that cause a generalized constriction of visual fields, which expands as the test distance lengthens, unlike hysterical field constriction, in which the narrowed field does not expand.

Cranial Nerve Palsies

General Considerations   Isolated cranial nerve (CN) palsies are typically localized distal to where the nerve fascicles exit the brainstem and proximal to their entry into the muscle. When there is involvement of more than one CN innervating the eye or a CN palsy with a Horner's syndrome, the lesion is generally in the ipsilateral cavernous sinus or superior orbital fissure. If there also is vision impairment caused by optic nerve involvement, the lesion is at the orbital apex. Regardless of whether the muscles innervated by a diseased CN are weak (paretic) or totally paralyzed (palsied), the anatomic localization of the lesion and its cause can be the same.

Frequency of Mayo Clinic Series of 881 Isolated Cranial Neuropathies

Cranial nerve VI: 48%
Cranial nerve III: 33%
Cranial nerve IV: 20%

Etiology

1. Idiopathic.
2. Ischemic (including diabetic): abrupt onset.

3. Tumor: gradually progressive.
4. Aneurysm: abrupt onset, affects pupil fibers on the periphery of CN III.
5. Trauma: abrupt onset.

Signs   Heterotropias detected with prism and cover testing in primary position, vertical and horizontal extremes of gaze and with head tilt to the right and left when a vertical eye muscle imbalance is present.

Differential Diagnosis   See Diplopia section, above. Clues suggesting a cranial neuropathy include the presence of ptosis and mydriasis (CN III), impaired corneal sensation (CN V), impaired hearing (CN VIII), Horner's syndrome, as well as the absence of exophthalmos, abnormal orbital resiliency, or abnormal forced ductions (orbital restrictive syndromes).

Workup

1. Blood pressure.
2. Laboratory tests: complete blood count, ESR, blood sugar, T_3, T_4, TSH, antinuclear antibody (ANA), acetylcholine receptor antibody (myasthenia).
3. MRI: suspected mass lesion.
4. Arteriography: an aneurysm may not show on MRI.

Cranial Nerve III Palsy

1. Anatomy: see Figure 9.8.
2. Signs: ptosis, mydriasis (95% of patients; Trobe 1988), exotropia greater in adduction (medial rectus weakness), hypotropia on upgaze (superior rectus weakness), hypertropia on downgaze (inferior rectus weakness).
3. A unilateral headache with an ipsilateral CN III palsy classically occurs with an aneurysm of the posterior communicating artery (compression of CN III near the cavernous sinus).
4. Older diabetic patients commonly develop a painful CN III palsy which spares the pupil. In this setting, arteriography to search for an aneurysm is not initially required as it usually resolves in 2 to 3 months. However, in persons aged 20 to 50 years, or in any person with only partial involvement of the extraocular muscles (EOMs) inverted by CN III, arteriography may be warranted.
5. An alert ambulatory person with a dilated fixed pupil and no other evidence of CN III dysfunction does not have a deteriorating neurologic condition that requires urgent attention. Patients who develop a fixed dilated pupil in the setting of a

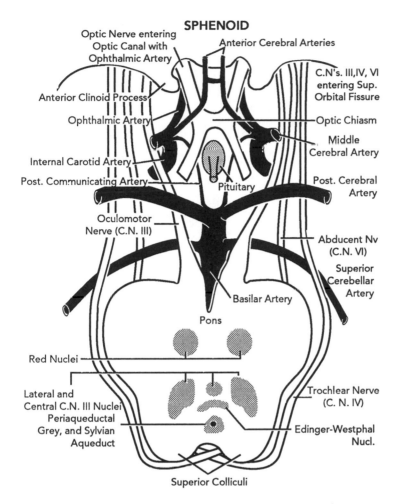

SPHENOID

Optic Nerve entering Optic Canal with Ophthalmic Artery

Anterior Cerebral Arteries

C.N's. III,IV, VI entering Sup. Orbital Fissure

Anterior Clinoid Process

Ophthalmic Artery

Optic Chiasm

Middle Cerebral Artery

Internal Carotid Artery

Post. Communicating Artery

Pituitary

Post. Cerebral Artery

Oculomotor Nerve (C.N. III)

Abducent Nv (C.N. VI)

Superior Cerebellar Artery

Basilar Artery

Pons

Red Nuclei

Lateral and Central C.N. III Nuclei Periaqueductal Grey, and Sylvian Aqueduct

Trochlear Nerve (C. N. IV)

Edinger-Westphal Nucl.

Superior Colliculi

FIGURE 9.8. Anatomy of Cranial Nerve III (Oculomotor)

herniating uncus of the temporal lobe of the brain caused by rising intracranial pressure are invariably obtunded (see Pupil Anomalies section, below).

6. A lesion involving only the nucleus of CN III in the midbrain is rare (must have a contralateral superior rectus palsy and bilateral levator palsy); most midbrain disorders also involve other pathways as in Weber's syndrome (ipsilateral CN III palsy and contralateral weakness—pyramidal tract) and Benedikt's syndrome (ipsilateral CN III palsy and contralateral tremor—red nucleus).

7. The most common manifestation of ophthalmoplegic migraine is a transient CN III palsy in children.
8. Aberrant regeneration of CN III fibers following compressive, traumatic, neoplastic, or aneurysmal damage can result, for example, in fibers initially destined to the medial rectus innervating the levator muscle, resulting in anomalous phenomena such as elevation of the eyelid on attempted adduction. Aberrant regeneration never occurs following ischemic insults to the nerve.

Cranial Nerve IV Palsy

1. Signs of a unilateral weakness of the superior oblique (mnemonic SO4) include a hypertropia that is worse in adduction, on downgaze, and on head tilt to the same side; and a compensatory head position with chin down and head tilted toward opposite shoulder. If bilateral, an esotropia in the primary position, worse in downgaze (V-esotropia), with a right hypertropia on leftward gaze and head tilt to the right and a left hypertropia on rightward gaze and on head tilt to the left, will occur.
2. Common etiologies are head trauma and congenital.
3. Anatomically, CN IV is unique in that it is the only cranial nerve that exits the brainstem dorsally and is completely crossed.

Cranial Nerve V

1. Anatomy: see Figure 9.9.
2. Important clinical conditions involving the first division of CN V:
   a) Tic douloureux (see Headache section, above).
   b) Raeder's trigeminal neuralgia—facial pain with an ipsilateral Horner's syndrome.
   c) Anesthetic cornea—chronic epithelial defects due to lack of corneal sensation.

Cranial Nerve VI Palsy

1. Anatomy: see Figure 9.10.
2. Signs of a weakness of the lateral rectus (mnemonic LR6) include an esotropia greater at distance than near and on lateral gaze to the ipsilateral side.
3. Etiologies can also include increased intracranial pressure, a pontine lesion when CN VII is also involved (CN VII fascicle wraps around CN VI nucleus), and metastases to the base of the skull where CN VI runs from the pons. Specific syndromes:
   a) Millard-Gubler syndrome includes a CN VII palsy plus contralateral hemiparesis.

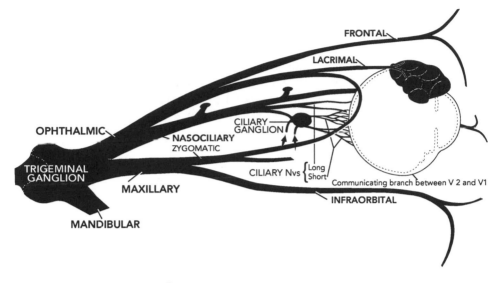

FIGURE 9.9. Anatomy of Cranial Nerve V (Trigeminal)

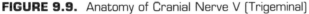

    b) Foville's syndrome includes CN V, VI, VII, VIII and Horner's syndrome.

    c) Gradenigo's syndrome includes CN V, VI, VII, VIII and otitis media.

  4. Must be differentiated from comitant esotropia of childhood and spasm of the near reflex.

FIGURE 9.10. Anatomy of Cranial Nerve VI (Abducens)

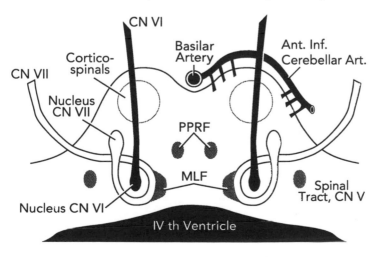

Cranial Nerve VII

1. Anatomy: see Figure 9.11.
2. The motor nucleus of CN VII splits in the pons, the upper facial muscles receive bilateral cortical innervation, the lower facial muscles receive contralateral and unilateral innervation. Therefore, a supranuclear facial palsy causes contralateral weakness of the lower half of the face.
3. Cerebellopontine angle (CPA) lesion will result in ipsilateral facial weakness, loss of hearing, hyperacusis, CN V, VI, VII palsy.
4. Ramsay Hunt's syndrome as a result of herpes zoster results in same deficits as CPA lesion except no other CN are involved and vesicles are present on the tympanic membrane.
5. "Crocodile tears" result from aberrant nerve regeneration between the chorda tympani and the lacrimal gland. Hence a patient will cry when presented with a stimulus to salivate.

Treatment

1. Specific etiologies (e.g., diabetes) should be treated.
2. Occlusion of one eye: temporary measure.
3. Prisms in glasses.
4. Botulinum, for example, inject the medial rectus in a case of CN VI palsy to prevent contracture.
5. Eye muscle surgery if deviation is unchanged for 6 to 12 months.

FIGURE 9.11. Anatomy of Cranial Nerve VII (Facial)

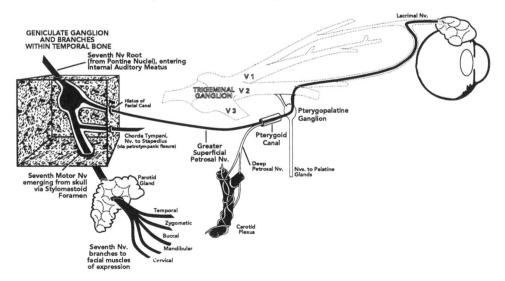

Nystagmus

Definition Nystagmus is an involuntary rhythmical oscillation of the eyes. Abnormalities of either the sensory or motor portions of the visual system can result in loss of steady visual fixation. Nystagmus can be described as horizontal, vertical, rotary, pendular (equal speed in both directions), or "jerk" (faster in one direction) and is said to "beat" in the direction of the fast movement. Observation of the nystagmus wave form may not enable one to identify the cause of the problem with certainty. The following are normal forms of nystagmus:

Optokinetic nystagmus results from vestibular stimulation (spinning chair or irrigation of water into an ear). Cold water irrigation of the ear will result in nystagmus beating in a direction away from the side of irrigation; warm water causes beating in a direction toward the ear. Hence the mnemonic "COWS."

Voluntary nystagmus is a rapid, low-amplitude oscillation of the eyes that can be sustained for only 20 to 40 seconds.

Endpoint nystagmus is a mild horizontal nystagmus, beating in the direction of gaze, on extreme horizontal gaze.

Abnormal forms of nystagmus can be separated into congenital (generally stable without oscillopsia) or acquired (indicating an active process involving the brainstem, cerebellum, or vestibular apparatus, with oscillopsia). The following are congenital forms:

Congenital sensory nystagmus is usually a horizontal pendular nystagmus. There is no null point (i.e., a direction of gaze that markedly reduces the condition). Vision is reduced and may be due to achromatopsia, albinism, aniridia, or congenital maculopathies.

Congenital motor nystagmus is usually a horizontal jerk nystagmus but occasionally is rotary. A null point exists where vision may be normal, whereas vision is poor if the patient is forced to look in the direction of gaze in which the nystagmus is more marked. The condition is often hereditary. The use of prisms or extraocular muscle surgery may be useful in therapy.

Latent nystagmus is a horizontal jerk nystagmus induced when one eye is occluded. It commonly occurs in children with strabismus. Monocular vision should be evaluated by fogging the fellow eye with a strong plus lens rather than an opaque occluder, which makes the nystagmus worse.

Etiology   The etiology behind acquired nystagmus may include neoplasm, demyelination (MS), infection, vascular occlusion, degenerations, CNS structural anomalies, or drug intoxication (sedatives, anticonvulsants). Workup may require MRI of the posterior fossa. There are several forms of acquired nystagmus:

Horizontal gaze nystagmus is a conjugate beating in the direction of attempted gaze, representing a weakness of horizontal gaze, occurring with lesions of the pons or cerebellum.

Vertical nystagmus can beat upward or downward. Upbeating nystagmus is usually caused by drug intoxication or disease of the brainstem or cerebellum. Downbeating indicates dysfunction of the cerebellum or brainstem at the junction of the medulla and cervical spinal cord. It commonly occurs as part of the Arnold-Chiari malformation (compression of the brainstem by the cerebellum) or platybasia, and may be improved by neurosurgery.

Rotary nystagmus indicates acquired disease of the vestibular system, and is especially prominent in young persons with presumably viral labyrinthitis.

Retraction–convergence nystagmus describes intermittent convergence of the eyes and retraction of the globes into the orbit with attempted upgaze. It is often seen in Parinaud's syndrome and is best seen with the optokinetic nystagmus drum moving downward.

Periodic alternating nystagmus is a horizontal jerk that cyclically changes the direction of its fast phase every 1 to 4 minutes. A lesion in the pontomedullary region ventral to the IV ventricle with involvement of the vestibular pathways is usually the cause. Baclofen can be beneficial in treatment (Weinstein et al. 1988).

Seesaw nystagmus describes the elevation and intorsion of one eye as the other eye depresses and extorts. Parasellar lesions (pituitary tumors, aneurysm, and craniopharyngiomas) are the cause, and a bitemporal hemianopia is common.

Spasmus nutans is an asymmetric (occasionally monocular), horizontal, low-amplitude motor nystagmus. It occurs in infants 3 to 13 months of age who display head nodding or an abnormal head position. This tends to resolve over 1 to 2 years. A similar picture can occur in children who have optic atrophy secondary to an optic nerve glioma, and MRI scanning should be performed to rule this out.

Several other excessive ocular motility syndromes are not truly forms of nystagmus because they lack regular rhythmicity:

Square wave jerks are small-amplitude, conjugate saccades first to the right and then to the left; between the saccades, the eyes are steady. They result from cerebellar dysfunction.

Ocular flutter occurs with impairment of cerebellar control and results in intermittent brief bursts of horizontal back-and-forth, small, conjugate ocular saccades.

Opsoclonus describes rapid, large-amplitude conjugate ocular saccades in all directions without any rhythmic patterns. This can occur with brainstem or cerebellar encephalitis or a neuroblastoma. Propranolol or baclofen may improve this condition.

Superior oblique myokymia is the idiopathic intermittent contraction of the superior oblique muscle causing subtle torsion of the eye with monocular oscillopsia. A slit lamp may be needed to see these fine movements. Carbamazepine or surgical tenectomy of the superior oblique muscle may be helpful in therapy; however, it may resolve spontaneously.

Pupil Anomalies

The pupil size is a balance of the autonomic nervous system's sympathetic stimulation enlarging the pupil and the parasympathetic stimulation constricting it. The pupillary light reflex has its afferent limb from the retina via the optic nerve and tract to the midbrain CN III nuclei, and the efferent limb via CN III and the ciliary ganglion in the orbit (Fig. 9.12).

Input from each eye is distributed equally to both CN III nuclei so that each pupil responds the same when either eye is stimulated (direct response = consensual response). Hence, total loss of vision in one eye does not cause anisocoria. Twenty percent of individuals have unequal pupil size without a structural disease (essential anisocoria, in which the pupil size difference is the same in the dark as in the light, and the reaction to light is normal).

Pupil Abnormalities

See Table 9.1.

Relative Afferent Pupil Defect [Marcus Gunn Pupil]

Requires substantial retinal or optic nerve disease, and does not occur with cataract or mild macular disease. Note that the consensual response of the other eye can indicate the integrity of the afferent limb in cases of pharmacologic mydriasis, cloudy cornea, etc.

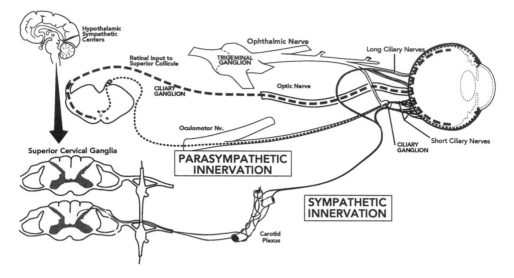

FIGURE 9.12. Parasympathetic and Sympathetic Pupil Pathways

Horner's Syndrome

An impairment of sympathetic innervation of the eye. Signs include miosis (more evident in dim light), mild ptosis of the upper lid and elevation of the lower lid, and facial anhidrosis when the first or second sympathetic neurons are involved. Congenital Horner's syndrome will result in decreased pigmentation of the iris and can be the initial sign of a thoracic neuroblastoma in an infant.

TABLE 9.1

Pupil flow chart

	Pupil Size Equal			**Pupil Size Unequal**		
Response to light	Normal	One is sluggish	Both sluggish	Both normal	Larger is sluggish	Smaller is sluggish
Diagnosis	Normal	Afferent lesion	1. Bilat. aff. lesion 2. Parinaud's 3. Bilat. Adie's 4. Argyll Robertson 5. Pharmacologic	1. Essential anisocoria 2. Horner's	Efferent lesion 1. CN III palsy 2. Adie's 3. Pharmacologic 4. Iris trauma	1. Adie's (longstanding) 2. Iritis 3. Iris trauma

The three-neuron sympathetic pathway is lengthy, extending from the hypothalamus via the brainstem and spinal cord to the chest and then reentering the skull along the internal carotid artery and passing via the cavernous sinus into the orbit. First neuron lesions generally have associated neurologic deficits. Second neuron lesions can be caused by thoracic disorders (Pancoast lung tumor), and third neuron lesions can occur with cavernous sinus pathology or Raeder's syndrome (migraine-like unilateral headache with an ipsilateral Horner's syndrome without anhidrosis).

The diagnosis is confirmed by failure of topical cocaine 5% to 10% (one drop in both eyes q. 5 min, three times) to effect pupil dilation. Cocaine blocks the reuptake of the norepinephrine into the sympathetic neuron after it acts on the iris muscle, thereby potentiating its effect. If the sympathetic system is defective, no norepinephrine is released, and the pupil does not dilate. Hydroxyamphetamine (Paredine) 1% normally stimulates the release of norepinephrine at the myoneural junction; therefore, in a complete third neuron lesion, topical Paredine will fail to cause mydriasis but will result in mydriasis in a first and second neuron lesion.

This test should be done 24 hours after a cocaine test. Workup should include a chest x-ray with apical views of the lung and possible MRI scan of the central nervous system.

Cranial Nerve III Palsy

Will result in anisocoria more evident in bright lighting (see Cranial Nerve Palsies section, above).

Adie's Tonic Pupil

An enlarged pupil that does not constrict or constricts poorly to light, but constricts better to the near stimulus. Later, the pupil may become smaller than the other. Irregular vermiform iris contractions may be evident on slit lamp examination. This commonly occurs in young women whose deep tendon reflexes of the lower extremities are diminished or asymmetric. Instillation of a weak miotic (pilocarpine 0.1%) will result in more miosis than the fellow normal eye owing to denervation hypersensitivity of the iris constrictor. Four percent of patients per year will sustain involvement of the fellow eye. Diagnostic studies are not needed.

Parinaud's Syndrome

Results in large pupils unreactive to light but constricting well to near stimuli (see Diplopia section, above).

Argyll Robertson Pupil

Secondary to CNS syphilis, pupils are small (owing to damage to supranuclear pathways inhibiting CN III nuclei) and constrict to a near stimulus but not to light. Cerebrospinal fluid test for syphilis (fluorescent treponemal antibody-absorption [FTA-ABS]) is needed to establish the diagnosis.

Pharmacologic Pupil Dilation

Secondary to inadvertent or intentional exposure to mydriatic eyedrops (even with a negative history of eyedrop use) results in unilateral or bilateral dilated and unreactive pupils. First use a weak miotic solution (pilocarpine 0.1%) to rule out Adie's pupil. Subsequent failure of miosis with pilocarpine 2% indicates pharmacologic blockade.

Iris Sphincter Trauma

Results in mydriasis that responds the same way as pharmacologic pupil dilation to miotic agents.

Paradoxic Pupil

Results in initial miosis upon onset of darkness, and has been reported with congenital stationary night blindness and congenital achromatopsia as well as patients with optic nerve anomalies, nystagmus, and strabismus. This sign appears not to have the specificity initially suspected (Frank et al. 1988).

Papilledema

Definition and Symptoms   Bilateral swelling of the optic discs caused by increased intracranial pressure (ICP). The mechanism is thought to be due to impairment of axoplasmic flow, though vascular and hydrostatic factors most likely play a role. There can be transient (5–10 s) obscurations of vision with positional change. Visual acuity is generally good unless the condition is severe and protracted. Associated symptoms are diplopia (due to CN VI paresis), headache, nausea, and vomiting. In pseudotumor cerebri, ICP is elevated, but the etiology is unknown. This typically affects young obese women.

Signs

1. Optic discs: early, hyperemic blurred margins, loss of spontaneous venous pulsation. Later, more elevation of disc, peripapillary retinal folds concentric with the disc margin, peripapillary hemorrhage and exudates.

2. Visual fields: enlarged blind spot early, with subsequent development of nerve fiber bundle defects, peripheral contraction, and blindness if raised ICP persists.

Etiology

1. Cerebral mass
2. Hydrocephalus
3. Encephalitis
4. Dural venous thrombosis
5. Unknown: pseudotumor cerebri
6. Hypoparathyroidism
7. Lead intoxication
8. Medications: corticosteroids, vitamin A, tetracycline, nalidixic acid, indomethacin
9. Pickwickian syndrome
10. Jugular venous obstruction

Workup

1. Neurology consultation.
2. MRI scan: in pseudotumor cerebri, ventricle size is normal.
3. Lumbar puncture (in absence of a focal mass lesion) to rule out meningoencephalitis and document the increased ICP.

Differential Diagnosis

1. Pseudopapilledema: optic disc drusen or congenital tortuosity of the retinal vessels.
2. Optic neuritis: mild disc swelling with marked vision impairment.
3. Ischemic optic neuropathy (acute onset, unilateral, nerve fiber bundle defects).
4. Diabetic papillopathy (Appen et al. 1980a): young juvenile diabetics.
5. Papillophlebitis/optic disc vasculitis (Appen et al. 1980b): unilateral, good vision, peripheral retinal venous congestion, and hemorrhage.
6. Accelerated hypertension.
7. Metastatic (i.e., leukemic) infiltration of the nerves.

Treatment   For severe headache or progressive vision loss:

1. Treat underlying cause (excision of neoplasm, etc.).
2. Medical therapy to lower ICP—acetazolamide, furosemide.

3. Lumbar peritoneal shunt (Corbet and Thompson 1989).
4. Optic nerve sheath decompression (Keltner 1988).

Prognosis Persistent elevation of ICP can result in permanent damage to the optic nerves, generally over months.

Carotid-Cavernous Fistula (CCF)

Etiology CCFs are either *direct* (a communication between the cavernous sinus and the internal carotid artery, generally following trauma), or *dural* (a communication between the cavernous sinus and smaller arterial branches, either from the internal or external carotid artery perfusing the dura, generally occurring spontaneously in middle-aged women).

Signs Direct: more severe, high flow disorder, causing

1. marked conjunctival congestion,
2. pulsating exophthalmos,
3. raised intraocular pressure,
4. limited eye movements,
5. orbital or cranial bruit.

Dural: findings are similar to direct but less pronounced.

Workup

1. CT or MRI scan: engorged superior ophthalmic vein or abnormality in the cavernous sinuses.
2. Cerebral angiography: selective injection of the external and internal carotid systems is required for definitive diagnosis.

Differential Diagnosis

1. Chronic conjunctivitis
2. Dysthyroid ophthalmopathy
3. Orbital cellulitis
4. Cavernous sinus thrombosis
5. Ischemic oculopathy

Treatment

1. Corneal lubrication for exposure keratitis.
2. Reduce elevated intraocular pressure.
3. Elevate head of bed to decrease exophthalmos.

4. Detachable intravascular balloon, for severe symptoms. A fistula arising from the internal carotid artery can be obliterated. Embolization of external carotid branches is more difficult but possible.
5. Dural fistulas more commonly close spontaneously or after angiography and less often require intravascular detachable balloons.

Prognosis An intracranial vascular catastrophe is a rare complication; therefore, the severity of the clinical signs and symptoms should dictate the need for angiography or invasive therapy.

Chronic Progressive External Ophthalmoplegia (CPEO)

Definition and Etiology A rare, gradually progressive, bilateral myopathy of the extraocular and levator palpebrae superioris muscles. Age of onset varies from childhood to midlife. The disorder may be part of a systemic condition affecting the retina, central nervous system, and cardiac conduction system (Drachman's ophthalmoplegia plus). A mutation of mitochondrial DNA resulting in abnormal mitochondrial protein synthesis is the underlying etiology.

Syndromes of CPEO For reference see Di Mauro et al. (1985) and Schapira (1989).

1. Kearns-Sayre syndrome: onset under 15 years of age, retinal degeneration, heart block, elevated CSF protein, cerebellar dysfunction.
2. MERRF (myoclonic epilepsy and ragged red fibers) syndrome: CNS involvement.
3. MELAS (mitochondrial myopathy, encephalopathy, lactic acidosis, stroke-like episodes) syndrome.

Signs

1. Bilateral ptosis.
2. EOM impairment: symmetric without diplopia.
3. Normal pupils.
4. Exposure keratopathy.
5. Pigmentary retinopathy: less pronounced than that seen in retinitis pigmentosa.

Workup

1. Goldmann perimetry.
2. Electroretinogram.
3. Tensilon test (rule out myasthenia).
4. Electrocardiogram.
5. Neurology referral.
6. Muscle biopsy: ragged red fibers result from abnormal accumulation of mitochondria.
7. Cardiology referral.
8. Genetic counseling.

Differential Diagnosis

1. Myasthenia gravis
2. Dysthyroid ophthalmopathy
3. Brainstem neoplasm
4. Guillain-Barré syndrome, Miller-Fisher variant
5. Basilar meningitis

Treatment

1. Ptosis: lid crutches—lid surgery should be approached cautiously owing to the risk of exposure keratitis from a poor Bell's phenomenon.
2. Corneal lubrication for exposure keratopathy.
3. Coenzyme Q-10 has been reported to be beneficial.

Prognosis   Varies depending on the timing of mutation of mitochondrial DNA following ovum fertilization, which influences extent of tissue involvement.

Myasthenia Gravis

Definition and Symptoms   Myasthenia gravis (MG) is an autoimmune disease of neuromuscular transmission in which antibodies to the acetylcholine (ACh) receptor sites in skeletal muscle block ACh action. Peak incidence for women is in their twenties, and for men in their sixties (more women are affected overall). Patients will have the following symptoms:

1. Variable muscle weakness that worsens as the day progresses or with exercise.
2. Diplopia: some patients will have only involvement of the eye muscles.
3. Difficulty chewing, swallowing, speaking, or breathing.

Signs

1. Normal vision and pupil function.
2. Ptosis: variable and worsens with sustained upgaze, and will improve with rest.
3. Cogan lid twitch: produced by having the patient perform extended downward gaze. When the eyes are quickly redirected to the primary position, an overshoot or twitch of the upper eyelid occurs.
4. EOM weakness of any combination with variability of measurements.

Workup

1. Tensilon (edrophonium HCl) is a rapidly acting anticholinesterase agent that potentiates ACh and tends to reverse the ptosis or diplopia in MG. Pretreatment with atropine will prevent its cholinergic side effects including bradycardia, intestinal cramps, vomiting, or vasovagal hypotension. A test dose of 1 mg (0.1 ml) is given intravenously and the patient is observed for a minute. If the ocular signs are not corrected (lasting for only 1–2 min) and no serious side effects occur, additional 3 mg (0.3 ml) boluses are given at 1 to 2 minute intervals until a total of 10 mg (1 ml) has been given. A false-negative test result can occur, but false-positive results are rare.
2. Prostigmin (Neostigmine) can be given intramuscularly (1.5 mg for adults, 0.04 mg/kg for children) when intravenous injection is not feasible, with assessment 30 minutes after injection.
3. Laboratory tests: serum ACh receptor antibody, thyroid functions, and ANA to look for associated autoimmune diseases.
4. Electromyography (EMG) of skeletal muscles will show a decreasing response with generalized MG but may be normal in patients with ocular MG.
5. CT of chest: 15% of patients will have a thymoma.
6. Neurology referral.

Differential Diagnosis

1. Ptosis
   a) Horner's syndrome (slight ptosis without variability)
   b) CPEO (symmetric ptosis without variability)
   c) Involutional ptosis (does not improve with rest)
   d) CN III palsy (possible mydriasis, consistent eye muscle imbalance)
2. Myasthenic (Eaton-Lambert) syndrome: occurs with oat cell carcinoma, causing an impaired release of ACh from the nerve

terminal, resulting in weakness that improves with exercise. Ptosis and EOM abnormalities are less common in this syndrome.

3. Guillain-Barré syndrome.
4. Botulism.

Treatment   Is generally managed by a neurologist. Mestinon (anticholinesterase) may help, along with corticosteroids for antibody suppression, thymectomy, or plasmapheresis.

Prognosis   Difficult to predict individually, but about 65% of patients with ocular signs will progress to develop systemic MG; 10% to 20% will enjoy spontaneous remission. A few patients will experience progressive disability and death from respiratory failure.

Myotonic Dystrophy

Definition and Symptoms   Myotonic dystrophy (MD) is an autosomal dominant disorder of muscle cell metabolism characterized by generalized muscle weakness and atrophy. The precise biochemical defect remains unknown. Onset usually begins between ages 10 and 20.

Ocular Signs

1. Variable ptosis
2. Weakness of orbicularis oculi muscles
3. Slowing of ocular saccades
4. Ocular hypotony
5. Peripheral pigmentary retinopathy
6. Cataract ("Christmas tree" crystalline deposits)

Systemic Signs

1. Delayed ability to relax the grip after shaking hands
2. Frontal baldness
3. Facial and temporal muscle atrophy
4. Intestinal and urinary smooth muscle dysfunction
5. Cardiac hypertrophy and valvular disease
6. Mental retardation
7. Testicular atrophy

Differential Diagnosis   See Myasthenia Gravis section, above.

Treatment   No specific therapy is available.

Course Slowly progressive. Descendants of an affected person develop manifestations of the disorder at progressively younger ages (phenomenon of "anticipation").

Optic Neuropathies

General Comments

If a person experiences unilateral vision impairment and there is no refractive error or ocular abnormality, an optic neuropathy is likely. If both eyes are impaired, another possible explanation is that the optic chiasm (bitemporal field defects) or cerebral visual pathways (homonymous defects) are affected. Several of the more common optic neuropathies are discussed below.

Optic Neuritis

Symptoms Abrupt onset of vision loss (unilateral in 85%; typically younger patients; female more than male) followed by variable improvement (75% recover to at least 20/40); light flashes or scintillations; pain with eye movement; transient worsening of vision with physical exertion or heat exposure (Uhthoff's symptom).

Etiology

1. Unknown
2. Multiple sclerosis

Signs

1. Impaired central visual acuity (central scotoma on visual field testing).
2. Impaired color vision.
3. Afferent pupil defect.
4. Optic disc can be normal 50% (retrobulbar neuritis), swollen 35% (papillitis), or pale 15% (optic atrophy).

Workup

1. Laboratory: complete blood count, ESR, ANA, FTA-ABS, Lyme titer.
2. Neurologic consultation including MRI scanning for mass lesions and demyelinated plaques. Lumbar puncture only in cases atypical of optic neuritis or when vision does not improve over several weeks' time.

Differential Diagnosis

1. Retinal disorders, especially central serous choroidopathy, will not have an afferent pupil defect.

2. Other causes of optic disc swelling such as compressive and ischemic optic neuropathies are discussed later in this section.

3. Leber's hereditary optic neuropathy is an uncommon bilateral condition often involving one nerve several weeks or months before the other. This typically affects men around 20 years of age who notice the sudden severe loss of central vision. A mutation of mitochondrial DNA is thought to be responsible. Characteristic small peripapillary telangiectatic vessels that *do not* leak with fluorescein angiography accompany hyperemic optic nerves. Optic atrophy generally results. No therapy has been definitely successful, although hydroxocobalamin and even craniotomy to lyse arachnoid adhesions around the optic nerves have been reported to be helpful.

4. Tobacco-alcohol amblyopia is a bilaterally symmetric condition occurring in malnourished alcoholics. It is unclear if the toxins from smoking, inadequate vitamin intake, or both are responsible. Vision loss is central and gradual, and the nerves are hyperemic early and pale later. Cessation of tobacco and alcohol use and multivitamin administration may improve the condition.

5. Autoimmune disorders: lupus can cause an optic neuritis mainly in young women who have an elevated ESR, abnormal ANA, and vasculitis on skin biopsy.

6. Basilar meningitis, secondary to syphilis, tuberculosis, Lyme disease, viral (varicella or postvaccination), and fungal infections (cryptococcal), can result in optic nerve dysfunction. Generally, other symptoms and signs will point to the underlying condition.

7. Functional vision loss is suggested by varying visual acuity measurements, normal pupils, and tubular constriction of visual fields.

8. Dominant optic atrophy: autosomal dominant inheritance, onset in first decade of life, mild vision impairment (20/50), which slowly declines with time, temporal pallor of the disc.

Treatment   Prednisone. In 1988, the Optic Neuritis Treatment Trial (ONTT) was begun to compare a 2-week course of oral prednisone; intravenous megadose methylprednisolone therapy for 3 days (I.V.M.P.) followed by prednisone; and a placebo. In 1992, Beck et al. reported that at 6 months from the onset there was no difference in visual outcome between the patients treated with oral prednisone and those treated with a placebo. Those patients receiving I.V.M.P. recovered more quickly, especially when the vision had initially been more severely impaired. Measurements of contrast sensitivity, color vision, and visual fields suggested a slight improvement in outcome for patients receiving I.V.M.P. compared with placebo at 6 months. The surprise finding was that those patients receiving oral prednisone alone had a higher incidence of subsequent recurrence of optic neuritis (27%) than did those receiving placebo (15%) and I.V.M.P. (13%). The study suggests that there is no role for oral prednisone therapy alone in the treatment of idiopathic or demyelinating optic neuritis. When the vision is substantially impaired it is uncertain whether there is cost-benefit justification to initiate treatment with 3 days of I.V.M.P. This decision is up to the physician and the patient. The results have not been revealed to date. In patients who have no contraindication to steroids and have substantial pain or vision loss, it may be reasonable to treat with prednisone, 60 to 80 mg per day for several days, followed by a 4 to 6 week taper.

Course Most patients with optic neuritis experience improvement of vision in the first few weeks of onset, and about 75% have recovery of at least 20/40 (Cohen et al. 1979). In the following 5 years, about 30% to 40% of patients experience a recurrence of optic neuritis in the same or other eye.

It is accepted that a third of patients with MS have optic neuritis at some time during their illness. Results of studies attempting to reveal what portion of persons experiencing isolated optic neuritis ultimately prove to have MS have been markedly variable. In a prospective study of patients with isolated optic neuritis followed for at least 5 years, Cohen, Lessell, and Wolf (1979) reported that 35% of the patients later showed evidence of definite or probable MS (curiously, 45% of the women compared to 11% of the men). In an update in 1988, after a mean follow-up of 15 years (range of 5–20 yrs), they found that the later diagnosis of MS applied to 58% (69% of women and 33% of men). They concluded that in the majority of cases, optic neuritis in New England Caucasian women is a harbinger of MS. However, only 6 of the original 60 members of the cohort were "moderately or severely disabled" because of MS (Rizzo and Lessell 1988).

It is likely that modern diagnostic methods (especially MRI scan) increase the sensitivity of diagnosing MS, but the numerous past references in the literature to a more "benign" variant of MS that begins as optic neuritis remain valid.

The ophthalmologist who treats a patient with optic neuritis must decide whether or not to discuss with the patient the possibility that the condition may be the first sign of MS. Although there is merit in alerting a patient to possible future developments, there is *not* certainty that the later diagnosis of MS automatically implies a disabling neurological affliction.

Because of (1) the probability that not all persons with optic neuritis eventually have MS, (2) the inappropriate public belief that MS is invariably disabling, (3) the prior reports of the "more benign" course of MS when optic neuritis is the initial manifestation, and (4) the lack of treatment for asymptomatic MS, it seems reasonable to defer that discussion until the patient asks about it or has neurologic symptoms.

Whenever the discussion might occur, it is of great importance that it not be casual or rushed. It is vital that the ophthalmologist spend the time necessary to educate the patient regarding the points noted above, and attempt to provide some reassurance regarding the diagnosis.

Compressive Optic Neuropathy

Symptoms   Gradual relentless loss of vision (central and/or color, unilateral or bilateral). Headache is rare.

Etiology

1. Pituitary adenoma: most common intracranial cause. Most that lead to vision loss are endocrinologically "silent," and those that secrete hormones rarely affect vision.
2. Meningioma: Foster Kennedy syndrome (rarely seen today) describes a condition due to a subfrontal lobe meningioma that compresses one optic nerve until optic atrophy and blindness ensue, with papilledema of the fellow eye due to increased intracranial pressure.
3. Craniopharyngioma.
4. Aneurysm.
5. Optic nerve tumors
   a) Optic glioma—composed of benign astrocytes, can affect one nerve in the orbit, the chiasm, or both nerves intracranially. Sixty percent of patients will have von Recklinghausen's neurofibromatosis (NF) while only 10% to 15% of patients with NF (café-au-lait spots, Lisch nodules of the iris) have an optic glioma. Gliomas in NF are more often of a benign nature.
   b) Optic nerve sheath meningioma—composed of arachnoidal tissue that can grow around the optic nerve, invade it, or extend intracranially through the optic canal. Typically affects middle-aged women.
   c) Leukemia or other metastatic infiltrates—generally rare.

Signs

1. Variable vision impairment.
2. Visual field defects may take any form, but early chiasmal compression may cause predominant impairment of the temporal field in the less involved eye despite normal central acuity.
3. Afferent pupil defect with unilateral nerve involvement.
4. Exophthalmos with intraorbital nerve involvement.
5. Optic discs are often normal with CNS disease early, but atrophy generally occurs months to years after symptoms. If the optic nerve is involved in the orbit, ipsilateral disc swelling can occur with collateral shunt vessels from the retinal venous circulation to the choroid (especially in nerve sheath meningiomas). A central retinal vein occlusion can occur.

Workup

1. Visual field measurement: defects may take any form, but early chiasmal compression may cause predominant impairment of the temporal field in the less involved eye despite normal central acuity.
2. MRI scan with gadolinium enhancement for suspected meningioma or contrast enhanced CT. Note orbit MRI scanning requires suppression of fat signals. Gliomas typically show smooth fusiform enlargement. Meningiomas show a thickened irregular nerve with calcium and parallel linear densities (railroad tracks) representing thickened meninges.
3. Arteriography: for possible aneurysm.
4. Endocrine consultation: for pituitary lesions.
5. Neurosurgery consultation.

Differential Diagnosis See "Optic Neuritis," above.

Treatment

1. Depends on the specific etiology, but in general neurosurgery, as indicated by the diagnosis. Radiation therapy may have value for incomplete excision or recurrences, but not if a benign lesion is believed to have been completely excised.
2. Optic nerve glioma: observation is indicated except in cases with marked proptosis or clear progression of unilateral disease where transfrontal craniotomy or radiation therapy (for chiasmal involvement) may be indicated.
3. Optic nerve meningioma: surgical excision will sacrifice any preoperative vision, as a result of interference with arterial perfusion of the nerve. Since the course is indolent in older

patients and it is uncommon for tumors to extend intracranially, observation is indicated. However, craniotomy and orbitotomy is advisable in patients under age 40, in whom the tumor is more aggressive, to prevent involvement of the contralateral nerve and chiasm.

Prognosis   Vision can improve after surgical excision of lesions, but depends on the severity and duration of preoperative vision loss. Optic gliomas in adults may be extremely malignant, resulting in rapid death. Meningiomas are generally aggressive in younger patients and more benign in older patients.

Follow-up   Patients need visual fields monitored at 6 to 12 month intervals as well as repeated neuroimaging.

Ischemic Optic Neuropathy: Nonarteritic

Symptoms   Sudden vision loss often noted upon awakening from sleep in patients older than 45 years who often have hypertension or diabetes or both. Symptoms suggestive of temporal arteritis should be elicited.

Etiology

1. Arteriosclerosis: compromise of small arteries perfusing the optic nerve at the optic disc
2. Idiopathic

Signs

1. Central vision impairment can be mild to severe (normal in 30% of patients). Temporal arteritis becomes more likely the more severe the initial vision impairment.
2. Afferent pupil defect.
3. Swollen optic nerve acutely; atrophy develops later. Rarely retrobulbar ischemic optic neuropathy can occur with a normal nerve appearance, but one should look closely for a compressive lesion.

Workup

1. Visual fields show altitudinal or nerve fiber bundle defects, and the inferior nasal field is especially commonly affected.
2. Stat sedimentation rate to consider temporal arteritis; with temporal artery biopsy when indicated (see Temporal Arteritis section, below).

3. CT or MRI is generally not initially required, as intracranial compression of the optic nerve does not cause swelling of the optic disc.
4. General medical examination: there can be an increased incidence of stroke and heart disease in these patients.

Differential Diagnosis

1. Optic neuritis (see section on this topic, above).
2. Metastasis to the optic disc.

Treatment   None definitively proven.

1. Prednisone: short course, unlike temporal arteritis.
2. Optic nerve sheath decompression: advocated by Sergott in 1989 for patients whose vision worsens during the first weeks after the onset of symptoms.
3. Aspirin: low dose.
4. Smoking cessation.
5. Lower intraocular pressure when elevated.

Course   Vision tends to remain stable; a small minority of patients can experience progression of the impairment over several weeks. Twenty-five percent of persons will have involvement of the fellow eye in the subsequent months or years, though the involved eye rarely sustains a second episode.

Temporal Arteritis

Definition and Symptoms   Idiopathic (possibly autoimmune) granulomatous arteritis of older adults fragmenting the internal elastic lamina and causing thickening of the intima and media. Involvement of the ophthalmic and posterior ciliary arteries results in vision loss. The aorta and vertebral arteries are often involved; the cerebral arteries are rarely involved (Wilkinson and Russel 1972). Patients are generally older than 55 years and may complain of headache, malaise, myalgias, anorexia, weight loss, jaw claudication, amaurosis, sudden painless severe vision loss, or diplopia.

Signs

1. Prominent, tender superficial temporal arteries.
2. Afferent pupil defect.
3. Pale swollen disc with hemorrhage.

4. Central retinal artery occlusion (a central retinal vein occlusion virtually never occurs due to temporal arteritis).
5. CN VI palsy.

Workup

1. Sedimentation rate: note that Wintrobe ESR has 55 mm/h as its maximum value; Westergren can be greater than 100 mm/h.
2. Temporal artery biopsy (Hall and Hunder 1984): warranted if the clinical setting strongly suggests arteritis even if the ESR is normal, as rarely the biopsy will be positive with a normal ESR (Wong and Korn 1986). False-negative biopsy results are less likely to occur if a 3 to 5 cm segment is obtained and multiple histologic sections studied. In the event of a negative biopsy, study of the contralateral artery can be helpful in accounting for an abnormal ESR. If both sides are negative, the diagnosis should be reconsidered unless the clinical findings are incontrovertible. A biopsy of the contralateral side may be useful 2 to 3 years following an original biopsy if there is uncertainty about the activity of the disease.

Differential Diagnosis

1. Nonartertic ischemic optic neuropathy secondary to arteriosclerosis.
2. Elevated ESR with malaise: multiple causes; consult with internist.
3. See "Optic Neuritis," above.

Treatment

1. Corticosteroids: oral prednisone (80–100 mg/d) has been a standard treatment when an eye has had marked vision loss. Recently, megadose intravenous methylprednisone (1–2 gr q.d. for 3–4 d), followed by oral prednisone, has been advocated (Rosenfeld et al. 1986). Do not wait for the biopsy results before beginning treatment if clinical suspicion is high. The dose can generally be reduced to 60 mg of prednisone daily 1 month later. There is no consensus regarding the best alternative immuno-suppressive agent in patients intolerant of corticosteroids.
2. For cases of second eye involvement, consider anticoagulation, ocular hypertensive agents, and inhalation of a mixture of oxygen and carbon dioxide (carbogen).

Course It is uncommon for the involved eye to regain vision once it has been lost. Systemic symptoms typically improve promptly once therapy is begun.

Follow-up Management is best directed by a rheumatologist or internist familiar with this disease with observation of the ESR and systemic symptoms. Prednisone is reduced if possible by 5 to 10 mg decrements at monthly intervals. Ophthalmic collaboration is helpful. The disease usually subsides in 1 to 3 years.

Selected Readings

Amaurosis Fugax

Amaurosis Fugax Study Group. Current management of amaurosis fugax. Stroke 1990;21:201–209. A general overview of the subject.
Trobe JD. Carotid endarterectomy—who needs it? Ophthalmology 1987;94:725–730. Questions the value of carotid surgery.
Poole CJM, Ross Russell RW. Mortality and stroke after amaurosis fugax. J Neurol Neurosurg Psychiatry 1985;48:902–905. A 6 + year follow-up of patients with AF.

Diplopia

Appen RE, Wendelborn D, Nolten WE. Diplopia in autoimmune thyroid disease. Arch Intern Med 1982;142:898–901. Reviews 12 patients with diplopia due to dysthyroidism.

Headache

Burde RM, Savino PG, Trobe JD. Clinical decisions in neuro-ophthalmology. St. Louis: CV Mosby, 1985, pp. 303–26.

Visual Fields

Riise D. The nasal fundus ectasia. Acta Ophthalmol 1975;Suppl 126:11–208. A lengthy review with many examples.
Nepple EW, Appen RE, Sackett, JF. Bilateral homonymous hemianopia. Am J Ophthalmol 1978;86:536–43. A review of 15 patients.

Cranial Nerve Palsies

Rush JA, Younge BR. Paralysis of cranial nerves III, IV, and VI. Arch Ophthalmol 1981;99:76–79. A review of 1000 cases seen at Mayo Clinic.
Trobe JD. Third nerve palsy and the pupil. Arch Ophthalmol 1988;106:601–2. Editorial discussion of the subject.

Nystagmus

Weiss AH, Biersdorf WR. Visual sensory disorders in congenital nystagmus. Ophthalmology 1989;96:517–23. A review of 81 patients.
Lavery MA, O'Neill JR, Chu FC, Martyn LJ. Acquired nystagmus in

childhood—a presenting sign of intracranial tumor. Ophthalmology
1984;91:425–35. A review of 10 patients.

Yee RD. Downbeat nystagmus characteristics and localization of lesions.
Trans Am Ophthalmol Soc 1989;87:984–1032. An extensive review of the
subject and of 91 cases.

Weinstein JM, France TD, France LW. Medically treatable forms of
nystagmus. Am Orthoptic J 1988;38:168–76. A discussion of several
entities.

Pupil Anomalies

Frank JW, Kushner BJ, France TD. Paradoxic pupillary phenomena: a review
of patients with pupillary constriction to darkness. Arch Ophthalmol
1988;106:1564–66. Notes lack of specificity of the sign.

Maloney WF, Young BR, Moyer NJ. Evaluation of the causes and accuracy
of the pharmacologic localization in Horner's syndrome. Am J
Ophthalmol 1980;90:394–402. A review of 450 cases and summary of the
subject.

Thompson HS. Adie's syndrome: some new observations. Trans Am
Ophthalmol Soc 1977;75:587–622. A review of the subject.

Thompson HS, Pilley SFT. Unequal pupils. A flow chart for sorting out the
anisocorias. Surv Ophthalmol 1976;21:45–48. A review of the subject.

Thompson HS, Corbet JJ. Swinging flashlight test. Neurology 1989;39:154–56.
A description of the test.

Thompson HS, Newsome DA, Loewenfeld IE. The fixed dilated pupil:
sudden iridoplegia or mydriatic drops? A simple diagnostic test. Arch
Ophthalmol 1971;86:21–27. A simplified schema for evaluation.

Papilledema

Green GJ, Lessell S, Lowenstein JI. Ischemic optic neuropathy in chronic
papilledema. Arch Ophthalmol 1980;98:502–4. A case report.

Appen RE, Chandra SR, Klein R, Myers FL. Diabetic papillopathy. Am J
Ophthalmol 1980;90:203–9. A description of two patients.

Appen RE, De Vencia G, Ferwerda J. Optic disc vasculitis. Am J Ophthalmol
1980;90:352–59. A clinicopathologic case report.

Corbet JJ, Thompson HS. The rational management of idiopathic intracranial
hypertension. Arch Neurol 1989;46:1049–51. An overview.

Keltner J. Optic nerve sheath decompression: how does it work? Has its time
come? Arch Ophthalmol 1988;106:1378–83. An editorial comment on
three reports of the operation in the same journal.

Corbett JJ, Savino PJ, Thompson HS, et al. Visual loss in pseudotumor
cerebri. Arch Neurol 1982;39:461–74. A follow-up study of 57 patients.

Carotid-Cavernous Fistula

Keltner JL, et al. Dural and carotid cavernous sinus fistulas. Ophthalmology
1987;94:1585–1600. A general review of the subject.

Feifarek MJ, et al. Carotid-cavernous fistulae and their current therapy. Wis Med J 1982;81:17–20. A case report and review of the subject.

Myasthenia Gravis

Miller NR. Walsh and Hoyt's clinical neuro-ophthalmology. Baltimore: Williams and Wilkins, 1985, vol. II, pp. 840–66.

Optic Neuritis

Cohen MM, Lessell S, Wolf PA. A prospective study of the risk of developing multiple sclerosis in uncomplicated multiple sclerosis. Neurology 1979;29:208–13. A description of the 5 + year follow-up of 60 patients.

Newman NJ, Wallace DC. Mitochondria and Leber's hereditary optic neuropathy. Am J Ophthalmol 1990;109:726–30.

Dutton JJ, Burde RM, Klingele TG. Autoimmune retrobulbar optic neuritis. Am J Ophthalmol 1982;94:11–17.

Beck RW. The optic neuritis treatment trial. Arch Ophthalmol 1988; 106:1051–53.

Beck RW, Cleary PA, Anderson MM Jr, et al. A randomized controlled trial of corticosteroids in the treatment of acute optic neuritis. N Engl J Med 1992;326:581–8.

Rizzo JF, Lessell S. Risk of developing multiple sclerosis after uncomplicated optic neuritis—a long-term prospective study. Neurology 1988;38:185–90.

Compressive Optic Neuropathy

Lessell S. Current concepts in ophthalmology—optic neuropathies. N Engl J Med 1978;299:533–36. A review of the most common optic nerve syndromes.

Knight CL, Hoyt WF, Wilson CB. Syndrome of incipient prechiasmal optic nerve compression. Arch Ophthalmol 1972;87:1–11. Several case reports.

Stern J, Jakobiec FA, Housepian EM. The architecture of optic nerve gliomas with and without neurofibromatosis. Arch Ophthalmol 1980;98:505–11. A comparison of the histopathology in the two groups.

Jakobiec FA, et al. Combined clinical and computed tomographic diagnosis of orbital glioma and meningioma. Ophthalmology 1984;91:137–55. A review of radiologic differences.

Hoyt WF, Baghdassarian SA. Optic glioma of childhood. Natural history and rationale for conservative management. Br J Ophthalmol 1969;53:793–98. A review of the course of 36 patients.

Hoyt WF, et al. Malignant optic glioma of adulthood. Brain 1973;96:121–32. A description of 15 patients.

Wright JE, et al. Primary optic nerve sheath meningiomas. Br J Ophthalmol 1987;73:960–66. A review of 50 patients and a guide for management.

Sibony PA, et al. Optic nerve sheath meningiomas: clinical manifestations. Ophthalmology 1984;91:1313–26. A review of 22 patients.

Hollenhorst RW Jr, Hollenhorst RW Sr, MacCarty CS. Visual prognosis of optic nerve sheath meningiomas producing shunt vessels on the optic disc. Mayo Clinic Proc 1978;53:84–92. Review of nine patients.

Ischemic Optic Neuropathy: Nonarteritic

Boghen DR, Glaser JS. Ischemic optic neuropathy: the clinical profile and natural history. Brain 1975;98:689–708. A review of 50 patients.

Guyer DR, Miller NR, Aver CL, Fine SL. The risk of cerebrovascular and cardiovascular disease in patients with anterior ischemic optic neuropathy. Arch Ophthalmol 1985;103:1136–42. A follow-up of 217 patients.

Borchert M, Lessell S. Progressive and recurrent nonarteritic anterior ischemic optic neuropathy. Am J Ophthalmol 1988;106:443–49. A description of 10 patients.

Hayreh SS. Anterior ischemic optic neuropathy. Arch Neurol 1981;38:675–78. A summary of the subject.

Sergott RC, Cohen MS, Bosley TM, Savino PJ. Optic nerve decompression may improve the progressive form of nonarteritic ischemic optic neuropathy. Arch Ophthalmol 1989;107:1743–54. A retrospective review of surgery on 17 patients with ION.

Temporal Arteritis

Wilkinson IMS, Russel RWR. Arteries of the head and neck in giant cell arteritis. Arch Neurol 1972;27:378–91. Report 4 cases plus 8 from literature who had autopsies.

Fauchald P, Rygvold O, Øystese B. Temporal arteritis and polymyalgia rheumatica. Ann Intern Med 1972;77:845–52. Compares 62 cases of TA and 32 of PMR.

Hall S, Hunder GG. Is temporal artery biopsy prudent? Mayo Clin Proc 1984;59:793–96. Concludes that biopsy of artery is warranted.

Wong RL, Korn JH. Temporal arteritis without an elevated erythrocyte sedimentation rate. Am J Med 1986;80:959–64. A case report and literature review.

Rosenfeld SI, Kosmorsky GS, Klingele TG, Burde RM, Cohn EM. Treatment of temporal arteritis with ocular involvement. Am J Med 1986;80:143–45. Case report and discussion of megadose intravenous methylprednisolone.

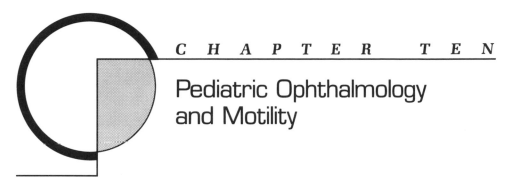

Pediatric Ophthalmology and Motility

Thomas D. France, M.D.

A/V Syndromes

Definition Horizontal incomitance in vertical gaze. An A pattern is an increasing esodeviation (eso) or decreasing exodeviation (exo) in up-gaze or a decreasing eso or increasing exo in downgaze, with the total difference being greater than 10^Δ from upgaze to downgaze. A V pattern is an increasing eso or decreasing exo in downgaze or a decreasing eso or increasing exo in upgaze, with the total difference being greater than 15^Δ from upgaze to downgaze. Variations would be an X pattern, a Y pattern, a Λ pattern or a diamond pattern.

Prevalence Twenty-five percent of all horizontal strabismus. Of the major A/V patterns:

> 41% are V esotropia,
> 25% are A esotropia,
> 23% are V exotropia, and
> 11% are A exotropia.

Examination

1. Measurement of horizontal deviation to include distance examination with head tilted up or down 25°. If near measurements are done, use +3.00 spheres to reduce accommodation.
2. Careful evaluation of versions.
3. An abnormal head position (chin elevation or depression) is a clue to the presence of an A/V pattern with binocularity: chin elevation in A eso or V exo or chin depression in V eso or A exodeviation.

Etiology Most commonly associated with overacting oblique muscles: inferior obliques (IO) in V patterns, superior obliques (SO) in A patterns. Occasionally associated with vertical rectus paresis or craniofacial abnormalities.

Differential Diagnosis Must ensure that accommodation is controlled during measurements. An accommodative esotropia with high AC/A ratio can mimic a V pattern esotropia and a divergence excess exotropia can mimic a V exotropia if allowed to accommodate during the measurements of the horizontal deviation.

Treatment Surgery is directed toward reducing the vertically acting horizontal incomitance without disrupting fusion in primary or downgaze.

In patients with oblique-muscle overaction (OA) i.e., an OA IO with a V pattern or OA SO with an A pattern, weaken the oblique at the same time as surgically correcting the horizontal deviation. Do *not* weaken the oblique muscles if the antagonist oblique is also overacting!

Patients with no oblique dysfunction can be improved by displacing the horizontal rectus muscles either upward or downward when correcting the horizontal deviation. The mnemonic MALE helps recall the direction the horizontal rectus muscles should be moved: "move the medials (M) toward the apex (A) and the laterals (L) toward the ends (E)." This means move the medial rectus muscles *downward* in V patterns or *upward* in A patterns, usually one–half to one full tendon width. The lateral rectus muscles are moved *upward* in V patterns or *downward* in A patterns. If performing a recess-resect procedure, the muscles can be moved in opposite directions without causing a torsional problem.

AC/A Ratio

Definition Refers to the amount of convergence resulting after a given level of accommodation. Purpose is to keep eyes aligned while focusing on objects close at hand. Normal AC/A ratio of 3.5 to 5 prism diopters/diopter (D) indicates that the eyes will converge $10.5^\triangle$ to $15^\triangle$ when focused on an object at $\frac{1}{3}$ meter (accommodating 3 D). AC/A ratios may be measured in two ways.

1. The most common way to determine the AC/A ratio is the *hetero-phoria* method in which measurements of horizontal deviations are made at a distance (6 m) and near ($\frac{1}{3}$ m), being careful to control accommodation at each distance by having the patient read a small line of letters with full refractive correction in place.

$$AC/A = PD + \left(\frac{Near\ deviation\ -\ Distance\ deviation}{3} \right)$$

Pupillary distance (PD) must be included in the formula.

2. The second method to determine the AC/A ratio is the *gradient* method. By this method the fixation distance is kept constant, at either $\frac{1}{3}$ or 6 m, and accommodation is changed by the addition of a minus or plus lens. If measured at $\frac{1}{3}$ m, a +3.00 D lens is used and it is anticipated that accommodation is relaxed by 3 D. The horizontal deviation is measured again with and without the lens in place.

$$AC/A = \left(\frac{Deviation\ with\ lens\ -\ Deviation\ without\ lens}{Dioptric\ power\ of\ lens} \right)$$

Normal AC/A ratios are slightly less by the gradient method than by the heterophoria method. The AC/A ratio is abnormal if greater than 10/1.

Miotics (echothiophate, diisopropylfluorophosphate) can be used to decrease the AC/A ratio. Cycloplegics (homatropine, tropicamide) have been said to increase the AC/A ratio.

The AC/A ratio must be considered when correcting accommodative esotropia or intermittent exotropia with glasses or surgery.

Amblyopia

Definition   A decrease in the best corrected vision in one or both eyes not due to an organic problem, usually considered to be a difference of two lines on the Snellen chart (e.g., 20/20 OD, 20/40 OS). Vision is worst when tested linearly, best when tested on single optotypes, owing to the "crowding" phenomenon.

Etiology

1. Strabismus, especially convergent
2. Anisometropia, especially hyperopic
3. Ametropia, high hyperopia or myopia
4. Deprivation of visual image during infancy, usually cataracts

Workup   Always test vision in the amblyopic eye first and on more than one occasion. Recheck refractive error with cycloplegic refraction using atropine if necessary. Careful examination to rule out any significant organic causes of low vision, especially tumors, and to detect conditions that are not treatable such as optic atrophy and optic nerve hypoplasia to avoid unnecessary occlusion.

Differential Diagnosis   Retinal detachment, glaucoma, and any other neurologic signs of central nervous system disease that might lead to decreased vision.

Treatment

1. In strabismic amblyopia, occlusion of the preferred eye until vision is equalized. To avoid inducing occlusion amblyopia, patch full-time for no longer than 1 week for each year of age (e.g., patch a 2–year-old full-time for 2 wks) and then reevaluate the vision. When equal vision is attained, surgery to align the eyes is indicated.
2. In anisometropic amblyopia, full-time wear of the refractive correction for at least 1 month to allow spontaneous improvement of vision, then occlusion as above with the correction in place.
3. In ametropic amblyopia, full-time wear of refraction. In high hyperopia, should consider reducing full correction by +1.50 initially to ensure the child will wear the glasses.
4. Deprivation amblyopia, once established, is not treatable at present. Prevention includes early correction of the obstruction to the visual image. In the case of monocular congenital cataracts, this means surgery by age 3 months; in bilateral cases, surgery may still be of benefit as late as 6 months. Beyond these ages, visual improvement is unlikely and the risks of surgery are not warranted.

Full-time occlusion should be continued until there has been no further improvement of vision for 3 months. Vision may again fall when occlusion is stopped, requiring part-time occlusion. This may have to be continued until the age of 8 or 9 years.

Part-time occlusion may be attained using patches, fogging of the refractive error with plus lenses, or tape applied to the glasses. These methods are used to *maintain* vision rather than to improve vision.

Abnormal Retinal Correspondence (ARC)

Definition   A *binocular* condition in which there appears to be a cortical realignment of localizing values of retinal images. It is associated with suppression and reduces diplopia in cases of long-standing childhood strabismus. It is most commonly seen in large-angle exotropias or in small-angle esotropias.

1. Harmonious ARC occurs when the objective angle of deviation equals the subjective angle of deviation on the synoptophore.
2. Nonharmonious ARC is present when the objective angle of deviation does not equal the subjective angle.

Examination   Testing on the synoptophore produces the most quantitative results. Testing with a red lens or with correcting prisms may give a qualitative response. Persistent diplopia with prism correction in a patient with long-standing strabismus may be a contraindication for surgical repair.

Brown's Syndrome (Superior Oblique Tendon Sheath Syndrome)

Definition   Limitation of elevation of the eye in adduction caused by a tightness of the superior oblique tendon.

Etiology

1. Congenital, most common cause
2. Rheumatoid arthritis (nodules) in adults
3. Trauma in the area of the superior oblique trochlea

Examination

1. Limitation of elevation of the eye in adduction with normal or nearly normal elevation in abduction.
2. Normal action of the ipsilateral superior oblique muscle, overaction of the contralateral superior rectus muscle.
3. May have an abnormal head position to attain binocularity: chin elevation with a head turn toward the affected eye and, in some cases, a head tilt away from the affected eye.
4. A V pattern (differentiates Brown's syndrome from paresis of the inferior oblique).
5. Widening of the palpebral fissure on adduction.
6. Positive forced duction test.
7. There may be a "clicking" sound associated with rheumatoid nodules and a temporary ability to elevate the eye in adduction.

Differential Diagnosis

1. Inferior oblique palsy (associated with a normal forced duction test and an A pattern)

2. Double elevator palsy
3. Orbital blow-out fracture
4. Thyroid ophthalmopathy

Treatment   Should be reserved for those patients with significant head positions, vertical deviations in the primary position, or diplopia.

1. Surgery to lengthen the superior oblique tendon via tenotomy or tenectomy will correct the condition. In about 50% of cases, a secondary overaction of the inferior oblique will develop, requiring further surgery. Parks has advocated recessing the inferior oblique muscle at the same sitting as the tenotomy of the superior oblique to avoid the second operation.
2. Injection of steroid into the area of the trochlea has been reported to be beneficial in adults with acquired Brown's syndrome associated with rheumatoid nodules.

Congenital Cataract

Definition   Significant lens opacity in one or both eyes present in the neonatal period, usually confined to those patients in whom vision is or will be impaired if the cataract is allowed to remain during the time of visual development.

Examination

1. Opacity noted on examination of the red reflex using the direct ophthalmoscope or the retinoscope.
2. May be associated with mild microphthalmos in the case of unilateral cataract secondary to persistent hyperplastic primary vitreous (PHPV).
3. If unable to see the posterior pole, ultrasound and electroretinography (ERG) or visual evoked response (VER) testing should be done to rule out significant retinal or optic nerve problems that would prevent visual function.
4. May be associated with other anterior segment anomalies: corneal opacities (Peter's anomaly), iris anomalies (Rieger's syndrome), glaucoma (Lowe's syndrome).
5. If bilateral, metabolic disease including galactosemia and galactokinase deficiency should be looked for on physical examination.

Workup

1. Careful family history to determine hereditary etiology.
2. If bilateral cataracts are present, then a systemic cause is more likely. Laboratory evaluation includes:

    a) blood sugar, calcium, phosphate, and galactokinase;
    b) a TORCH screen;
    c) urine amino acids, ketones, reducing substances (galactose); and
    d) chromosomal analysis if two or more organ systems are involved.
  3. Pediatric consultation.

Associated Conditions

1. PHPV with retinal involvement
2. Congenital glaucoma
3. Maternal infection
4. Trauma

Treatment

1. Surgical removal of lens if seen before onset of deprivation amblyopia.
2. Correction of refractive error by contact lens or glasses.
3. Amblyopia treatment if unilateral or if one eye preferred in bilateral case.

Follow-up

1. Frequent (monthly) evaluation of vision, refractive error, and fundus examination during first year of life.
2. Continued evaluation at 3–month intervals after first year until able to evaluate vision by Snellen chart.
3. Glaucoma evaluation (under anesthesia if necessary) if signs of rapidly decreasing hyperopia or increasing myopia, increasing corneal diameter, optic nerve cup changes, or photophobia.
4. Refractive correction with glasses and bifocals over contact lenses by school age.
5. Surgical correction of significant strabismus.

Convergence Insufficiency (CI)

Definition   An exodeviation greater near than at a distance.

Etiology   Can include any of the following:

1. Large pupillary distance (PD)
2. Paresis of medial rectus (e.g., weakness secondary to medial rectus recessions)
3. Presbyopia corrected for first time
4. Convergence paralysis due to trauma or tumor

5. Accommodation/convergence dyssynergy where convergence is less than required (low AC/A ratio)

Symptoms

1. Visual fatigue with near work
2. Headaches
3. Blurred vision with near work
4. Diplopia
5. Confusion following lines or letters

Examination   Measure the following:

1. Near point of convergence (NPC) using an accommodative target and red filter.
2. Near point of accommodation (NPA), one eye at a time on an accommodative target, wearing correction.
3. Vergences (measure divergence amplitudes at distance and near first, before convergence and vertical amplitudes): use an accommodative target and note blur point, point of diplopia (break), and recovery (can use rotary prism, prism bar, or single prisms). Normal values are as follows (divergence amplitudes should be about one–third of convergence amplitudes):

	Convergence (blur/break)	Divergence	Vertical
At 6 m	$25/20^\Delta$	$8/7^\Delta$	2.5^Δ
At 33 m	$40/35^\Delta$	$15/10^\Delta$	2.6^Δ

Clinically, convergence amplitudes at distance = $25/20^\Delta$ (recovery should be within 5^Δ); near = $35/40/30^\Delta$ (blur/break/recovery).

Differential Diagnosis

1. Convergence paralysis: usually history of trauma or illness. Rapid onset. Diplopia worsens within 5 to 6 feet. NPA is normal. Normal versions. Pupils are normal.
2. Accommodative insufficiency: may be combined with true CI or occur as an isolated condition. Not treatable with exercises. Remote NPA for age. Symptoms are better with +3.00 lenses and worse with −3.00 lenses. Treatment is reading glasses.
3. Combined accommodative and convergence insufficiency: the symptoms include blurred vision for near. Near point of convergence and NPA are poor. Convergence amplitudes are low. Minus lenses do not act beneficially. Treatment consists of plus lenses, convergence exercises, or base-in prisms.
4. Accommodative effort syndrome: symptoms are of asthenopia

and diplopia. Findings show an esophoria at near, normal NPA, normal NPC, and benefit from +3.00 lenses. Divergence amplitudes are poor. Treatment includes plus lenses, exercises, and occasionally miotics.

5. Accommodative spasm: this tends to be a functional problem. Symptoms are blurred distance vision and myopia on manifest refraction. A cycloplegic examination must be done as this shows the true refractive error. The pupils tend to be miotic. No benefit from +3.00 or −3.00 lenses.

Treatment

1. Eliminate suppression using physiologic diplopia exercises, red filters, synoptophore in the office, stereograms.
2. Improve fusional amplitudes with prisms, the synoptophore, the Tibbs binocular trainer for near problems, or the Orthofusor.
3. Improve NPC by jump convergence, dot card, push-up exercises, red filter and light.
4. Improve accommodation/convergence synergy using stereograms, the diploscope, and framing.
5. In cases of true convergence insufficiency orthoptics is 90% effective within 8 weeks if treatment is carried out as directed.

Convergence Spasm

Definition   Increased tone of accommodation or convergence or both.

Etiology   Almost exclusively secondary to hysteria, but has been reported following trauma.

Examination

1. Decreased distance vision; myopia on manifest refraction.
2. Miosis.
3. Improved distance vision and no myopia on cycloplegic refraction.
4. No other neurologic signs.

Differential Diagnosis

1. Parinaud's syndrome (midbrain syndrome)
2. Trauma
3. Malingering

Treatment   Cycloplegics (atropine, homatropine), bifocals.

Duane's Syndrome (Stilling-Turk-Duane Syndrome)

Definition   Oculomotor imbalance due to abnormal innervation of one or more of the ocular muscles, usually associated with cocontraction and retraction of the globe.

Examination

1. Three types of Duane's syndrome are recognized. See Table 10.1.
2. Definite preference to affect the left eye (65%).
3. Bilaterality uncommon—perhaps 10% to 15%.
4. Girls more common than boys (3:2).
5. Amblyopia in 10% to 30% (anisometropia in two–thirds).
6. Abnormal head position: usually associated with an esotropia less than 30^Δ. Therefore, head position (to fuse) is toward the affected eye (L head turn with OS affected). In type II can see an exotropia—head turn is away from the affected eye. (R head turn with OS affected.)
7. Duane's syndrome has been found to be associated with skeletal and auditory abnormalities.

Etiology   At first thought to be due to fibrosis of the lateral rectus (LR) muscle. Later, Blodi showed that on abduction there was no recruitment of action potentials in the LR while on adduction there was an

TABLE 10.1

Duane's syndrome categories	
Type I	Poor abduction.
	Slight restriction of adduction.
	Retraction of the eye on attempted adduction frequently with an upshoot or downshoot.
	Narrowing of the palpebral fissure due to the cocontraction and retraction.
	Deficiency of convergence of the affected eye(s).
Type II	Good abduction.
	Poor adduction.
	Slight retraction with adduction.
Type III	Poor abduction.
	Poor adduction.
	Marked retraction.
	Poor convergence.

increase in action potentials in both the medial rectus (MR) and the LR muscles. He felt this was due to a supranuclear abnormality in the central nervous system. Hotchkiss and associates have shown that a patient with bilateral Duane's syndrome had a total absence of the sixth cranial nerves (CN VI), both peripheral and nuclear, with innervation of the LR muscles by CN III.

Workup

1. Traction tests.
2. Saccadic velocities.
3. Binocular (diplopia) fields.
4. In a young child, newly diagnosed, a hearing test is indicated to rule out significant hearing loss.

Differential Diagnosis

1. CN VI nerve palsy: a very common mistake
2. Myasthenia gravis
3. Thyroid ophthalmopathy
4. Congenital esotropia

Treatment   Observation if not cosmetically significant; otherwise, surgery to improve the head position or significant strabismus in the primary position. One cannot improve the innervational pattern with surgery. Recession of a contracted MR muscle is the most common approach. Recession of both MR and LR may be indicated to relieve significant retraction. Never resect the LR more than 4 mm if there is moderate to marked cocontraction in adduction. In exotropic Duane's syndrome, recess the LR, and perhaps resect the MR.

Dissociated Vertical Deviations (DVD)

Definition   Vertical deviation, either manifest or latent, without an associated hypotropic movement of the contralateral eye on alternate cover. Other names: alternating sursumduction, alternate hyperphoria, alternate hypertropia, occlusion hypertropia, double dissociated hypertropia, and double hypertropia. The main distinction is a latent versus manifest appearance of a dissociated deviation.

Examination

1. The eye extorts on elevation and intorts on depression.
2. The downward movement is often a slow, floating movement compared to the smooth redress of a hyperdeviation (true hyper).

3. Often associated with latent nystagmus.
4. There may be a small vertical deviation manifest on the cover-uncover test and an asymmetric vertical response to the alternate cover test. One eye may deviate upward more, while the contralateral eye manifests more torsion.
5. Bielschowsky phenomenon: the occluded eye will show an upward deviation due to a dissociated vertical divergence and will then make a gradual downward movement if a neutral density filter wedge is placed before the fixing eye and the image gradually darkened (von Noorden 1990).
6. DVD occurs in 70% to 90% of congenital esotropia. It may also occur in congenital exotropia and in patients with orthophoria, but not as frequently. It is often noted after surgical correction and in nonoperated patients after age 2 years. It is uncommon after age 8 years.

Workup

1. Measurement of angle with prisms, neutralizing the downward, refixating movement of the elevated eye.
2. Look for Bielschowsky phenomenon.
3. Sensory testing to determine binocular function.

Differential Diagnosis

1. Inferior oblique overaction
2. Skew deviation

Treatment   Usually for cosmetic improvement. Large recession of the superior rectus muscle, anteriorization of the inferior oblique muscle, and resection of the inferior rectus muscle have all been suggested. Surgery on one eye often leads to significant DVD in the other eye.

Prognosis   Surgical results not uniformly successful. DVDs may be less apparent as the child grows. Usually associated with poor binocular function.

Esodeviations

Definition   A convergent strabismus that may be

1. manifest, an esotropia (ET),
2. intermittent, E(T), or
3. latent, an esophoria (E).

Classification

Accommodative (50% of total esodeviations)

1. Refractive $(\frac{1}{3})$.
2. High AC/A $(\frac{1}{3})$.
3. Combined $(\frac{1}{3})$.

Nonaccommodative

1. Infantile esotropia.
2. Nystagmus compensation esotropia (see "Nystagmus Compensation" Syndrome section, below).
3. Acquired esotropia (i.e., trauma).
4. Monofixation syndrome (see section on this topic, below).
5. Neurologic (i.e., CN VI palsy).

Accommodative Esotropia

Definition   A convergent strabismus that is due to secondary convergence associated with accommodation. May be one of two basic types:

1. Refractive: due to high ($\geq$ +4.00) hypermetropia.
2. High AC/A: due to an overconvergence for a given degree of accommodation (see AC/A Ratio section, above).

Etiology   The near reflex includes a convergent response to accommodation to normally keep the eyes aligned as objects are brought closer to the face. In patients with significant hypermetropia the accommodation needed to view near objects is so great as to increase the convergence beyond that necessary. This results in an esotropia with diplopia and secondary suppression. The onset may be related to an acute febrile illness that lessens the ability of the patient to both accommodate and keep the eyes aligned.

Children with high AC/A ratios develop esotropias with otherwise normal refractive errors under similar circumstances.

Examination

1. Measurement of convergent deviations at distance and near, with and without refractive correction.
2. Use a +3.00 lens near to determine AC/A ratio.
3. Visual acuity testing reveals amblyopia due to early suppression. Loss of sensory fusion occurs with suppression as well.
4. Refraction using cyclopentalate or atropine to fully determine hyperopic refractive error.

Differential Diagnosis

1. Esotropia with nystagmus compensation
2. Infantile esotropia, nonaccommodative acquired esotropia

Treatment

1. *Full* correction of any hypermetropic error in infants and young children. Use of flat-top bifocal lenses (+3.00 in infants, +2.50 in older children) in cases with high AC/A ratio type.
2. Anticholinesterase drops may be used as a diagnostic aid in accommodative esotropia but are not widely used as long-term therapy owing to their frequent side effects.
3. The identification and treatment of any amblyopia present.
4. Surgical correction of the *residual* esotropia after full refractive correction.

Follow-up   Careful following of visual acuity (amblyopia), sensory testing (fusion, stereopsis), and refractive error, as well as the degree of strabismus present to age 12 to 15 years. Frequent changes of glasses are necessary as the refractive error changes with age. Surgical intervention for the *nonaccommodative* convergent strabismus is common.

Infantile Esotropia

Definition   A convergent strabismus that has been present since soon after birth and has been documented by an ophthalmologist before 6 months of age.

Signs

Early

1. Equal vision
2. Crossed fixation
3. Large-angle strabismus
4. Normal refraction
5. Poor lateral rectus function

Later

6. Dissociated hypertropias (72%)
7. Overaction of inferior obliques (64%)
8. Latent nystagmus (16%)

9. Accommodative component (50%)
10. Amblyopia (late)

Examination and Workup

1. Fixation pattern: look for amblyopia.
2. Motor examination.
3. Measure angle of deviation:
   a) Hirschberg, Krimsky light reflexes
   b) Simultaneous prism and cover test
   c) Alternate cover test
   d) Distance-versus-near deviation and with +3.00 spheres
4. Ductions and versions: look for
   a) CN VI paresis and
   b) A or V pattern.
5. Sensory testing (when possible)
   a) Worth four dot test
   b) Stereo acuity testing
   c) Bagolini, 4$^\Delta$ test, Maddox rod, etc.
6. Cycloplegic refraction: look for hyperopia using:
   a) Cyclogyl 1%, 2%, or
   b) Atropine 1% (b.i.d. for 3 d).
7. Ophthalmoscopic examination: look for
   a) tumor (rule out retinoblastoma) and
   b) inflammation (toxoplasmosis, *Toxocara*, Coats' disease).
8. Neurologic evaluation: look for cerebral palsy.

Differential Diagnosis

1. Pseudostrabismus
2. Accommodative esotropia
3. Late onset acquired esotropia
4. Nystagmus compensation syndrome

Treatment

1. Occlusion
   a. Monocular for amblyopia.
   b. Alternate to improve lateral rectus function.
2. Refractive error
   a. Glasses if greater than +2.00.
   b. Miotic therapy if less than 1 year old.
3. *Early* surgery (before age 2 yrs):
   a. To produce peripheral fusion.
   b. To provide long-term stability.

Exodeviations

Definition   A divergent strabismus that may be defined on the basis of fusion as follows:

1. Manifest: an exotropia, XT
2. Intermittent: X(T)
3. Latent: an exophoria, X

Exodeviations may also be defined on the basis of measurements:

1. Basic exotropia: the measurement at 6 m equals that at $\frac{1}{3}$ m (XT = XT').
2. Divergence excess exotropia: the measurement at 6 m is greater than at $\frac{1}{3}$ m (XT > XT').
3. Simulated divergence excess exotropia: XT > XT', but XT = XT' with +3.00 lenses to reduce accommodation or following occlusion for 1 hour.
4. Convergence insufficiency exotropia: the measurement near is greater than at 6 m (XT < XT').

Exotropias may also be identified as

1. alternating or monocular (R or L XT),
2. consecutive, when a previously *esotropic* patient becomes XT without surgery, and
3. secondary (following an operation for ET).

Etiology

1. Innervational (imbalance of tonic convergence-divergence), either primary (good vision OU) or secondary (unilateral anomaly impairing visual function).
2. Anatomic, due to congenital skeletal abnormality (Crouzon's disease, etc.), or secondary to hypertrophy of the lateral rectus or an anomalous insertion of muscles.

Examination

1. Exophoria (X) *usually* asymptomatic, but patients may complain of asthenopia, momentary diplopia, or blurred vision.
2. Intermittent exotropia, or X(T), usually appears after 6 months of age, is worse at distance (divergence excess or simulated divergence excess), and is worse when aggravated by fatigue, illness, upon first awakening, or when visually inattentive. Patients are annoyed by bright illumination, with monocular eye

closure common. It may deteriorate to constant XT and is frequently hereditary. The principal difference between X and X(T) is the presence of suppression and the larger angle seen in X(T).

3. Exotropia (XT) is usually of the acquired type, with congenital exotropia being rare. Acquired XTs may be deteriorated intermittent exotropias or are secondary to an anomaly impairing vision in one eye.

Workup

1. Measurements of deviation at distance (both 6 and 60 m), and near, with and without +3.00 lenses, using an accommodative target. Look for lateral gaze incomitance and A or V patterns. Occlusion of one eye for 1 hour or longer to detect simulated divergence excess.
2. Sensory testing should include the following:
   a. A red lens test to determine suppression
   b. Worth four dot test to find suppression and ARC
   c. Stereo acuity testing
   d. Vergence amplitudes in cases of convergence insufficiency

Treatment

1. Exophoria: none unless symptoms are present. Orthoptic therapy in the office or at home may benefit. Can undercorrect hyperopia, overcorrect myopia. Base-in prisms are not recommended.

2. Intermittent exotropia: the objective is to prevent suppression, which reduces the prognosis for a successful result. Orthoptics can be used preoperatively for antisuppression and postoperatively to improve fusional vergence amplitudes. Surgery is designed to correct the distance measurement (basic deviation), usually disregarding the near measurement, which is dependent on the AC/A ratio. Undercorrect if less XT on side gaze. Bilateral recession of the LR muscle is usually the primary procedure, with the best results if there is initially a slight 10$^\Delta$) overcorrection. Undercorrections are reoperated at 6 weeks and overcorrections at 6 months.

3. Exotropia: must treat amblyopia first if present and not organic. A functional result is the goal if vision is good in each eye. Surgery at any age after 6 months. If amblyopia is organic and XT is a cosmetic problem, surgery can be done at 3 to 4 years of age. Usually do a recession-resection of the amblyopic eye and try to overcorrect about 10$^\Delta$ to 15$^\Delta$ since the eyes may tend to diverge.

Extraocular Muscles

1. Six muscles attached to each eye to effect ocular movements (see Table 10.2).
2. Spiral of Tillaux: medial rectus attaches closest to the cornea (4.7 mm), followed by the inferior rectus (5.9 mm), lateral rectus (6.3 mm), and superior rectus (6.7 mm).
3. Herring's law of equal innervation: yoke muscles receive equal innervation in each of the nine cardinal positions of gaze.
4. Sherington's law of reciprocal innervation: antagonist ocular muscles are inhibited in equal fashion as their agonist muscles are innervated.

Juvenile Xanthogranuloma

Definition   Benign histiocytic inflammation of infants and children. Onset is usually during infancy.

Examination   Usually presents as spontaneous hyphema with glaucoma, heterochromia, and typical eyelid lesions. These are elevated,

TABLE 10.2

Actions of the extraocular muscles

| Muscle | Muscle Action in Various Globe Positions | | |
	Abducted	Primary	Adducted
Superior rectus	Elevation Adduction	Elevation Adduction Intorsion	Elevation Intorsion
Inferior rectus	Depression Adduction	Depression Adduction Extorsion	Depression Extorsion
Superior oblique	Intorsion	Intorsion Depression Abduction	Intorsion Depression
Inferior oblique	Extorsion	Extorsion Elevation Abduction	Elevation Extorsion
Medial rectus	Adduction	Adduction	Adduction
Lateral rectus	Abduction	Abduction	Abduction

round, nonulcerated yellowish nodules, composed of lipid-filled histiocytes.

Differential Diagnosis   Neurofibromatosis, other histiocytosis X conditions.

Treatment   Low-dose steroids, radiation.

Prognosis   Benign; lesions may spontaneously resolve.

Monofixation Syndrome

Definition   A *sensory* condition in which only one eye is used for central fixation, usually associated with a small angle of strabismus, peripheral fusion, and present but reduced stereopsis. Other names: fixation disparity, monofixational phoria, microtropia, retinal slip, flicker cases, strabismus spurious, and microstrabismus.

Etiology

1. With strabismus, 66%
2. With strabismus and anisometropia, 8%
3. With anisometropia alone, 6%
4. With "primary" monofixation, 20%

Of 615 consecutive strabismus patients, 134 (22%) had monofixation syndrome in Parks' series.

Examination

1. Good vision OU: usually one line difference between the two eyes (e.g., 20/15 OD, 20/20 OS). Amblyopia, if present, is usually mild.
2. No or small ($< 8^\Delta - 10^\Delta$) deviation on cover-uncover test; 37% have no shift on cover-uncover test.
3. A phoria may be superimposed on the small tropia. (Alternate cover test yields a larger total deviation than cover-uncover test.) Of patients with a shift on cover-uncover test 41% show a phoric component.
4. Normal fusional amplitudes.
5. Suppression of one eye when fixing on the Worth lights at distance (Worth lights subtend 1.25° at 6 m); fusion on the near Worth lights at 13 inches (Worth lights subtend 6° at 12 inches).

6. Gross stereopsis is present but is not better than 60 seconds of disparity at either distance or near.
7. Bagolini lenses will reveal a facultative scotoma in good observers. This can be mapped out with the Lancaster red–green lights.
8. Four prism diopter base-out test will usually be positive except in rapid alternators or patients with straight eyes.

Treatment   None, as monofixation usually indicates a stable ocular pattern and results may be the best obtainable in patients with acquired strabismus or anisometropia.

Nystagmus Compensation Syndrome

Definition   Esotropia with early (infantile) onset associated with nystagmus. Most will exhibit an abnormal head position toward the uncovered eye with occlusion of the other eye. The nystagmus can be latent or manifest and is best seen on abduction with the fast phase toward the direction of gaze. Frequency is reported to be 4.8% (von Noorden 1976) to 10.2% (Adelstein and Cüppers 1966).

Examination

1. Large-angle, variable esotropia in infancy with variable head turn
2. Amblyopia early
3. Nystagmus, either large or small amplitude, in primary gaze and abduction (see Tables 10.3 and 10.4)

Etiology   Convergence is thought to eliminate nystagmus (tonic or accommodative vs. voluntary or mechanical).

TABLE 10.3

Congenital esotropia *versus* nystagmus compensation syndrome

Congenital Esotropia	Nystagmus Compensation Syndrome
No nystagmus in primary position.	Nystagmus in primary and abduction.
Primary position only one eye adducted.	Both eyes adducted in primary position.
No amblyopia.	Amblyopia is present early.

TABLE 10.4

Cranial nerve VI palsy versus nystagmus compensation syndrome

CN VI Palsy	Nystagmus Compensation Syndrome
Abduction limited.	Abduction limited.
Head turn present with one eye occluded.	Head turn present with one eye occluded.
Under anesthesia ET present.	Under anesthesia ET absent.
No nystagmus following anesthesia.	Nystagmus present following anesthesia.
Positive forced duction.	Negative forced duction (with time can become positive).

Treatment

1. Alternate occlusion
2. Surgery (recess medial rectus OU vs. recess medial rectus and resect lateral rectus of same eye) with posterior fixation suture (Faden procedure)

Persistent Hyperplastic Primary Vitreous (PHPV)

Definition   A congenital condition usually associated with monocular cataracts.

Etiology   A developmental, congenital, nonhereditary condition of unknown origin. May involve both anterior and posterior segments of the eye. Almost never bilateral (may be confused with Norrie's syndrome if bilateral).

Examination   Presents at birth with the following:

1. Microcornea and microphthalmus
2. Cataract
3. Posterior lenticular membranes
4. Elongated ciliary processes
5. Retinal folds (may at times involve the macula)

Workup   If monocular and obvious microcornea with elongated ciliary processes, should rule out retinal involvement before removing the cataract. Ultrasonography and ERG/VER testing should be done.

Treatment Removal of the cataract within the first 3 months of life gives the opportunity for vision to develop if the refractive error is corrected by a contact lens and amblyopia is vigorously treated. After 3 months of age removal of the congenital cataract may prevent acute uveitis or intraocular hemorrhage but cannot be expected to restore vision. If the cataract forms late, vision may be attained at a later time. Retinal folds through the macula have not been correctable surgically.

Retinoblastoma

Definition The most common ocular tumor of childhood. It is a highly malignant congenital tumor of embryonal cells of the photoreceptor elements of the retina. Often present at birth, it may be inherited in an autosomal dominant manner.

Etiology Retinoblastoma is known to be related to specific genetic abnormalities of chromosome 13. It is inherited in 5% to 10% of the cases, the remaining being sporadic in origin. When bilateral, it is always hereditary.

Examination White tumors of the retina extending into the vitreous (exophytic), or beneath the retina (endophytic), of one or both eyes. May present with the following:

1. Leukocoria (white pupil).
2. Strabismus (due to poor vision if the macula is involved).
3. Uveitis.
4. Glaucoma.
5. Retinal detachment: ultrasound will demonstrate calcium in the tumor mass and may be diagnostic.

Differential Diagnosis

1. Leukocoria
2. Coats' disease
3. Retinopathy of prematurity (ROP)
4. Persistent hyperplastic primary vitreous (PHPV)

Workup

1. Family history.
2. Examination of parents and siblings.
3. Examination under anesthesia, with careful examination of *both* eyes.

4. Ultrasound: will demonstrate calcium in the tumor mass and may be diagnostic.
5. Computed tomography (CT) scan to detect extraocular extension.
6. Pediatric genetic and oncology consultations. Second neoplasms (e.g., osteogenic sarcomas) are common in patients with bilateral retinoblastoma, so careful evaluation for other cancers is necessary.

Treatment Enucleation if the tumor has destroyed visual integrity. Radiation and chemotherapy may preserve useful vision if the tumor is not advanced. Cryotherapy may be useful for tumors anterior to the equator.

Follow-up Children should be examined under anesthesia frequently for the first 4 to 6 years to detect recurrences of the tumor.

Prognosis If the tumor has extended beyond the eye, mortality is nearly 100%. With earlier diagnosis the 5–year survival rate is 92%.

Retinopathy of Prematurity (ROP)

Previously called retrolental fibroplasia (RLF).

Definition ROP is a proliferative vascular retinopathy. It is seen almost exclusively in premature infants, especially those weighing less than 1000 g at birth.

Etiology The developing retina is poorly vascularized until term. The premature infant's retina, therefore, has not fully vascularized at the time of birth. When exposed to high levels of oxygen (or even ambient oxygen), the newly forming vessels retract and are later replaced by new vessels that are abnormal in their permeability. As these new vessels proliferate, they leak fluid and cells into the retina and vitreous, resulting in the formation of a fibrovascular scar, which can lead to complete retinal detachment and permanent loss of vision. Although most commonly seen in premature infants, ROP has been reported in full-term infants not exposed to high levels of oxygen.

Examination Careful evaluation of premature babies in the newborn nursery has become a standard practice. The infant should be examined by an ophthalmologist using an indirect ophthalmoscope. Classifi-

TABLE 10.5

Proliferative ROP classification

Location:

    Zone I—posterior retina, 60° circle around the optic disc.

    Zone II—from zone I to nasal ora serrata.

    Zone III—zone II outward (temporal retina).

Extent: described by number of clock hours involved.

Severity:

    Stage I—demarcation line between vascularized and nonvascularized retina.

    Stage II—elevated demarcation line with ridge.

    Stage III—ridge with extraretinal fibrovascular proliferation; mild, moderate, or severe.

    Stage IV—stage III with serous retinal detachment.

"Plus" disease is any of the above with vascular dilation, vitreous haze, or pupillary involvement.

cation of the disease process has been divided into proliferative and cicatricial stages. Proliferative ROP is defined by location, extent, and severity (Table 10.5). Cicatricial ROP is classified as in Table 10.6.

Treatment   Has been directed at prevention and early diagnosis. Recently, cryotherapy has been shown to be helpful. Vitamin E therapy has not received widespread acceptance.

TABLE 10.6

Cicatricial ROP classification

Stage I—mild peripheral changes including retinal pigmentation and vitreous opacification.

Stage II—temporal vitreal retinal fibrosis with dragging of the posterior retina.

Stage III—peripheral fibrosis with falciform retinal folds.

Stage IV—partial retinal detachment with partial ring of retrolental fibrovascular tissue.

Stage V—complete retinal detachment and complete ring of retrolental fibrovascular tissue.

Sensory System

Definition   That portion of the visual system that coordinates binocular function to blend the images from each eye into a single mental image. Other important terms:

Binocular vision: with both eyes open and functioning, the perception of a single image with stereopsis.

Fusion: the reflex involved in *cortical* integration of similar images into a unified perception (Table 10.7).

Corresponding retinal areas: those receptive fields in the two eyes that have the same visual direction.

Horopter: that portion of space in which objects will form images on the two retinas on corresponding retinal areas.

Pannum's space: an area lying slightly in front of or behind the horopter, in which objects can still be fused but will induce the perception of depth.

Tests of the Sensory System

1. Worth four dot test
   a) A test of fusion. An eye will see only red lights through the red lens and only green lights through the green lens. Distance test (at 6 m) subtends 1° and is a test of central fusion. Near test at $\frac{1}{3}$ m subtends 6° and is a test of peripheral fusion.
   b) Results (red lens over the right eye):

   Four lights = fusion
   Two lights = suppression of OS
   Three lights = suppression of OD
   Five lights = diplopia
   Red lights on right = homonymous diplopia
   Red lights on left = crossed diplopia

TABLE 10.7

Differences between fusion and stereopsis

Fusion	Stereopsis
Eliminates disparity	Demands disparity
Horizontal, vertical, torsional	Horizontal only
Has a motor component	No motor component
Two-dimensional	Three-dimensional
	Requires good visual acuity

2. Red lens test: a diplopia test with interpretation similar to Worth four dot test.
3. Stereo testing: Titmus stereo acuity test, a polaroid vectorgraphic test that measures stereopsis in seconds of disparity. Normal binocular vision allows excellent stereopsis to at least 60 and often to 20 seconds. In monofixation syndromes, stereopsis is reduced to worse than 60 seconds, usually in the 3000 to 80 second range (peripheral fusion only). Using random dot patterns to detect stereopsis further increases the sensitivity of this test.
4. Four prism diopter base-out test: evaluates the presence of a facultative scotoma in one eye (e.g., monofixation syndrome). A four prism diopter prism is placed in front of one eye, base-out, while the patient watches a distant target. The other eye is observed for any movement. Possible results:
   a) The uncovered eye abducts and then adducts: the expected response, indicating no scotoma in either eye.
   b) No movement of the uncovered eye: a scotoma is present in the prism covered eye or that eye has converged without a preliminary version. The prism is then placed in front of the second eye and the first eye is observed for movement.
   c) The uncovered eye abducts and remains abducted: there is a facultative scotoma in the uncovered eye which prevents the perception of diplopia and the corrective convergence (seen as adduction) that diplopia would induce. The test is always done in front of each eye to ensure consistency of results. It is positive in only 50% of patients with monofixation syndrome owing to alternation of fixation.
5. Bagolini striated lens test: a test of sensory fusion using striated lenses to induce an oblique streak of light when viewing a fixation light at distance or near. The lenses are positioned such that the streaks are oriented at 45° and 135° to avoid hemiretinal suppression scotomas. Results are shown in Figure 10.1.

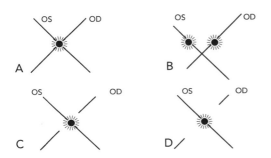

FIGURE 10.1 Several Possible Responses with Bagolini Lenses [A] Normal response. [B] Uncrossed diplopia. [C] Central scotoma. [D] ARC with esotropia.

Vertical Strabismus

Definition Vertical muscle imbalance with one eye higher or lower than the fixing eye. Usually defined according to the higher eye (e.g., hypertropia, HT; right hypertropia, RHT; left hypertropia, LHT). One should name the lower eye in restrictive conditions (e.g., hypotropia) such as double elevator palsy, blow-out fracture of the orbit, and thyroid myopathy. Vertical strabismus may by constant, intermittent, or phoric, depending on the sensory status. Vertical strabismus is often associated with vertical muscle weakness and is more complex due to the multiple actions of these muscles (vertical, horizontal, and torsional; incyclotorsion, excyclotorsion).

Examination

1. Abnormal head position: turn, tilt, chin up, chin down. In the absence of nystagmus, an abnormal head position indicates the presence either of binocular function or of restricted ocular movement of the preferred eye.

2. Ductions and versions in eight fields of gaze. The vertical recti act primarily as depressors or elevators with secondary torsional and horizontal actions. The obliques act as primary tortors of the eye with secondary vertical and horizontal actions. (See Extraocular Muscles section, above.) Ductions are often normal in mild paresis. Look for primary and secondary deviations, overactions, and underactions during version examination.

3. Cover test: measurements in nine positions with each eye fixing. Three-step test:
- a) Step one—determine right or left hypertropia (RHT or LHT).
- b) Step two—determine where greatest deviation occurs in horizontal gaze (R or L?).
- c) Step three—Bielschowsky head tilt; determine greatest deviation on right and left head tilt.

A hypertropia is considered to be secondary to a paresis of either a depressor in the higher eye or an elevator in the lower eye. Therefore, a RHT could be due to a weakness either of one of the right eye depressors (RIR or RSO) or of a left eye elevator (LSR or LIO). If the greatest deviation is in *left* gaze, this would indicate that a muscle that acts in that field is most likely to be affected (RSO or LSR). Head tilting induces incyclotorsion or excyclotorsion. In each eye, the two muscles that effect a torsional movement have opposite vertical actions (e.g., the two incyclotortors in the right eye are the RSO and the RSR). A weakness of one will allow the other to overact vertically, increasing the vertical deviation. So the presence of a greater deviation on right head tilting

O.D. FIXING

0$^\Delta$	5$^\Delta$	10$^\Delta$
0$^\Delta$	RHT = 10$^\Delta$	15$^\Delta$
0$^\Delta$	10$^\Delta$	20$^\Delta$

Head Tilting Right
RHT = 15$^\Delta$

O.S. FIXING

0$^\Delta$	0$^\Delta$	5$^\Delta$
0$^\Delta$	RHT = 5$^\Delta$	5$^\Delta$
0$^\Delta$	0$^\Delta$	10$^\Delta$

Head Tilting Left
RHT = 0$^\Delta$

FIGURE 10.2. Pattern of Extraocular Muscle Deviations in a Patient with a Right Superior Oblique Palsy.

(induces incyclotorsion of the right eye), would indicate a weakness of the RSO (allowing the RSR, the other incyclotorter of the OD to act vertically and elevate the OD) (see Fig. 10.2.)

4. Torsion testing is carried out using the double Maddox rod test. Using a trial frame or the phoropter, a red Maddox rod is placed in front of one eye and a white Maddox rod in front of the other. The patient is asked to align one streak with the other, which is set to a vertical position. The type and amount of torsion (excyclotorsion, incyclotorsion) is read off the cylinder scale on the trial frame. Excyclotorsion greater than 10° is usually associated with *bilateral* superior oblique palsies while a unilateral palsy measures less than 10°.

5. Consideration of neurologic evaluation must be part of the workup of patients with sudden onset of vertical or torsional diplopia.

Differential Diagnosis

1. Trauma, affecting one CN IV or both, is the most common cause of a vertical muscle paresis.
2. Cerebrovascular accidents.
3. Tumors of the brainstem.
4. Myasthenia gravis: common cause for an isolated vertical rectus muscle weakness.

Treatment When the etiology is established and the deviation is stable, surgical intervention to correct the deviation is indicated. Weakening the overacting antagonist muscle (e.g., the inferior oblique in the case of a superior oblique palsy) is often the primary method of treatment. Combined weakening of the antagonist and the yoke (e.g., the inferior rectus in the case of a superior oblique palsy) when the deviation is large or has been long-standing with secondary contraction of the yoke muscle is common. In the case of a superior oblique palsy, a strengthening procedure of the paretic muscle, a tuck, may be indicated if there is little overaction of the antagonist inferior oblique. With bilateral superior oblique paresis and significant torsional diplopia but only a small vertical imbalance, bilateral strengthening of the anterior half of each superior oblique tendon (the Harada-Ito procedure) has been found to be useful.

Visual Assessment in Infants and Children

Definition The assessment of vision in infants and children before they can read is an important step in any evaluation of development or suspected ocular or visual abnormality. Both qualitative and quantitative methods are available.

Examination
Infants

1. Initial testing of infants and children should include the Brückner test to determine the presence of any abnormality in the visual axes of either eye. This is done by simply observing the red reflex from both eyes simultaneously through the direct ophthalmoscope. Each eye should have the same color and intensity of red reflex, a "twin" or "Gemini" reflex. Any abnormality of the ocular media (cataracts, corneal leukoma, vitreous hemorrhage, etc.), refractive error (anisometropia), oculomotor imbalance (strabismus), or retina (tumor, myelinated nerve fibers, etc.) will result in significant differences in the two red reflexes. Identification of this difference requires careful evaluation including refraction and examination of the posterior pole of the eye to determine the cause.

2. Visual function
  a) Fixation behavior: newborn infants, when alert, will prefer to fix on a face as opposed to a light or a colored toy. Following movements develop soon after fixation and should be present by age 3 months. Oculomotor control should be intact by the same age.

  Poor vision in one eye can be detected by noting a fixation preference. Covering of the preferred eye will result in objection to the cover or change in fixation to another object.

  Record fixation as C, S, and M. Fixation should be noted to be *central* (C), that is, not eccentric, when looking at the target. Fixation should be *steady* (S), without sign of nystagmus or wandering eye movements during fixation. Fixation should be *maintained* (M) by either eye when the other eye is uncovered. In the absence of any strabismus to help determine maintenance of fixation, a deviation can be induced by a 10^Δ prism held base-down in front of first one eye and then the other and noting if fixation is maintained by the non-prism-covered eye after cover testing the other eye.

Free alternation of fixation is an indication of normal vision in each eye. Immediate return of fixation to the preferred eye usually indicates significantly reduced visual function in the nonpreferred eye. Nystagmus and eccentric fixation are usually associated with vision less than 20/200.

b) Preferential looking techniques can provide a more quantitative evaluation of vision in infancy. Teller acuity card (TAC) testing is a clinically relevant method of testing that has been used successfully in the office. The targets used are spatial frequency grids, which test the infant's ability to differentiate between a blank screen and a grid. The results are reported in cycles per degree but have been occasionally converted to Snellen letter equivalents. Unfortunately, the results of TAC testing tend to overestimate vision as compared to Snellen letter testing. This test does, however, allow comparison between one examination and another, quantitatively, and has been found useful in detection and treatment of amblyopia in infants.

Vision assessment in children Older children can be tested using the above methods of testing as well. Other tests that can be used in children 2 to 4 years of age:

1. (HOTV or STYCAR) or Sheridan-Gardiner test. This is a matching test in which the child holds a card with four to nine letters on it and is asked to point out (match) the letter that is presented at 10 or 20 feet by the examiner. The presented letters may be single or linear optotypes and are Snellen-sized. Results of this testing, if presented linearly, are equivalent to the usual Snellen letter testing in older children and adults. If the letters are presented as single optotypes, vision may be overestimated in cases of amblyopia.

2. Allen pictures consist of pictures of varying sizes that are identified by the child (horse, telephone, etc.). Testing is done at 10 feet and is reported in Snellen equivalents. Allen cards have been shown to overestimate vision in amblyopia.

3. E game testing allows the child to identify orientation of the letter E, which is usually presented at 20 feet in a linear mode. Young children (age 3 or 4 yrs) often have trouble with right/left orientation but do well with vertical presentations. Results are presented as Snellen equivalents and, if presented linearly, are consistent with Snellen letter testing.

Selected Readings

A/V Syndromes

Knapp P. Vertically incomitant horizontal strabismus: the so–called "A" and "V" syndromes. Trans Am Ophthalmol Soc 1959;57:666–99.

Metz HS, Schwartz L. The treatment of A and V patterns by monocular surgery. Arch Ophthalmol 1977;95:251–53.

Jampolsky A. Oblique muscle surgery of the A-V patterns. J Pediatr Ophthalmol 1965;2:31–36.

AC/A Ratio

von Noorden GK. Binocular vision and ocular motility, 4th ed. St. Louis: CV Mosby, 1990, pp. 89–96.

Amblyopia

von Noorden GK. Classification of amblyopia. Am J Ophthalmol 1967;63:238–44.

Burian HM. Amblyopia. Am J Ophthalmol 1969;67:1–12.

France TD. Amblyopia update: diagnosis and therapy. Am Orthopt J 1984;34:4–12.

Hess RF, Campbell, FW, Zimmern R. Differences in the neural basis of human amblyopias: the effect of mean luminance. Vision Res 1980;18:931–36.

Abnormal Retinal Correspondence

Lyle TK, Wybar KC. Lyle and Jackson's practical orthoptics in the treatment of squint, 5th ed. London: HK Lewis, 1967, pp. 205–58.

Brown's Syndrome [Superior Oblique Tendon Sheath Syndrome]

Brown HW. Congenital structural muscle anomalies. In: Allen JH, ed. Strabismus: Ophthalmology Symposium I. St. Louis: CV Mosby, 1950, p. 205.

Scott AB, Knapp P. Surgical treatment of the superior oblique tendon sheath syndrome. Arch Ophthalmol 1972;88:282–86.

Parks MM, Brown M. Superior oblique tendon sheath syndrome of Brown. Am J Ophthalmol 1975,79:82–86.

Crawford JS. Surgical treatment of true Brown's syndrome. Am J Ophthalmol 1976;81:289–95.

Congenital Cataract

Kohn BA. The differential diagnosis of cataracts in infancy and childhood. Am J Dis Child 1976;130:184–92.

Parks MM. Visual results in aphakic children. Am J Ophthalmol 1982;94:441–49.

Helveston EM, Saunders RA, Ellis FD. Unilateral cataracts in children. Ophthalmic Surg 1980;11:102–8.

Convergence Insufficiency

Raskind R. Problems at the reading distance. Am Orthopt J 1976;26:53–9.

Hugonnier R, Hugonnier S. Strabismus, heterophoria, ocular motor paralysis. St. Louis: CV Mosby, 1969, p. 519.

von Noorden GK, Brown D, Park M. Associated convergence and accommodative insufficiency. Document Ophthalmol 1973;34:393–403.

Convergence Spasm

Miller NR, ed. Clinical neuro-ophthalmology. Baltimore: Williams and Wilkins, 1985, vol. 2, pp. 533–35.

Guiloff RJ, Whitely A, Kelly RE. Organic convergence spasm. Acta Neurol Scand 1980;61:252–59.

Moore S, Stockbridge L. Another approach to the treatment of accommodative spasm. Am Orthoptic J 1973;23:71–72.

Duane's Syndrome

Blodi FC, van Allen MW, Yarbrough JC. Duane's syndrome: a brain stem lesion. Arch Ophthalmol 1964;72:171–77.

Isenberg S, Urist MJ. Clinical observations in 101 consecutive patients with Duane's retraction syndrome. Am J Ophthalmol 1977;84:419–25.

Metz HS, Scott AB, Scott WE. Horizontal saccadic velocities in Duane's syndrome. Am J Ophthalmol 1975;80:901–6.

Pfaffenbach D, Cross HH, Kerns TP. Congenital anomalies in Duane's retraction syndrome. Arch Ophthalmol 1972;88:635–39.

Hotchkiss MG, Miller NR, Clark AW, Green WR. Bilateral Duane's retraction syndrome: a clinical pathologic case report. Arch Ophthalmol 1980;98:870–74.

Dissociated Vertical Deviations

Helveston E. 'A' exotropia, alternating sursumduction, and superior oblique overaction. Am J Ophthalmol 1969;67:377–80.

von Noorden GK. Binocular vision and ocular motility, 4th ed. St. Louis: CV Mosby, 1990, pp. 341–44.

Parks MM. Ocular Motility and Strabismus. Hagerstown, Maryland: Harper and Row, 1975, pp. 149–52.

Harley RD. Pediatric Ophthalmology, Philadelphia: WB Saunders, 1975, p. 167.

Accommodative Esotropia

Raab EL. Etiologic factors in accommodative esotropia. Trans Am Ophthalmol Soc 1982;80:657–94.

Parks MM. Ocular motility and strabismus. Hagerstown, Maryland: Harper and Row, 1975, pp. 99–105.

von Noorden GK, Morris J, Edelman P. Efficacy of bifocals in the treatment of accommodative esotropia. Am J Ophthalmol 1978;85:830–34.

Swan KC. Accommodative esotropia long range follow-up. Ophthalmology 1983;90:1141–45.

Infantile Esotropia

Costenbader FD. Infantile esotropia. Trans Am Ophthalmol Soc 1961;59:397–429.

Taylor DM. Early surgery for strabismus. Arch Ophthalmol 1963;80:752–56.

Ing MD, Costenbader FD, Parks MM, Albert DG. Early surgery for congenital esotropia. Am J Ophthalmol 1966;61:1419–27.

Fisher NF, Flom MC, Jampolsky AJ. Early surgery of congenital esotropia. Am J Ophthalmol 1968;65:439–43.

Symposium: infantile esotropia. Am Orthoptic J 1968;18:5–22.

Ing MR. Early surgical correction for congenital esotropia. Trans Am Ophthalmol Soc 1981;79:625–63.

Exodeviations

Burian HM. Exodeviations: their classification, diagnosis and treatment. Am J Ophthalmol 1966;63:1161–66.

Burian HM, Franceschetti AT. Evaluation of diagnostic methods for the classification of exodeviations. Am J Ophthalmol 1971;71:34–41.

Jampolsky A. Ocular divergence mechanisms. Trans Am Ophthalmol Soc 1970;68:730–822.

Hiles DA, Davies GT, Costenbader FD. Long-term observation unoperated intermittent exotropia. Arch Ophthalmol 1968;80:436–42.

Moore S. The prognostic value of lateral gaze measurements in intermittent exotropia. Am Orthopt J 1969;19:69–71.

Carlson MR, Jampolsky A. Lateral incomitancy in intermittent exotropia. Arch Ophthalmol 1979;97:1922–25.

Hardesty HH, Boynton JR, Keenan JP. Treatment of intermittent exotropia. Arch Ophthalmol 1978;96:268–74.

Extraocular Muscles

von Noorden GK. Binocular vision and ocular motility, 4th ed. St. Louis: CV Mosby, 1990, pp. 289–92.

Juvenile Xanthogranuloma

Zimmerman LE. Ocular lesions of juvenile xanthogranuloma. Trans Am Acad Ophthalmol Otolaryngol 1965;65:412–39.

Gass JDM. Management of juvenile xanthogranuloma of the iris. Arch Ophthalmol 1964;71:344–47.

Monofixation Syndrome

Parks MM, Eustis AT. Monofixational phoria. Am Orthoptic J 1961;11:38–45.
Parks MM. The monofixation syndrome. Trans Am Ophthalmol Soc 1969;67:609–57.
Jampolsky A. Retinal correspondence in patients with small degree strabismus. Arch Ophthalmol 1951;45:18–26.
Ogle KN, et al. Fixation disparity and fusional processes in binocular single vision. Am J Ophthalmol 1949;32:1069–87.
Ogle KN. Fixation disparity and oculomotor imbalance. Am Orthoptic J 1958;8:21–36.
Lang J. Microtropia. Arch Ophthalmol 1969;81:758–62.

Nystagmus Compensation Syndrome

von Noorden GK. The nystagmus compensation (blockage) syndrome. Am J Ophthalmol 1976;82:283–90.
Adelstein F, Cüppers C. Zum problem der echten und scheinbaren abducenslähmung (das sogenannte "Blockierungs-syndrom"). Büch. d. Augenarzt, 1966;46:271–78.
Frank JW. Diagnostic signs in the nystagmus compensation syndrome. J Pediatr Ophthalmol Strabismus 1979;16:317–20.

Persistent Hyperplastic Primary Vitreous

Haddad R, Font RL, Reeser F. Persistent hyperplastic primary vitreous. A clinicopathologic study of 62 cases. Surv Ophthalmol 1978;23:123–34.
Karr DJ, Scott WE. Visual acuity results following treatment of persistent hyperplastic primary vitreous. Arch Ophthalmol 1986;104:662–67.

Retinoblastoma

Pendergrass TW, Davis S. Incidence of retinoblastoma in the United States. Arch Ophthalmol 1981;98:1204–10.
Rosenbaum A, Falk P, Parker RG. Neoplasms of the eye: retinoblastoma. In: Haskell CM, ed. Cancer treatment. Philadelphia: WB Saunders, 1980, pp. 569–85.
Ellsworth RM. The practical management of retinoblastoma. Trans Am Ophthalmol Soc 1969;67:462–534.
Howard GM, Ellsworth RM. Differential diagnosis of retinoblastoma: a statistical survey of 4500 children: II. Factors relating to the diagnosis of retinoblastoma. Am J Ophthalmol 1965;60:618–21.
Sparkes RS, Murphree AL, Lingua RW, et al. Gene for hereditary retinoblastoma assigned to human chromosome 13 by linkage to esterase D. Science 1983;219:971–73.

Retinopathy of Prematurity

The Committee for the Classification of Retinopathy of Prematurity. An international classification of retinopathy of prematurity. Arch Ophthalmol 1984;102:1130–34.

Cryotherapy for Retinopathy of Prematurity Cooperative Group. Multicenter trial of cryotherapy for retinopathy of prematurity: preliminary results. Arch Ophthalmol 1988;106:471–79.

Phelps DL, Phelps CE. Cryotherapy in infants with retinopathy of prematurity: a decision model for treating one or both eyes. JAMA 1989;261:1751–56.

Hittner HM, Rudolph AJ, Kretzer FL. Suppression of severe retinopathy of prematurity with vitamin E supplementation. Ophthalmology 1984;12:1512–23.

Sensory System

von Noorden GK, Maumenee AE. Atlas of Strabismus. St. Louis: CV Mosby, 1973, pp. 62–107.

Vertical Strabismus

Parks MM. Isolated vertical muscle palsy. Arch Ophthalmol 1958;60:1027–35.

Knapp P. Diagnosis and surgical treatment of hypertropia. Am Orthopt J 1971;21:29–37.

Hardesty HH. Diagnosis and treatment of paretic vertical muscle. Arch Ophthalmol 1967;77:147–56.

Herrman JS. Masked bilateral superior oblique paresis. J Pediatr Ophthalmol Strabismus 1981;18:43–48.

Harada M, Ito Y. Surgical correction of cyclotropia. Jpn J Ophthalmol 1964;8:88–96.

Visual Assessment in Infants and Children

Teller DY, McDonald MA, Preston K, Sebris SL, Dobson V. Assessment of visual acuity in infants and children: the acuity card procedure. Dev Med Child Neurol 1986;28:779–89.

Moseley MJ, Fielder AR, Thompson JR, Minshull C, Price D. Grating and recognition acuities in young amblyopes. Br J Ophthalmol 1988;72:50–54.

Sheridan MD. Vision screening of very young or handicapped children. Br Med J 1960;2:453–56.

Allen JF. Testing visual acuity in preschool children: norms, variables and a new picture test. Pediatrics 1957;19:1093–1100.

Cibis-Tongue AB, Cibis GW. Brückner test. Ophthalmology 1981;88:1041–44.

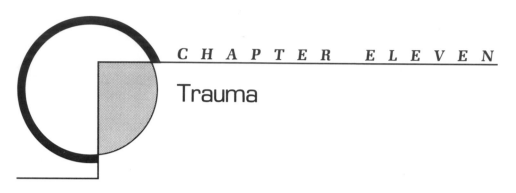

Trauma

Michael P. Vrabec, M.D.
Vincent S. Reppucci, M.D.
Gregory L. Skuta, M.D.
Keith D. Carter, M.D.
Gene R. Howard, M.D.

Evaluation of the Trauma Patient

A thorough history and physical examination are required for every trauma patient because of potential serious injuries that may not be initially apparent, the possibility of multiple injuries, and medical-legal considerations. The physician may be asked to testify in court (either as an expert witness or possibly in his or her own defense), making accurate and legible notes a must.

History   Special emphasis should be placed on the following:

1. Exactly when and how did the accident occur? Try to get a detailed description and picture the incident clearly in your mind. This is especially true of high-speed projectiles (striking metal on metal), which may not cause much pain on impact. If an object was involved in the injury is it available (for culture or metallurgic evaluation)?
2. What was the previous visual acuity of the eye? Is there a history of past ocular trauma or amblyopia?

3. Did this occur at work?
4. Were safety glasses being worn at the time of the injury?
5. What and when was the patient's last meal? This can determine when a patient may be taken to the operating room.
6. Was the injury self-inflicted?
7. Is tetanus vaccination up-to-date?
8. Are there medical conditions (e.g., severe emphysema) that could make a general anesthetic a significant risk?

Physical Examination A complete eye examination should be performed to avoid missing occult or multiple injuries. In cases of obvious severe trauma, minimal manipulation is recommended to avoid further damage. An examination under anesthesia will be required in these cases and will be part of the surgical repair. This is also true with injuries in uncooperative children.

1. Visual acuity: always assess except in incidences of chemical burns, in which copious irrigation will preclude and precede determination of vision. This must always be recorded in the chart.
   a) Pinhole vision is acceptable when glasses are absent or broken.
   b) A facial nerve block may be required for excessive lid squeezing.
   c) Children are especially prone to peeking with the fellow eye on visual examinations, so it should be covered completely with occlusive tape.
2. Confrontation visual fields.
3. Versions: limitations may indicate cranial nerve or extraocular muscle damage.
4. Pupils: look for and note the presence of a relative afferent pupillary defect. Even if the traumatized eye has a fixed and dilated pupil one can still look for an afferent defect based on the reaction of the fellow pupil.
5. External or slit lamp examination:
   a) Palpate orbital rims for signs of fracture.
   b) Auscultate orbit for bruits if indicated.
   c) Lid eversion and double lid eversion with a paper clip in search of foreign bodies. Desmarres lid retractors are useful to retract swollen lids.
   d) One may carefully explore areas of a conjunctival laceration with cotton-tipped applicators if there is no obvious uveal prolapse.

e) Seidel testing: best performed by initially anesthetizing the eye with a topical anesthetic. A 2% fluorescein strip is then moistened and placed on the area of question. A bright green stream of aqueous through a pool of dark fluorescein indicates a leak. The rate of aqueous loss is important to note as small beveled corneal wounds with a slow leak of aqueous and a deep chamber may not need to be repaired.

f) Gonioscopy for anterior chamber injury and foreign bodies that may have settled in the inferior anterior chamber angle.

6. Intraocular pressure evaluation should be performed if the globe is intact. A normal or even slightly elevated intraocular pressure does not rule out a scleral rupture.

7. Mydriasis: avoid if extremely narrow angles are present or if there is iris prolapse in a corneal wound (iris may be pulled out of a laceration if the pupil is dilated, resulting in a flat anterior chamber, and having the iris within the cornea may limit contamination into the eye).

8. Posterior segment evaluation as soon as possible as blood or cataract formation may obscure the view. Careful attention for a second perforation site should be noted.

9. Consider photographic documentation for medical-legal purposes.

Initial Workup

1. A Fox shield should be placed over the injured eye for protection.

2. Patient should be made N.P.O.—make sure this is emphasized to a referring physician before the patient is sent.

3. A general physical examination must be performed to treat other injuries in an organized, multispecialty team approach, thus avoiding multiple anesthetics.

4. Notify the operating room and the anesthesia department of the potential case early on to avoid delays. Note that general anesthesia is nearly always preferred over local anesthesia to avoid the retrobulbar pressure associated with a local block. Succinylcholine should be avoided (a depolarizing agent that can cause extraocular muscle contraction during induction, possibly causing loss of intraocular contents). Nitrous oxide may also have to be avoided if intraocular gas is to be used.

5. Always assume an intraocular foreign body is present until proven otherwise. Hence, computed tomography (CT) scans of the eye and orbit are often indicated. Avoid magnetic resonance imaging (MRI) scans because of the possibility of a foreign body being metallic.

6. A general discussion with the patient and family should be extremely guarded. The serious nature of the injury and unknown future course for the eye should be emphasized. This avoids unrealistic expectations on the patient's part and highlights the potential for secondary sight-threatening processes to develop in the future. In severe injuries a discussion of sympathetic ophthalmia should be mentioned (see Sympathetic Ophthalmia section, Chapter 6).
7. Pain management is often required, but have the patient sign the informed consent for surgery before administering any pain medications.
8. Update tetanus toxoid vaccination if necessary.

Anterior Segment Trauma
Chemical Burns

General   Although the cornea may be the main attention of focus with chemical burns, damage may be more extensive and involve the lid and adnexal structures (see "Chemical and Thermal Burns" in Adnexal and Orbital Trauma section, below). Alkaline solutions tend to be more destructive than acid solutions as they saponify corneal proteins and induce collagen breakdown. Acids tend to precipitate with corneal proteins and therefore cause less damage. The following are common chemicals in ocular chemical burns:

1. Acids: sulfuric (from battery explosions), sulfur dioxide, hydrochloric.
2. Alkalis: lye (sodium hydroxide or potassium hydroxide), household ammonia (ammonium hydroxide), lime (calcium hydroxide.
3. Mace (chloroactetophenone).

Treatment

1. Acute: this is one of only several true ophthalmic emergencies, and no time should be wasted with a history or examination; treatment must begin immediately, at the scene if possible, even with unsterile water. Test vision only after copious irrigation is completed with normal saline, lactated Ringer's solution, or sterile water. Do not delay irrigation waiting for a "more appropriate" irrigation solution. This is best administered through sterile intravenous tubing or with a special irrigating contact lens. One to two liters of fluid should be used (at least 20 or 30 min of irrigation or until the pH is neutralized). It may be difficult to get the pH back to 7, but a trend toward neutralization is important to document. One can use litmus paper or the pH indicator in a urine dip stick to determine pH.

Topical anesthetic applied each 15 minutes with a lid speculum and possibly a facial nerve block will aid in the irrigation. Carefully check and swab the fornices for foreign particles (especially lye) which can be a continual source of the toxic agent. Any necrotic tissue should be debrided.

2. After initial treatment, the eye history should be taken. This should include identification of the substance. A label of the chemical solution is often available. Poison Control Centers often have specific descriptions of multi-ingredient chemicals.

3. Examination should assess the damage from the chemical agent. One can roughly describe burns as mild, moderate, or severe based on the findings (see Table 11.1). The prognosis for chemical burns generally is dependent on the initial severity of the injury.

TABLE 11.1

Severity of chemical burns

	Mild	**Moderate**	**Severe**
Eyelids	Unaffected	Slight swelling	Loss of tissue with malposition
Conjunctiva	Mild injection and chemosis	Surface defects; moderate injection and chemosis	Symblepharon, necrosis
Sclera	Mild injection	Moderate inflammation	Extensive blanching from severe ischemia
Cornea	Mild SPK	Surface defects; mild-moderate stromal edema & haze	Severe edema, melting, opacification, vascularization
Anterior chamber	Normal (can see iris)	Mild iritis (can see iris)	Severe iritis (hypopyon)
IOP	Normal	Normal or elevated	Elevated

SPK, superficial punctate keratopathy; IOP, intraocular pressure.

Management

1. Patients with moderate to severe chemical burns should be hospitalized for careful observation and a complete evaluation. A burn specialist may have to be consulted. This also helps the patient realize the serious nature of the injury. The conjunctiva should be carefully followed for symblepharon formation. Frequent (at least b.i.d.) lysis of adhesions may be necessary. This can be performed with Desmarres retractors lubricated with ophthalmic ointment, a glass rod, or the end of a glass thermometer. A methyl methacrylate ring can be placed in the fornix.

2. The cornea should be encouraged to heal and secondary infection should be prevented. Patients must be watched carefully for the development of corneal melts. Epithelial defects will often heal with antibiotic ointments, cycloplegia, and pressure patching. One should avoid epithelial toxic agents such as gentamicin. Bilateral patching will help keep the eye still. Bandage soft contact lenses may also be required. Moist chambers or Saran Wrap may be required to protect the globe if there is extensive lid injury and the globe cannot be covered. If there is any evidence of corneal melting, consider using acetylcysteine 10% to 20% (Mucomyst). Ascorbic acid has also been helpful in corneal melting. A corneal perforation may require cyanoacrylate tissue glue (for defects $\leq$ 1 mm diameter) or a patch graft. Topical steroids are indicated in moderate to severe burns when there is iritis and edema. In the initial phase of the injury, glucocorticoids (prednisone) are helpful, but after a week of treatment consideration should be given to changing to anabolic steroids (progesterone), which have an anti-inflammatory action like prednisone with less collagenase activity (and therefore are less likely to result in stromal melting).

3. Elevations of intraocular pressure should be treated with beta-blockers and carbonic anhydrase inhibitors. With a severe alkaline burn, a paracentesis of the anterior chamber with reformation using Tris buffer may be indicted.

4. Long-term rehabilitation of the eye is typically achieved with a multidisciplined, multistaged approach. These procedures are best undertaken 6 months to 1 year after the initial injury to allow for stabilization of the eye.
   a) Artificial tears or punctal occlusion if a dry eye develops.
   b) Conjunctival resection may be necessary in severe cases of corneal melting.
   c) Lid reconstruction with mucous membrane grafts for entropion; correction of ectropion.
   d) Epilation or cryotherapy for trichiasis. Any anomalies of the eyelids or eyelashes should be corrected prior to corneal surgery.

e) Conjunctival autotransplantation: the uninvolved eye may be used as a donor site for conjunctival epithelium, but the graft may not take if there is extensive ischemia of the host bed.

f) Corneal transplantation may be considered if there is significant scarring and the eye has remained quiet for at least 6 months to 1 year. The prognosis is generally poor because of recurrent corneal epithelial erosions, dry eye, and corneal neovascularization. A liberal tarsorrhaphy should be considered.

g) Keratoprothesis (e.g., Kardona) may be necessary for visual rehabilitation in severe cases with good macular function.

h) Glaucoma surgery.

Penetrating Trauma

History   See Evaluation of the Trauma Patient, above.

Physical Examination   See Evaluation of the Trauma Patient, above.

1. Chemosis, a subconjunctival hemorrhage, or a conjunctival laceration may obscure a scleral rupture.
2. Always assume a corneal laceration extends past the limbus until proven otherwise.
3. Posterior scleral rupture may occur with anterior segment chemosis, a subconjunctival hemorrhage, or in an eye with a deeper than normal anterior chamber.

Workup   See Evaluation of the Trauma Patient, above.

1. CT scan may show a "flat tire" (depressed globe with thickened sclera and intraocular air). MRI scanning is best avoided.

Management   In the operating room:

1. Conjunctival and corneal cultures should be taken at the wound site before preparation for surgery. Bacillus organisms are of particular concern with lacerations involving organic material. Cultures may help to identify an agent if postoperative endophthalmitis develops.
2. Repair principles and primary goals:
   a) Water-tight closure with restoration of normal intraocular pressure. In cases of a small beveled corneal laceration with a slow Seidel leak and a formed anterior chamber, a bandage contact lens or a pressure patch with or without glue may be enough to seal the wound. In general, however, err on the side of suture repair. Cyanoacrylate glue is typically effective

for perforations less than or equal to 1 mm in diameter with concomitant loss of tissue, making suture repair difficult if not impossible.

b)   Avoid iatrogenic damage to surrounding ocular structures.

c)   Protect the visual axis without jeopardizing goals (a) and (b).

3. Repair steps:

a)   Remove any foreign material and debride nonviable tissue, except uvea. Cutting uvea may result in severe bleeding.

b)   If the chamber is flat, consider a paracentesis to reform the anterior chamber with either a viscoelastic substance or saline and sweep the iris away if incarcerated in the wound. It is best to try to save the iris if it appears viable and the injury is less than 24 hours old.

c)   Consider traction sutures at the limbus in two sites for positioning and eye control. Using 5-0 vicryl on a spatula needle works well. A conjunctival peritomy is performed for 360° if there is any question about the extent of injury. Observation should be made posterior to the equator and under muscles with their removal if necessary.

d)   In corneal/scleral lacerations, one should approximate the limbus first. The corneal laceration should then be closed preferably with 10-0 nylon. Start in the middle of the wound and continually bisect until closed. Loose suture should be replaced. Temporary sutures may be needed to approximate the wound initially which are later removed. Deep bites (three-fourths depth) ensure a water-tight closure. Sutures usually have to be tied rather tightly to prevent leakage from an irregular wound. Knots should be buried away from the visual axis. Purse-string suturing techniques may be required for stellate wounds.

4. Scleral lacerations: extraocular muscles may have to be removed with fixation by 5-0 vicryl sutures. It is best to close in an anterior-to-posterior direction and reposit all iris tissue. Cut extruded vitreous at the sclera with scissors; do not use sponges to pull vitreous out of the wound. One must always watch for retina in lacerations behind the ora serrata. Cryotherapy is indicated only for a visualized retinal tear; blind cryotherapy could produce proliferative vitreoretinopathy. Small lacerations behind the equator may not have to be closed.

5. With significant tissue loss, glue or a patch graft will be needed.

6. It is best to defer to a second operation other procedures such as lensectomy, or vitrectomy except in the presence of an intraocular foreign body, suspected endophthalmitis, or obvious cataract formation.

7. Subconjunctival antibiotics (e.g., cefazolin and gentamicin) are given prophylactically at the end of the case.

Follow-up   Patients must be watched carefully for postoperative infection and elevations in intraocular pressure. Sutures in the cornea should remain at least 6 months unless they erode or the wound appears well healed with vascular or avascular scars.

Blunt Trauma

Always suspect an occult globe rupture and perform a careful history and physical examination as discussed in Evaluation of the Trauma Patient, above. The following are some of the more common blunt injuries (other than hyphema, which will be discussed separately).

Corneal Abrasions

Abrasions, if large enough, can result in secondary lid swelling, corneal edema, endothelialitis, and iritis. Treatment should include topical antibiotic drops or ointment and cycloplegia. Firm pressure patching is indicated except in patients who wear contact lenses, in whom patching is contraindicated as it can create an environment more suitable for corneal ulceration. Topical steroids may be added when the epithelium heals if there is a significant inflammatory component to the injury and no evidence of an uncontrolled infection. Epithelial debridement of necrotic edges should be considered to encourage more rapid healing and prevent recurrent erosions. Follow-up should be daily until the epithelium heals, then weekly until the iritis resolves. Consideration should be given to hypertonic saline (5% sodium chloride) drops three times a day and ointment just before sleep for 4 to 6 weeks in the hope of preventing recurrent erosion syndrome.

Angle Contusion Glaucoma

This injury is often associated with a hyphema. Findings on examination may include iridodialysis (tear at the iris root), cyclodialysis (separation of the ciliary body from the scleral spur), and angle recession (irregular widening of the ciliary band or tear of the trabecular meshwork). Four to nine percent of eyes with greater than 180° of angle recession eventually develop chronic glaucoma. Angle recession itself is not the cause of decreased outflow but indicates past injury to the outflow system. Fellow eyes may eventually develop increased intraocular pressure and may be steroid-responsive, suggesting that the same eyes with contusion injury may have already had an underlying predisposition to pressure elevation.

Treatment includes standard medical therapy including miotic agents. Argon laser trabeculoplasty is not highly successful but may be attempted before filtering surgery.

Ghost Cell Glaucoma

This condition results from degenerated red blood cells (secondary to vitreous hemorrhage from trauma, retinal disease, or other causes) originating from the vitreous cavity entering the anterior chamber through a disrupted vitreous face and obstructing outflow. Signs include tan or khaki-colored ghost cells in the anterior chamber; one may also see a pseudohypopyon with a layer of fresher red blood cells on top. Intraocular pressure elevations are often transient and are secondary to obstruction of the meshwork by rigid red blood cells (ghost cells), which are empty except for clumps of denatured hemoglobin (Heinz bodies). These are best seen with phase contrast microscopy. Treatment initially includes medical therapy with aqueous suppressants. If this is ineffective, an anterior chamber washout with or without vitrectomy is indicated.

Subluxation of the Lens

Signs include phakodonesis or iridodonesis, sudden astigmatic shifts in refraction, and pupil block. Treatment includes correction of the refractive error (possibly an aphakic refraction). A lensectomy will be required for pupil block or visual impairment.

Lens Capsule Rupture

Signs include cataract formation. Typically, the posterior capsule is involved in blunt trauma while the anterior capsule (and possibly the posterior capsule) is involved in a perforating injury. The intraocular pressure may rise dramatically with lens leakage (phacolytic glaucoma). Treatment includes control of elevated intraocular pressure and inflammation prior to lensectomy.

Hyphema

The mechanism for hyphema is typically blunt trauma with associated anterior chamber hemorrhage from a tear in the iris root or ciliary body.

Always consider child abuse as a possible etiology in hyphema.

Findings include blood in the anterior chamber, which is quantified as the percentage of the anterior chamber that it occupies. Hyphemas may be microscopic, in which there is no layering of blood but red cells are floating throughout the anterior chamber.

Complications

1. Elevations in intraocular pressure: secondary glaucoma is directly related to the size of the hyphema and is due to obstruction of the meshwork by red blood cells, plasma, fibrin, and other debris. In an eight-ball hyphema (100%) the clot can directly obstruct the meshwork or produce pupillary block in the presence of a mushroom-like clot. With sickle cell hemoglobinopathy, sickled cells are less likely to pass through the meshwork, and the optic nerve is more sensitive to an increase in intraocular pressures.
2. Corneal blood staining: usually secondary to a prolonged hyphema and increased intraocular pressure. Seen as a central and diffuse rust-colored opacity that clears from the periphery toward the center.
3. Rebleeding: most hyphemas clear spontaneously, although 4% to 35% will rebleed in the first 5 days. The major concern is that the rebleed may be larger than the initial hyphema.

Workup   Other ocular injuries must be ruled out. However,

1. do not perform scleral depression or gonioscopy in the first 3 to 4 weeks as this manipulation can increase the chance of a rebleed; and
2. a sickle cell preparation is required in black patients to rule out sickle cell disease. If the preparation is positive, confirm the diagnosis with a hemoglobin electrophoresis.

Differential Diagnosis   In nontraumatic hyphemas, one must consider blood vessel wall fragility, rubeosis, blood dyscrasias, and leukemia. A spontaneous hyphema in children should lead one to suspect child abuse, retinoblastoma, leukemia, and juvenile xanthogranuloma.

Treatment

1. Avoidance of rebleeding in the first 5 days is paramount. This may be accomplished as follows:
   a) Bed rest with possible hospitalization—which may be indicated in certain social situations. However, in compliant patients, outpatient management is usually acceptable.
   b) Aspirin should not be given to the patient.
   c) Elevate the head of the bed.
   d) Television viewing is permitted; reading should be avoided.
   e) Antiemetics as needed.

f) Patching of the eye; possibly bilateral.

g) Amicar, an antifibrinolytic agent, may be given in a dosage of 50 mg/kg p.o. q. 4 h for 5 days. This is half of the recommended dosage, resulting in less nausea and vomiting. The maximum dose should be 50 g per day. Amicar comes in 500 mg tablets and a 1.25 g/5 ml syrup. It must not be given to patients who are pregnant or have liver or renal disease, and generally should be reserved for hyphemas larger than 75%.

h) Topical atropine and steroids; steroids may help decrease other injuries such as macular edema.

If a rebleed does occur, continue these treatments for 5 more days.

2. Treat elevations in intraocular pressure. The pressure should not be so low as to induce a rebleed. The goal is to keep the pressure less than 30 mmHg, and in sickle cell disease, less than 20 mmHg.

a) Aqueous suppressants (beta-blockers, acetazolamide, or methazolamide). Avoid carbonic anhydrase inhibitors in sickle cell disease as this can increase the tendency toward sickling.

b) Mannitol intravenously. Avoid glycerin by mouth as this may induce nausea, vomiting, and a rebleed.

c) Avoid epinephrine as it takes 2 weeks to work and pilocarpine as this causes vascular congestion. Intraocular pressure may increase after the discontinuation of Amicar. A rise or persistent elevation in intraocular pressure may be due to ghost cell glaucoma or angle recession.

3. An anterior chamber washout or clot expression may be necessary. This is best performed under general anesthesia and can be achieved with either a manual irrigation and aspiration cannula or a vitrectomy instrument. This is generally reserved for intraocular pressure elevations unresponsive to medical therapy in the following situations: a pressure of 60 mmHg for 3 days, 50 mmHg for 5 days, 35 mmHg for 10 days, or blood staining in patients less than 7 years old. A trabeculectomy with a peripheral iridectomy may be required in some cases of poor pressure control after a clot has been expressed.

Follow-up Patients should be followed each day for 5 days, then several days later after discharge. Physical activity should be limited for the first 2 to 3 weeks with full activities after 4 weeks. These patients need to be checked for angle recession at a later date.

Posterior Segment Trauma

Penetrating trauma and blunt trauma can result in multiple injuries to the posterior segment. The evaluation of such cases is discussed in Evaluation of the Trauma Patient, above. Some of the more common traumatic entities involving the posterior segment will be discussed below.

Vitreous Hemorrhage

Symptoms of vitreous hemorrhage include floaters and blurred vision. The etiology can include posterior scleral perforation, a retinal tear, or can be unrelated to the trauma, as with a preexisting disease such as proliferative diabetic retinopathy. Workup should include ultrasound if the posterior pole cannot be adequately visualized to rule out a retinal detachment. Treatment of a moderate to severe vitreous hemorrhage includes bed rest with the head of the bed elevated and bilateral patching. With time most vitreous hemorrhages will resolve spontaneously. A vitrectomy may be indicated if the blood does not resolve within 3 to 4 weeks or if a retinal detachment is developing.

Choroidal Rupture

Signs of choroidal rupture include a yellow to white crescent-shaped choroidal defect concentric to the optic disc. Subretinal or intraretinal hemorrhage may initially cover this defect. One must rule out preexisting conditions such as angioid streaks or the "lacquer cracks" of high myopia prior to making this diagnosis. Treatment involves careful observation each week until the hemorrhage resolves. Patients should be followed with an Amsler grid and watched carefully and treated for choroidal neovascular membranes that may develop. Fluorescein angiography plays a vital role in the follow-up management.

Retinal Trauma

Commotio Retina or Berlin's Edema

Signs and symptoms include a decrease in vision with a confluent discrete region of retinal whitening. This may look similar to a retinal artery occlusion, but such an event is rare after trauma. This usually resolves spontaneously and may clear faster with steroids. One must always rule out other associated injuries, especially a retinal detachment.

Retinal Dialysis and Tears

Symptoms include floaters and photopsia. Signs include an avulsed or detached vitreous or vitreous base. These injuries typically involve the superior temporal quadrant. Treatment involves laser photocoagulation, cryopexy to seal the tear, and scleral buckling for localized retinal detachment. Note that these patients must be followed carefully as an unrecognized dialysis or tear can later lead to retinal detachment.

Adnexal and Orbital Trauma

Eyelid Lacerations and Reconstruction

Etiology Lacerations can occur from a puncture or avulsion to the eyelid. Such injuries can adversely affect the structure and function of the lid. Always suspect a globe injury especially with a full-thickness laceration of the lid with prolapse of orbital fat. If a bite injury occurred, inquire if it was an animal or human bite. This is important as potential pathogens differ. Common organisms in bite injuries:

1. In human bites, consider *Streptococcus viridans*, *Staphylococcus aureus*, group A *Streptococcus*, *Bacteroides*, and *Fusobacterium*.
2. In dog bites, consider *S. aureus*, *Pasteurella multocida*, *S. viridans*, *Fusobacterium*, and *Bacteroides*.
3. In cat bites, consider *S. aureus*, *Pasteurella multocida*.

Evaluation A thorough eye examination, with special attention to

1. the extent of penetration of the lid and position of ocular and adnexal structures,
2. the function of the levator, and
3. probing and irrigation of the canalicular system if the injury might possibly involve the system.

Treatment Consider ice packing of the lid with repair within 12 to 18 hours if the proper operating room assistance and equipment are not available in the middle of the night.

1. Irrigation of the wound with copious amounts of normal saline after induction of appropriate anesthesia. Forceful irrigation with a large syringe and 19 gauge needle can be used if the globe is protected and is not ruptured. This is particularly important in puncture and bite wounds.
2. Do not remove eyelid tissue prior to surgical repair, but debride all foreign material to prevent infection or tattooing. Wrap

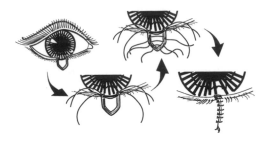

FIGURE 11.1. Technique for primary eyelid closure involving the loss of a small amount of the lid

amputated tissue in cool saline-soaked gauze, but do not immerse in saline solution.

3. If possible, attempt primary closure of tissue. This holds true for animal and human bites. Close tissue in appropriate anatomic layers. Primary reconstruction, which is possible for human bites, includes (Fig. 11.1) reapproximation of the gray line with two or three 4-0 silk sutures. Initially, leave these sutures long to prevent corneal exposure, and they should be left in place for 10 to 14 days before removal. The tarsal plate is the next layer closed with 5-0 vicryl, followed by closure of the skin layer with 7-0 nylon, silk, or vicryl. Skin in children should be closed with vicryl or fast absorbing gut.

4. More extensive injuries may have occurred. Periosteal tears should be closed with 4-0 vicryl. Orbital septum tears should not

TABLE 11.2

Management of lid lacerations treatment

Lid Loss	Treatment
Upper Lid	
Less than $\frac{1}{3}$	Lateral canthotomy and cantholysis (Fig. 11.2)
Less than $\frac{2}{3}$	Lateral canthotomy and cantholysis with Tenzel advancement flap (Fig. 11.3)
Greater than $\frac{2}{3}$	Cutler-Beard procedure
Lower Lid	
Less than $\frac{1}{3}$	Lateral canthotomy and cantholysis
Less than $\frac{2}{3}$	Lateral canthotomy and cantholysis plus Tenzel flap
Greater than $\frac{2}{3}$	Hughes' procedure (Fig. 11.4) Mustarde flap

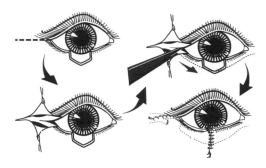

FIGURE 11.2. Technique for eyelid closure involving less than one-third of the upper lid using a lateral canthotomy and cantholysis approach

be closed. If the levator is disinserted, reattach with 5-0 vicryl. The orbicularis should also be repaired with 5-0 vicryl sutures.

5. Secondary reconstruction is generally required with more tissue loss (Table 11.2).

6. Silicone intubation of lacerated canaliculi is necessary to prevent chronic epiphora. The upper and lower system is usually cannulated but monocanalicular intubation is also possible. The canaliculus itself should be repaired with 8-0 vicryl sutures. Canthal avulsions or lacerations must be resutured to the periosteum.

7. Prophylactic antibiotics are usually not necessary for clean lacerations seen shortly after injury. Dirty or infected wounds may require antibiotic coverage. Antibiotic options include amoxicillin/clavulanate, penicillin, cefalosporins (Keflex, Cefoxitin, Ceftriaxone), and tetracycline in patients who are allergic to penicillin.

Complications

1. Eyelid malposition
2. Lacrimal drainage system obstruction
3. Infection

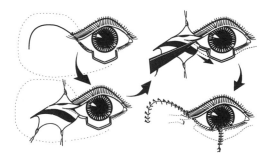

FIGURE 11.3. Technique for eyelid closure involving less than two-thirds of the upper lid using a lateral cantholysis and Tenzel flap

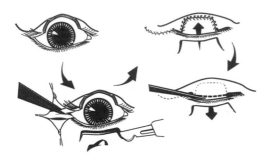

FIGURE 11.4. Technique for eyelid closure involving more than two-thirds of the lower lid using a lid-sharing technique

Chemical and Thermal Burns

Thermal burns are typically classified as follows:

> *First degree:* damage to the epidermis; redness, blistering.
> *Second degree* (partial thickness): damage to the dermis and epidermis.
> *Third degree* (full thickness): damage to the dermis as well as subcutaneous tissues.

Chemical and electrical burns may cause similar tissue destruction.

Evaluation   Please see "Chemical Burns" in Anterior Segment Trauma section, above, for discussion of chemical burns of the anterior segment. With regard to the lids, careful observation is required to watch for and break symblepharon with glass rods several times daily. Cicatricial ectropion and entropion may develop and require treatment.

Thermal Burns   Other ocular injuries must be ruled out. In the management of such burns, one must be careful to avoid extensive debridement of lid tissue. Antibiotic ointments on corneal or conjunctival abrasions are required, and one should cover for pseudomonas. Bland ocular ointments are also used for corneal exposure. Eyelid skin should be covered with "wet to dry dressings." Avoid silver sulfadiazine ointment on the eyelid skin. A suture tarsorrhaphy may be required for persistent corneal exposure. Surgically lyse cicatricial bands. Cover exposed skin with a full-thickness or split-thickness skin graft. Grafting may be initiated during the first few weeks after injury. Note that full-thickness grafts are better cosmetically but may shrink to 30% of their initial size. Split-thickness grafts have a poorer cosmetic result and may shrink to 50% of their initial size.

Close follow-up is required for repeated evaluation of symblepharon, ectropion, entropion, trichiasis, graft failure, and recurrent scarring. Patients should be made aware that skin grafting may have to be repeated on multiple occasions secondary to contractures and poor cosmetic results.

Orbital Fractures

Etiology Midfacial fractures resulting from blunt force may result in injury to one or more of the orbital bones.

Presentation Signs and symptoms may include visual loss, diplopia, pain on extraocular muscle (EOM) movement, EOM restriction due to muscle entrapment or edema, enophthalmos from the eye sinking into the sinus, hypesthesia of periorbital skin and ipsilateral cheek, hypesthesia of oral structures, cerebrospinal fluid leakage, displacement of zygomatic arches, periorbital edema, and epistaxis.

Evaluation A thorough ophthalmic examination includes Hertel exophthalmometry, palpation of the orbital bony rim, evaluation of skin hypesthesia in the area of the infraorbital nerve, forced duction testing, orbital skull film series, and orbital CT scanning with axial and coronal views.

Differential Diagnosis

1. Le Fort fracture I: low transverse maxillary fracture, this does not involve the orbit.
2. Le Fort fracture II (the most common): pyramidal fracture involving the maxilla, nasal bones, and medial orbital wall.
3. Le Fort fracture III: cranial facial dysjunction—orbits are extensively involved.
4. Zygomatic fracture.
5. Tripod fracture.
6. Orbital apex fracture.
7. Orbital roof fracture.
8. Orbital medial wall fracture.
9. Orbital floor (blow-out) fracture can be from a direct orbital rim fracture or indirect. In a true blow-out fracture the orbital rim is intact.

Treatment

1. Initially cold compresses, decongestants, and oral antibiotics (especially with a history of chronic sinusitis).

2. Le Fort I and II fractures: intermaxillary fixation or open reduction and fixation by wiring in fixation plates.
3. Le Fort III fractures: generally involve intracranial injuries and require neurosurgical intervention.
4. Zygomatic fractures: may require open reduction and fixation if they are markedly displaced. No treatment is required if the zygoma is not displaced.
5. Orbital apex fractures: observation if no visual loss occurs. Visual loss or encroachment of a bony spur on the optic nerve, however, may require surgical decompression of the optic nerve.
6. Orbital roof fractures: observation if no cerebrospinal fluid leakage or herniation of intracranial contents occurs; otherwise, neurosurgical intervention is necessary. Surgical obliteration of the frontal sinus may prevent a mucocele.
7. Medial wall fractures: usually not treated unless entrapment of the orbital tissue occurs with restrictive motility or enophthalmos. Orbital emphysema is common with medial wall fractures.
8. Orbital floor fractures (treatment is controversial): the primary indications for surgical intervention are enophthalmos greater than 2 mm, persistent diplopia in primary or downgaze with positive forced ductions, or fractures involving more than half of the orbital floor. Surgical correction may occur 2 to 3 weeks after the injury if no resolution of symptoms occurs, which requires close observation. Intervention after 1 month may reduce globe ptosis or enophthalmos but usually does not resolve diplopia. Common implant materials are Supramyd, bone grafts, and fascia.

Traumatic Optic Neuropathy

Definition and Symptoms   Blunt or sharp trauma resulting in damage to the optic nerve. Patients typically notice a sudden profound loss of vision, althouth other injuries may result in a patient's being unable to offer this history. Damage can result from compression or laceration of the nerve by bone fracture. Ischemic injury from a sheering force is also possible.

Signs

1. Poor central and peripheral vision typically at the hand motions, light perception, or no light perception level.
2. Relative afferent pupillary defect.

3. The optic nerves may appear normal or give the appearance of an avulsion.

Workup

1. Rule out other causes of severe vision loss such as vitreous hemorrhage and retinal detachment.
2. CT scanning of the orbits: request small cuts of 1 mm. Coronal and axial views with bone windows looking for impingement on the optic nerve.

Treatment   Must be undertaken in the first 24 hours to be effective. High-dose intravenous steroids (e.g., methylprednisolone i.v. 30 mg/kg body weight followed in 2 h by 15 mg/kg q. 6 h for 48 h) has been recommended, as well as surgical decompression of the optic nerve by releasing pressure from fractured bones or decompression of the nerve sheath.

Foreign Bodies

General Considerations

Always assume an ocular injury involves a foreign body until proven otherwise. The tolerance of the eye to foreign bodies varies. In general:

1. Poorly tolerated—wood, copper, iron, steel.
2. Moderately well tolerated—nickel, lead, zinc.
3. Inert (if not coated with another material)—glass, carbon, lead, silver, stone.

BB's and pellets are composed of lead and iron of various grades. These as well as organic materials are poorly tolerated.

Missing a foreign body can lead to loss of vision, infection, or tetanus. Deferral of a foreign body removal usually increases fibrosis and increases the difficulty in removing the foreign body at a later date.

CT scanning with 1 mm cuts is the best method of detecting foreign bodies, both metallic and nonmetallic. MRI scanning should be avoided because of the potential metallic nature of foreign bodies. However, wood will show up much better with an MRI than a CT scan. Orbital plain films are less expensive, but many times futher radiographic studies are required to better locate and identify the foreign body. Ultrasound can be utilized to identify a foreign body which is suspected but not detected by other methods.

Anterior Segment Foreign Bodies

Conjunctival Foreign Bodies

External foreign bodies may be hidden by mucus or a fold in the conjunctiva. Associated signs may include vertical scratches on the cornea and subconjunctival hemorrhage. Examination should include double lid eversion with Desmares retractors to examine the conjunctival fornices. Multiple conjunctival foreign bodies can be irrigated out of the eye or removed with a cotton-tipped applicator by sweeping the fornices.

Corneal Foreign Bodies

Look for associated infiltrates around a foreign body, which could be the start of a secondary infection. Removal of a foreign body can be achieved with a spud or 25 gauge needle at the slit lamp with topical anesthesia. In general, corneal foreign bodies should be removed because of secondary toxic effects on the epithelium and possible infection. A rust ring is generally best removed at a later time, especially if it is deep into the stroma, as it tends to soften with time. Treatment includes patching, topical antibiotic ointment, cycloplegia, and follow-up in 24 hours.

Anterior Segment Foreign Bodies

Usually associated with a perforation of the cornea. Inferior edema of the cornea may be secondary to a foreign body in the inferior anterior chamber angle. Removal is usually easiest through a limbal approach, constricting the pupil preoperatively to avoid lens damage.

Posterior Segment Foreign Bodies

1. Signs of a possible posterior foreign body are iris transillumination defects, irregular pupils, and vitreous hemorrhage.
2. Various techniques have been described for removing the foreign body from the posterior segment. Options include removal through the entrance wound, a transcleral cut down with diathermy of the choroid to prevent intraocular bleeding, a pars plana vitrectomy with forceps removal, or external magnets (Table 11.3).
3. Intravitreal antibiotics for prophylaxis should be considered but at a lower dose than those used for infectious endophthalmitis.
4. Patients with a retained foreign body should be followed with electroretinography for signs of toxic retinal reactions.

TABLE 11.3

Management of posterior segment foreign bodies (FB)

Methods of Removal of FB from Posterior Segment	Indications	Advantages	Disadvantages
1. Through eye wall where FB is located.	Magnetic FB that is embedded at least partially in eye wall > 2 mm from disc.	Minimal vitreous trauma.	Choroidal hemorrhage possible. Posteriorly located FB requires excessive manipulation of globe.
2. Through pars plana a. With electromagnet applied outside of eye.	Magnetic FB that is not embedded or only slightly embedded in eye wall.	FB drawn out through least vascular portion of uvea & area of retina least likely to detach.	Additional vitreous trauma.
b. With "rare earth" magnet introduced into eye after vitrectomy.	Same.	Same.	No capability of releasing FB once it is engaged.
c. With forceps after doing vitrectomy.	a. Any FB. b. Any large or very irregular FB. c. Any FB ≤ 2 mm from optic disc.	Only method for nonmagnetic FB. Allows maximal control of eye pressure. Allows direct visualization of FB.	Requires considerable technical support.
3. Through limbal wound or corneal trephine wound.	Very large or very irregular FB.	Least vascular area of eye wall. Includes simultaneous management of extensive corneal damage.	Poor control of eye pressure. Requires extensive technological support.
4. Through entry wound.	Considered for small, usually magnetic FB.	No other eye incisions.	Entry wound often irregular & in vascular area so control of eye pressure is difficult, hemorrhage is likely.

Adapted from trauma lecture series by Thomas S. Stevens, M.D., University of Wisconsin.

Orbital Foreign Bodies

Signs and Symptoms   May include proptosis, pain with eye movement, diplopia, cellulitis, or a chronic draining fistula. Blunt trauma or an occult tumor may cause similar signs and symptoms.

Management

1. Inert foreign bodies easily located in the anterior orbit may be removed. Objects located in the posterior orbit not encroaching on vital structures (ophthalmic nerve, ophthalmic artery, sclera) may be observed. However, watch for infection with secondary extrusion or fistula formation, loss of vision, progressive pupil anomalies, and elevations of intraocular pressure.
2. Organic materials should be removed.
3. Intravenous antibiotic prophylaxis with cefazolin, gentamicin, and clindamycin may be warranted, especially with organic foreign bodies.

Prognosis   Generally depends on structures injured and composition of the foreign body. If the globe or optic nerve has not been injured, the prognosis is generally good.

Selected Readings

Burns CL, Chylack LT. Thermal burns—the management of thermal burns of the lids and globes. Ann Ophthalmol 1979;11(9):1358–68.

Campbell DG, Shields MB, Liebmann JM. Ghost cell glaucoma. In: Ritch R, Shields MB, Krupin T, eds. The glaucomas. St. Louis: CV Mosby, 1989, vol. 2, chap. 69, pp. 1239–47.

Deutsch TA, Feller DB. Paton and Goldberg's management of intraocular injuries, 2nd ed. Philadelphia: WB Saunders, 1985, pp. 93–107.

Divine RD, Anderson RL. Techniques in eyelid wound closure. Ophthalmic Surg 1982;13:283–87.

Dortzbach RK. Orbital floor fracture. Ophth Plast Reconstr Surg 1985;1:149–50.

Flanagan JC, McLachlan DL, Shannon GM. Orbital roof fractures: neurologic and neurosurgical considerations. Ophthalmology 1980;87:325–29.

Frank DH, Wachtel T, Frank HA. The early treatment and reconstruction of eyelid burns. J Trauma 1983;23:874–77.

Green BF, Kraft SP, Carter KD, et al. Magnetic resonance imaging of intraorbital wood. Ophthalmology 1990;97(5):608–11.

Herschler J. Trauma and elevated intraocular pressure. In: Ritch R, Shields MB, Krupin T, eds. The glaucomas. St. Louis: CV Mosby, 1989, vol. 2, chap. 68, pp. 1225–37.

Hoskins HD Jr, Kass MA. Secondary open-angle glaucoma. In: Becker-Shaffer's diagnosis and therapy of the glaucomas, 6th ed. St. Louis: CV Mosby, 1989, chap. 19, pp. 324–30.

Kulwin D. Treatment of periorbital burns. In: Advances in ophthalmic
    plastic and reconstructive surgery. New York: Pergamon Press, 1987.
Kulwin DR, Leadbetter MG. Orbital rim trauma causing a blowout fracture.
    Plast Reconstr Surg 1984;73(6):969–70.
Manson PN, Crawley WA, Yaremchuk MJ, Rochman GM, Hoopes JE, French
    JH. Midface fracture: advantages of immediate extended open reduction
    and bone grafting. Plast Reconstr Surg 1985;76:1–10.
Ralph RA, Slansky HH. Therapy of chemical burns. Int Ophthalmol Clin
    1974;14(4):171–91.
Tenzel RR, Stewart WB. Eyelid reconstruction by the semicircle flap
    technique. Ophthalmology 1978;85:1164–69.
Waller RR. Treatment of acute eyelid trauma to prevent late complications.
    Trans Am Acad Ophthalmol Otolaryngol 1976;81:556–59.
Walters M, Lowell G. Corneal problems in burned patients. J Burn Care
    Rehab 1982;3:367.
Zinreich SJ, Miller NR, Aguayo JB, et al. Computed tomographic three-
    dimensional localization and compositional evaluation of intraocular
    and orbital foreign bodies. Arch Ophthalmol 1987;104:1477–82.

INDEX